T0205578

Benign Esophageal Disease

Natan Zundel • W. Scott Melvin
Marco G. Patti • Diego Camacho
Editors

Benign Esophageal Disease

Modern Surgical Approaches and Techniques

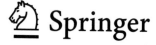 Springer

Editors
Natan Zundel
Jackson North Medical Center
University at Buffalo
Miami, FL
USA

W. Scott Melvin
Montefiore Medical Center
Albert Einstein College of Medicine
Bronx, NY
USA

Marco G. Patti
Department of Surgery and Medicine
University of North Carolina
Chapel Hill, NC
USA

Diego Camacho
Montefiore Medical Center
Albert Einstein College of Medicine
Bronx, NY
USA

ISBN 978-3-030-51491-4   ISBN 978-3-030-51489-1   (eBook)
https://doi.org/10.1007/978-3-030-51489-1

This Springer imprint is published by the registered company Springer Nature Switzerland AG
The registered company address is: Gewerbestrasse 11, 6330 Cham, Switzerland

Preface

Over the past few decades, minimally invasive techniques have evolved and changes in esophageal surgery have been dramatic. Due to the improvements in diagnosis, the surgical community became more aware of these diseases and better procedures are being developed.

Changes from open surgery to laparoscopic, robotic, and endoscopic procedures brought remarkable improvements in outcomes and decreased the morbidity and mortality of esophageal surgery.

As is expected with an evolution, and as our capacity to resolve problems increases, we face new challenges such as reoperations and complications from endoscopic procedures among others.

This book focuses on the diagnosis and treatment of benign esophageal disorders. A large number of world-renowned authors collaborated to develop what we consider a magnificent compilation of amazing, state-of-the art chapters.

Particular emphasis has been placed on gastroesophageal reflux disease (GERD), a highly prevalent problem. This book describes the different diagnostic tools available as well as the therapeutic approaches for the management of GERD and its potential complications such as Barrett's esophagus or strictures and the associated anatomical abnormalities such as hiatal hernia or short esophagus. We also discussed the primary motility disorders of the esophagus such as achalasia and esophageal diverticula. Different devices and approaches can be used to treat these diseases and they will be covered and explained in different chapters of the book.

It is an honor for me to edit this book with Dr. Camacho, Dr. Melvin, and Dr. Patti since they are all leaders in the field of foregut surgery in the USA and all around the world. An amazing group of people to work with, whom I am honored to call friends.

I would like to thank first and foremost our families for all their support to make this book a reality, to all the authors that agreed to participate in this project with us, and last but not least to Richard Hruska, Lillie Gaurano, Kevin Wright, and Daniel Dominguez from the editorial team for all their hard work.

Miami, FL, USA   Natan Zundel
Bronx, NY, USA   W. Scott Melvin
Chapel Hill, NC, USA   Marco G. Patti
Bronx, NY, USA   Diego Camacho

Contents

1 Gastroesophageal Reflux Disease: Workup and Evaluation. 1
   Marco Di Corpo, Kamil Nurczyk, and Marco G. Patti

2 Endoscopic Therapies for GERD 11
   John Cole Cowling, Shinil K. Shah, Erik B. Wilson, and Melissa
   M. Felinski

3 Magnetic Sphincter Augmentation 25
   Kathleen L. Lak and Jon C. Gould

4 Surgical Therapy for GERD 31
   Ariel Shuchleib, Elias Chousleb, and Natan Zundel

5 Recurrence of Symptoms After Surgical Therapies 43
   Sammy Ho and Sara Welinsky

6 Short Esophagus: Its Relationship with Fundoplication
   Failure and Postoperative Recurrence of the Hiatal Hernia. 47
   Italo Braghetto and Owen Korn

7 Hiatal Hernia. 59
   Kamil Nurczyk, Marco Di Corpo, and Marco G. Patti

8 Redo Antireflux Surgery 71
   Brett Parker and Kevin Reavis

9 Motility Disorders: Workup and Evaluation 91
   Samuel Szomstein, Alejandro Cracco, and Jose Melendez-Rosado

10 Motility Disorders: Medical Modalities 103
   Andrew M. Brown and Aurora D. Pryor

11 Esophageal Motility Disorders. 113
   Michael Jureller and Erin Moran-Atkin

12 The Endoscopic Treatment of Esophageal Motility Disorders 137
   Vitor Ottoboni Brunaldi and Manoel Galvao Neto

13 Redo Interventions in Failed Procedures 149
Kelly R. Haisley and Lee L. Swanström

14 Diverticulum: Workup and Evaluation. 165
Juan S. Barajas-Gamboa and Matthew Kroh

15 Esophageal Diverticula. 173
Andrew T. Strong and Jeffrey L. Ponsky

16 Surgical Techniques for Lower Esophageal Diverticula 211
Francesca M. Dimou and Alfons Pomp

17 Medical Evaluation of Barrett's Esophagus. 219
Brian Hodgens, Reid Sakamoto, and Dean Mikami

18 Ablative Therapies in Barrett's Esophagus 225
Audrey C. Pendleton and W. Scott Melvin

19 Endoscopic Mucosal Resection 233
Terence Jackson, David Faugno-Fusci, Aric Wogsland, and
Jeffrey Marks

**20 Surgical Management of Esophageal Strictures After Caustic
Ingestion**. 243
Derek Moore, Georgios Orthopoulos, and John R. Romanelli

21 Endoscopic Management of Esophageal Perforations. 259
Naomi Berezin

22 Surgical Treatment of Esophageal Perforation 267
Thomas C. Tsai, Christopher R. Morse, and David W. Rattner

Index. 275

Contributors

Juan S. Barajas-Gamboa Department of General Surgery, Digestive Disease Institute, Cleveland Clinic Abu Dhabi, Abu Dhabi, United Arab Emirates

Naomi Berezin General Surgery, Montefiore Medical Center/Albert Einstein College of Medicine, Bronx, NY, USA

Italo Braghetto Department of Surgery, Hospital "Dr. José J. Aguirre", University of Chile, Santiago, RM, Chile

Andrew M. Brown Department of Surgery, Stony Brook University Hospital, Stony Brook, NY, USA

Vitor Ottoboni Brunaldi Gastrointestinal Endoscopy Unit, Gastroenterology Department, University of São Paulo Medical School, Sao Paulo, Brazil

Elias Chousleb Department of General Surgery, The Bariatric and Sleeve Gastrectomy Center at Jackson North, Miami, FL, USA

John Cole Cowling Division of Minimally Invasive and Elective General Surgery, Department of Surgery, McGovern Medical School, University of Texas Health Science Center at Houston, Houston, TX, USA

Alejandro Cracco Cleveland Clinic Florida – Weston, Weston, FL, USA

Marco Di Corpo Department of Surgery, University of North Carolina, Chapel Hill, NC, USA

Francesca M. Dimou Department of Surgery, Weill Cornell Medicine/New York Presbyterian Hospital, New York, NY, USA

David Faugno-Fusci Department of General Surgery, University Hospitals of Cleveland, Cleveland, OH, USA

Melissa M. Felinski Division of Minimally Invasive and Elective General Surgery, Department of Surgery, McGovern Medical School, University of Texas Health Science Center at Houston, Houston, TX, USA

Jon C. Gould Department of Surgery, Medical College of Wisconsin, Milwaukee, WI, USA

Kelly R. Haisley Gastrointestinal and Minimally Invasive Surgery, The Oregon Clinic, Portland, OR, USA

Brian Hodgens Department of Surgery, University of Hawaii, Honolulu, HI, USA

Sammy Ho Montefiore Medical Center, Bronx, NY, USA

Terence Jackson Department of General Surgery, University Hospitals of Cleveland, Cleveland, OH, USA

Michael Jureller, MD General Surgery, Montefiore Medical Center/Albert Einstein College of Medicine, Bronx, NY, USA

Owen Korn Department of Surgery, Hospital "Dr. José J. Aguirre", University of Chile, Santiago, RM, Chile

Matthew Kroh Department of General Surgery, Digestive Disease Institute, Cleveland Clinic Abu Dhabi, Abu Dhabi, United Arab Emirates

Cleveland Clinic Lerner College of Medicine, Cleveland Clinic, Cleveland, OH, USA

Kathleen L. Lak Department of Surgery, Medical College of Wisconsin, Milwaukee, WI, USA

Jeffrey Marks Department of General Surgery, University Hospitals of Cleveland, Cleveland, OH, USA

Jose Melendez-Rosado Eisenman & Eisenman M.D., Advanced Gastro Consultants, Lake Worth, FL, USA

W. Scott Melvin, MD Department of Surgery, Montefiore Medical Center, Bronx, NY, USA

Dean Mikami Department of Surgery, The Queen's Medical Center, Honolulu, HI, USA

Derek Moore University of Massachusetts Medical School – Baystate Medical Center, Springfield, MA, USA

Erin Moran-Atkin, MD General Surgery, Montefiore Medical Center/Albert Einstein College of Medicine, Bronx, NY, USA

Christopher R. Morse Division of Thoracic Surgery, Department of Surgery, Massachusetts General Hospital, Boston, MA, USA

Manoel Galvao Neto Surgery Department, ABC University, Sao Paolo, Brazil

Kamil Nurczyk Departments of Surgery and Medicine, University of North Carolina, Chapel Hill, NC, USA

Georgios Orthopoulos University of Massachusetts Medical School – Baystate Medical Center, Springfield, MA, USA

Brett Parker Providence Portland Medical Center, The Oregon Clinic GMIS, Portland, OR, USA

Marco G. Patti Departments of Surgery and Medicine, University of North Carolina University of North Carolina, Chapel Hill, NC, USA

Audrey C. Pendleton, MD Department of Surgery, Montefiore Medical Center, Bronx, NY, USA

Alfons Pomp Department of Surgery, Weill Cornell Medicine/New York Presbyterian Hospital, New York, NY, USA

Jeffrey L. Ponsky Digestive Disease and Surgery Institute, Cleveland Clinic, Cleveland, OH, USA

Cleveland Clinic Lerner College of Medicine of Case Western Reserve University, Cleveland, OH, USA

Aurora D. Pryor Department of Surgery, Stony Brook University Hospital, Stony Brook, NY, USA

David W. Rattner Division of General and Gastrointestinal Surgery, Massachusetts General Hospital, Boston, MA, USA

Kevin Reavis Division of Minimally Invasive Surgery, The Oregon Clinic, Portland, OR, USA

John R. Romanelli University of Massachusetts Medical School – Baystate Medical Center, Springfield, MA, USA

Reid Sakamoto Department of Surgery, John A. Burns School of Medicine, Honolulu, HI, USA

Shinil K. Shah Division of Minimally Invasive and Elective General Surgery, Department of Surgery, McGovern Medical School, University of Texas Health Science Center at Houston, Houston, TX, USA

Michael E. DeBakey Institute for Comparative Cardiovascular Science and Biomedical Devices, Texas A&M University, College Station, TX, USA

Ariel Shuchleib Department of General Surgery, ABC Medical Center, Mexico City, Mexico

Andrew T. Strong Digestive Disease and Surgery Institute, Cleveland Clinic, Cleveland, OH, USA

Cleveland Clinic Lerner College of Medicine of Case Western Reserve University, Cleveland, OH, USA

Lee L. Swanström Gastrointestinal and Minimally Invasive Surgery, The Oregon Clinic, Portland, OR, USA

Samuel Szomstein Cleveland Clinic Florida – Weston, Weston, FL, USA

Thomas C. Tsai Division of General and Gastrointestinal Surgery, Massachusetts General Hospital, Boston, MA, USA

Sara Welinsky Columbia University Medical Center, New York, NY, USA

Erik B. Wilson Division of Minimally Invasive and Elective General Surgery, Department of Surgery, McGovern Medical School, University of Texas Health Science Center at Houston, Houston, TX, USA

Aric Wogsland Department of General Surgery, University Hospitals of Cleveland, Cleveland, OH, USA

Natan Zundel Department of Surgery, University at Buffalo, Miami, FL, USA

Gastroesophageal Reflux Disease: Workup and Evaluation

Marco Di Corpo, Kamil Nurczyk, and Marco G. Patti

General Considerations

Gastroesophageal reflux disease (GERD) is the most frequent gastrointestinal disorder with an increasing incidence likely due to the rising obesity epidemic [1]. GERD is secondary to the backflow of gastric contents through an incompetent gastroesophageal junction (GEJ), causing symptoms and/or complications [2]. The most common GERD symptom is heartburn, often associated with regurgitation and dysphagia. However, some patients may present with atypical or extraesophageal symptoms such as laryngitis, hoarseness, cough, or asthma.

Clinical Findings

Symptoms

GERD patients may present with typical "esophageal" symptoms or atypical "extraesophageal" symptoms (Table 1.1).

There is some evidence about the value of empiric medical therapy with proton pump inhibitors (PPI) for GERD patients presenting with heartburn and regurgitation, the so called "PPI trial," which consists of a 14-day course of high-dose PPI, on the assumption that a response would confirm the diagnosis of GERD. In the American College of Gastroenterology (ACG) guidelines published in 2013, the PPI trial strategy was proposed as a diagnostic method, based on the extent of symptom relief [3].

M. Di Corpo
Department of Surgery, University of North Carolina, Chapel Hill, NC, USA

K. Nurczyk · M. G. Patti (✉)
Departments of Surgery and Medicine, University of North Carolina, Chapel Hill, NC, USA
e-mail: marco_patti@med.unc.edu

© Springer Nature Switzerland AG 2021
N. Zundel et al. (eds.), *Benign Esophageal Disease*,
https://doi.org/10.1007/978-3-030-51489-1_1

Table 1.1 Symptoms associated with gastroesophageal reflux disease (GERD)

Clinical presentation of GERD	
Esophageal	Heartburn
	Regurgitation
	Dysphagia
Gastric	Bloating
	Early satiety
	Belching
	Nausea
Pulmonary	Aspiration
	Asthma
	Wheezing
	Cough
	Dyspnea
Ears, nose, throat	Globus
	Water brash
	Hoarseness
Cardiac	Chest pain

Conversely, it has been shown by Patti et al. [4] that 30% of ~800 patients with symptom and endoscopy-based GERD diagnosis (excluding patients with biopsy-proven Barrett's esophagus) referred for esophageal function testing had a normal esophageal acid exposure as determined by esophageal manometry and 24-hour pH monitoring. These results were later confirmed by Bello et al. [5] in a similar study, showing that among 134 patients referred for laparoscopic anti-reflux surgery (LARS) with a diagnosis of GERD based on symptoms and endoscopy, 24-hour pH monitoring showed that 42% (56 patients) had a normal reflux score. Two of those patients were found to have type II achalasia by high-resolution manometry.

Based on these and similar data, the World Gastroenterology Organization (WGO) guidelines, published in 2017 [6], have discouraged the use of the PPI trial as a diagnostic method due to the lack of sensitivity and specificity.

Clinical Evaluation

Given this evidence, GERD patients should undergo a thorough objective evaluation prior to surgical treatment.

Endoscopy

Often this is the first test done, particularly when dysphagia is present, to rule out complications (such as a stricture) or other conditions such as eosinophilic esophagus or cancer [7, 8]. However, EGD presents two major limitations: [1] about 2/3 of GERD patients do not have esophagitis and [2] there is major inter-observer variability for the low grade of esophagitis [9]. In order to classify the EGD findings, the "Los Angeles" (LA) classification was introduced by Lundell et al. [10]. Mucosal breaks were graded as A, B, C, or D based on the severity of the erosions (Table 1.2).

Table 1.2 Los Angeles classification system for esophagitis

Los Angeles grading system for esophagitis	
Grade A	Mucosal breaks ≤5 mm long, none of which extends between the tops of the mucosal folds
Grade B	Mucosal breaks >5 mm long, none of which extends between the tops of two mucosal folds
Grade C	Mucosal breaks that extend between the tops of ≥2 mucosal folds, but that involve <75% of the esophageal circumference
Grade D	Mucosal breaks that involve ≥75% of the esophageal circumference

Unfortunately, there is evidence of high inter-observer discrepancy among lower LA grades [11], and due to this observation, the Esophageal Diagnostic Advisory Panel recommends further studies such as 24-hour pH monitoring in order to certify GERD [12].

Barium Swallow

The barium swallow is used to assess anatomical and functional characteristics of the swallowing process (pharynx, esophagus, and GEJ), while the sensitivity and specificity for the diagnosis of GERD is low. Bello et al. [6] confirmed these data by finding positive radiological reflux signs in less than 50% of GERD patients (whose diagnosis was obtained by pH monitoring). Furthermore, a study from the Netherlands [13] found similar results when comparing barium swallow to 24-hour pH-impedance monitoring for GERD diagnosis (sensitivity 46% and specificity 44%).

On the other hand, barium swallow gives valuable information about esophageal and GEJ anatomy, and helps to determine the presence, size, and type of hiatal hernias. Moreover, it can assess GERD complications such as ring or strictures [3, 14] (Fig. 1.1).

Esophageal Manometry

This study provides information about the exact location of the LES (important for the correct positioning of the pH catheter), and about LES pressure and relaxation. In addition, it characterizes esophageal peristalsis, rules out achalasia, and allows the choice of the proper anti-reflux operation (Fig. 1.2).

Ambulatory pH Monitoring

Ambulatory 24-hour pH monitoring is considered the gold-standard test for GERD diagnosis, having a reported sensitivity and specificity around 90% [3, 15]. It is the only study that can determine objectively the esophageal acid exposure; thus, having a normal pH study of acid control medications strongly suggests the absence of

Fig. 1.1 Hiatal hernia in
barium swallow

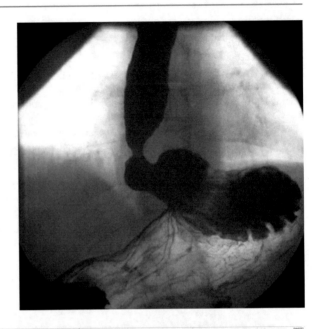

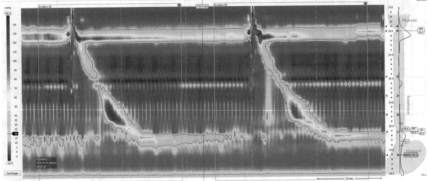

Fig. 1.2 Normal HRM.

GERD [14]. Esophageal pH assessment can be done with a trans-nasal probe for 24 hours or with a wireless probe for 48 hours [16]. Six parameters are considered: number of reflux episodes, duration of the longest one, number of episodes lasting >5 minutes, total percentage of time the pH is <4 in total, and in the supine and upright positions. On the basis of these data, the DeMeester score is generated, and it is considered abnormal when the final composite score is more than 14.7 (Table 1.3) [17]. In addition, the study allows the determination of a temporal correlation between symptoms experienced by the patient and episodes of reflux. While analyzing the tracings, it is considered positive when the reported symptom occurs within 2 minutes of the reflux episode [18]. Moreover, a positive correlation is a predictor for treatment success after LARS [19], being more sensitive for patients with typical symptoms rather than atypical ones [20].

Table 1.3   Normal values for pH monitoring

Normal values for ambulatory 24-hour pH monitoring	
Percentage of total time pH < 4.0	5%
Percentage of upright time pH < 4.0	8%
Percentage of supine time pH < 4.0	4%
Number of episodes of reflux	47
Number of episodes >5 minutes	3.5
Longest episode (minutes)	20
Composite score[a]	14.7

[a]The composite score indicates the extent to which the patient's values deviate from the normal means of the six variables. It allows one to express in a single figure the degree of the patient's abnormality

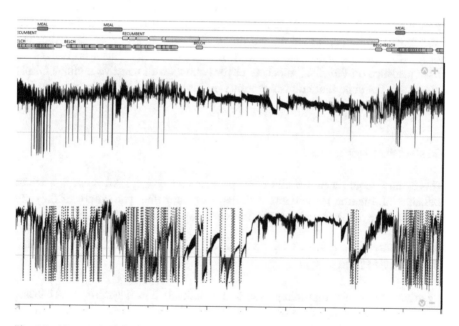

Fig. 1.3   Abnormal pH. Orange spots indicate symptoms reported by the patient, used for analyzing symptom correlation with reflux episodes

Due to the fact that the pH catheter should be placed 5 cm proximal to the upper border of the LES and with the aim to diminish the false-positive and false-negative rates, the best-case scenario is to perform this study after having manometric knowledge of the exact position of the LES. Molena et al. [21] confirmed these data showing only 25% of accuracy when positioning the pH probe using the "step" technique (placing the pH catheter into the stomach through the nose and after confirming the intra-gastric pH value, the probe was progressively withdrawn until obtaining pH values >4). Patients should hold anti-acid medications prior to the study (7 days for PPI and 3 for H_2 blockers) and they are encouraged to continue with their normal lifestyle and meals. (Fig. 1.3).

Based on the evidence from The Esophageal Diagnostic Advisory Panel [12] and the ACG guidelines [3], the ambulatory pH monitoring is recommended for the following:

- Patients with refractory GERD.
- Patients with GERD symptoms and negative EGD findings.
- Patients with EGD findings compatible with LA "A" or "B".
- Patients scheduled for LARS.
- Patients with persistence or recurrence of symptoms after LARS.

Interestingly, a combination of conventional pH monitoring and impedance technology allows a comprehensive evaluation of esophageal reflux events, either for non-acidic, weakly, or acidic episodes, providing key information particularly for refractory GERD patients [19, 22]. Contrary to conventional pH monitoring, pH-impedance can be performed on anti-reflux medications. However, the indication for LARS is not clear for patients with non-acidic reflux events who underwent pH-impedance on PPI or H_2 blockers or for patients with negative findings on pH monitoring but abnormal number of reflux events measured by pH-impedance [12, 23] (Fig. 1.4a,b).

Gastric Emptying Study

This is not a requirement for all GERD patients undergoing LARS, but it provides valuable information for patients with nausea or bloating, particularly if they are known to have diabetes mellitus of connective tissue disorders [12] (Fig. 1.5).

Differential Diagnosis

Heartburn can be the presenting symptom of irritable bowel syndrome, achalasia, cholelithiasis, coronary artery disease, or psychiatric disorders. Esophageal manometry and pH monitoring are essential to determine with certainty if GERD is present and if reflux is the cause of the symptoms.

Complications

Esophagitis is the most common complication. Peptic strictures are uncommon, particularly in the era of proton pump inhibitors. Barrett's esophagus is found in about 10–15% of patients with reflux documented by pH monitoring. Some patients may eventually progress to high-grade dysplasia and adenocarcinoma. Respiratory complications vary from chronic cough to asthma, aspiration pneumonia, and even pulmonary fibrosis. Vocal cord and dental damage can also occur.

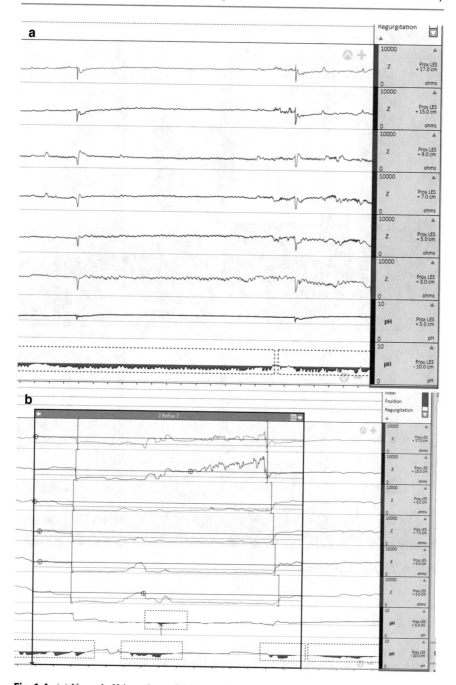

Fig. 1.4 (**a**) Normal pH-impedance (**b**) Abnormal pH-impedance

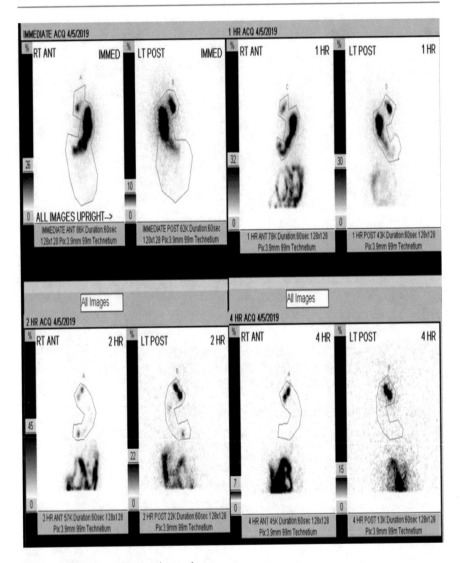

Fig. 1.5 Normal gastric emptying study

References

1. El-Serag HB, Sweet S, Winchester CC, Dent J. Update on the epidemiology of gastro-oesophageal reflux disease: a systematic review. Gut. 2014;63(6):871–80.
2. Vakil N, van Zanten SV, Kahrilas P, Dent J, Jones R. The Montreal definition and classification of Gastroesophageal reflux disease: a global evidence-based consensus. Am J Gastroenterol [Internet]. 2006;101(8):1900–20.
3. Katz PO, Gerson LB, Vela MF. Guidelines for the diagnosis and management of gastroesophageal reflux disease. Am J Gastroenterol. 2013;108(3):308–28.

4. Patti MG, Diener U, Tamburini A, Molena D, Way LW. Role of esophageal function tests in diagnosis of gastroesophageal reflux disease. Dig Dis Sci. 2001;46(3):597–602.
5. Bello B, Zoccali M, Gullo R, Allaix ME, Herbella FA, Gasparaitis A, et al. Gastroesophageal reflux disease and antireflux surgery-what is the proper preoperative work-up? J Gastrointest Surg. 2013;17(1):14–20.
6. Hunt R, Armstrong D, Katelaris P, Afihene M, Bane A, Bhatia S, et al. World gastroenterology organisation global guidelines. J Clin Gastroenterol. 2017;51(6):467–78.
7. Vakil NB, Traxler B, Levine D. Dysphagia in patients with erosive esophagitis: prevalence, severity, and response to proton pump inhibitor treatment. Clin Gastroenterol Hepatol. 2004;2(8):665–8.
8. Shaheen NJ, Weinberg DS, Denberg TD, Chou R, Qaseem A, Shekelle P. Upper endoscopy for gastroesophageal reflux disease: best practice advice from the clinical guidelines committee of the American College of Physicians. Ann Intern Med. 2012;157(11):808–17.
9. Ates F, Vaezi MF. New approaches to management of PPI-refractory gastroesophageal reflux disease. Curr Treat Options Gastroenterol. 2014;12(1):18–33.
10. Lundell LR, Dent J, Bennett JR, Blum AL, Armstrong D, Galmiche JP, et al. Endoscopic assessment of oesophagitis: clinical and functional correlates and further validation of the Los Angeles classification. Gut. 1999;45(2):172–80.
11. Nasseri-Moghaddam S, Razjouyan H, Nouraei M, Alimohammadi M, Mamarabadi M, Vahedi H, et al. Inter- and intra-observer variability of the Los Angeles classification: a reassessment. Arch Iran Med. 2007;10(1):48–53.
12. Jobe BA, Richter JE, Hoppo T, Peters JH, Bell R, Dengler WC, et al. Preoperative diagnostic workup before antireflux surgery: an evidence and experience-based consensus of the esophageal diagnostic advisory panel. J Am Coll Surg. 2013;217(4):586–97.
13. Saleh CMG, Smout AJPM, Bredenoord AJ. The diagnosis of gastro-esophageal reflux disease cannot be made with barium esophagograms. Neurogastroenterol Motil. 2015;27(2):195–200.
14. SAGES Guidelines Committee. Guidelines for surgical treatment of gastroesophageal reflux disease (GERD). www.sages.org. 2001 [cited 2019 Apr 4]. pp. 1–44.
15. Fuchs KH, DeMeester TR, Albertucci M. Specificity and sensitivity of objective diagnosis of gastroesophageal reflux disease. Surgery. 1987;102(4):575–80.
16. Lacy BE, Dukowicz AC, Robertson DJ, Weiss JE, Teixeira P, Kelley ML. Clinical utility of the wireless pH capsule. J Clin Gastroenterol. 2011;45(5):429–35.
17. Johnson LFDT. Twenty-four-hour pH monitoring of the distal esophagus. A quantitative measure of gastroesophageal reflux. Am J Gastroenterol. 1974;62(4):325–32.
18. Savarino E, Bredenoord AJ, Fox M, Pandolfino JE, Roman S, Gyawali CP. Expert consensus document: advances in the physiological assessment and diagnosis of GERD. Nat Rev Gastroenterol Hepatol. 2017;14(11):665–76.
19. Vela MF. Non-acid reflux: detection by multichannel intraluminal impedance and pH, clinical significance and management. Am J Gastroenterol. 2009;104(2):277–80.
20. Patel A, Sayuk GS, Kushnir VM, Chan WW, Gyawali CP. GERD phenotypes from pH-impedance monitoring predict symptomatic outcomes on prospective evaluation. Neurogastroenterol Motil. 2016;28(4):513–21.
21. Molena D, Patti MG, Diener U, Way LW. Esophageal manometry is a prerequisite for pH monitoring. Gastroenterology. 2000;118(4):A1228.
22. Frazzoni M, de Bortoli N, Frazzoni L, Tolone S, Savarino V, Savarino E. Impedance-pH monitoring for diagnosis of reflux disease: new perspectives. Dig Dis Sci. 2017;62(8):1881–9.
23. Francis DO, Goutte M, Slaughter JC, Garrett CG, Hagaman D, Holzman MD, et al. Traditional reflux parameters and not impedance monitoring predict outcome after fundoplication in extra-esophageal reflux. Laryngoscope. 2011;121(9):1902–9.

Endoscopic Therapies for GERD

2

John Cole Cowling, Shinil K. Shah, Erik B. Wilson,
and Melissa M. Felinski

Introduction

Gastroesophageal reflux disease (GERD) has multiple causes including increased intra-abdominal pressure, hiatal hernia causing anatomical failure of the gastro-esophageal junction (GEJ), and dysfunction of the lower esophageal sphincter (LES). The clinical presentation of GERD can range from mild heartburn to erosive esophagitis. Chronic reflux may lead to histologic changes such as Barrett's esophagus, with the subsequent increased risk of esophageal cancer.

The treatment of GERD remains multifactorial. First-line treatment generally consists of diet, lifestyle modification, and weight loss. Medical therapy consists primarily of acid-reducing medications including proton pump inhibitors (PPIs). The use of PPIs has increased significantly in recent years [1]. Despite advances in medical therapy, as many as 40% of patients on PPIs continue to have persistent GERD symptoms [2]. Operative intervention with laparoscopic partial (Toupet) or complete (Nissen) fundoplication (with hiatal hernia repair, if indicated) is generally considered to represent the gold standard surgical option for the treatment of GERD, and exists for those who fail medical treatment or desire to stop taking daily

J. C. Cowling · E. B. Wilson · M. M. Felinski
Division of Minimally Invasive and Elective General Surgery, Department of Surgery, McGovern Medical School, University of Texas Health Science Center at Houston, Houston, TX, USA

S. K. Shah (✉)
Division of Minimally Invasive and Elective General Surgery, Department of Surgery, McGovern Medical School, University of Texas Health Science Center at Houston, Houston, TX, USA

Michael E. DeBakey Institute for Comparative Cardiovascular Science and Biomedical Devices, Texas A&M University, College Station, TX, USA
e-mail: shinil.k.shah@uth.tmc.edu

© Springer Nature Switzerland AG 2021
N. Zundel et al. (eds.), *Benign Esophageal Disease*,
https://doi.org/10.1007/978-3-030-51489-1_2

medications. Newer surgical options, including magnetic sphincter augmentation, are discussed in other chapters.

Within this spectrum of patients with GERD, there exists a subset who desire to eliminate medications due to concerns about side effects (osteoporosis, infectious complications, or impact on vitamin and mineral absorption [3]) from long-term PPI use, but are also concerned about the invasiveness or side effects of a surgical procedure (risk of anesthesia, bleeding, incisional hernia, and/or postoperative dysphagia and gas bloat). An endoscopic (incisionless) intervention aimed at addressing GERD and avoiding the consequences of the treatments mentioned above may be a reliable option for such patients. In this chapter, we will examine and evaluate the available endoscopic therapies for GERD, including transoral fundoplication techniques, radiofrequency (RF) therapies, as well as newer investigational procedures. While magnetic sphincter augmentation is sometimes included in a discussion of endoscopic therapies for GERD, it is covered in detail in a separate chapter.

Transoral Incisionless Fundoplication (TIF)

EsophyX (EndoGastric Solutions, Redmond, Washington) is a single-use endoscopic device that is used to perform a transoral incisionless fundoplication (TIF) procedure. The EsophyX device was approved by the US Food and Drug Administration (FDA) in 2007 and has since been revised as the EsophyX2 device and subsequent advanced models (EsophyX Z device). The technical aspects of the procedure have also evolved since the introduction of the device.

The device functions to create a posterior 180–270 degrees fundoplication to restore the angle of His. It is thought to resemble a surgically created partial fundoplication. The gastric cardia is approximated to the distal esophagus with SerosaFuse® polypropylene "H" shaped fasteners placed at 1–3 cm above the gastroesophageal junction. The fasteners are delivered with a squeeze and release of the trigger mechanism operated by the endoscopist. In creating the wrap, approximately 18–20 fasteners are deployed [4]. The procedure requires an experienced endoscopist to operate the EsophyX device, and an assistant to operate the endoscope. The procedure is generally performed in the operating room under general endotracheal anesthesia. The device is approved for patients with sliding hiatal hernias <2 cm as the device can be used to reduce a small sliding hernia during creation of the fundoplication by advancing the scope caudally before firing the fasteners. Contraindications to the TIF procedure include obesity (BMI >35 kg/m^2), esophageal ulcers, strictures, Barrett's esophagitis >2 cm in length, hiatal hernia >2 cm, LA grade C or D esophagitis, significant esophageal dysmotility, previous esophageal or gastric surgery, peptic ulcer disease, gastric outlet obstruction, gastroparesis, pregnancy (or plans for pregnancy in 12 months), immunosuppression, portal hypertension, and coagulopathy. Prior esophageal/gastric surgery is a relative contraindication, as there are reports of using the TIF device for recurrent reflux after formal surgical fundoplication [5]. Additionally, hiatal hernias should be reducible (sliding); fixed hiatal hernias of any size, including <2 cm, should represent a relative contraindication to the procedure.

The TIF procedure using the EsophyX2 device has been studied in several randomized controlled trials. The TEMPO study examined regurgitation and extraesophageal symptoms of GERD such as laryngitis, asthma, cough, and dental erosions by randomizing patients who were previously partial responders to PPI therapy, TIF, or maximum-dose PPI. While PPI therapy may address heartburn symptoms, medication typically does not affect regurgitation or extraesophageal symptoms. All patients in the study experienced GERD symptoms for >1 year, were on PPI therapy for >6 months, had hiatal hernias <2 cm, and an abnormal 48-hour pH studies while off PPI. At 6-month follow-up, elimination of regurgitation or extraesophageal symptoms were seen in 62% (24/39) patients undergoing TIF and 5% (1/21) in the PPI group. Furthermore, 90% (35/39) patients who had TIF were off PPIs. When evaluating esophageal acid exposure, the results were equivalent, with 54% (21/39) of patients in the TIF group having normal esophageal acid exposure post procedure as compared to 52% (11/21) of patients in the maximum-dose PPI group. This underscores the fact that endolumenal therapies can help improve GERD symptoms, but, similar to PPIs, they do not always normalize esophageal acid exposure. At the end of the trial, the 21 patients in the PPI group were crossed over to subsequently undergo TIF. In these patients, 6 months after their TIF, 71% of patients were off PPI (compared to the 90% mentioned above) and 33% (7/21) had normalized esophageal acid exposure [6]. In this subset of patients, 65% (13/20) had resolution of regurgitation and extraesophageal symptoms. Follow-up at 5 years showed only 34% (15/44) of patients who underwent TIF were on daily PPIs and overall Gastroesophageal Reflux Disease—Health-Related Quality of Life (GERD-HRQL) scores for all patients in the study had decreased from 22.2 to 6.8 ($p < 0.001$) [7].

The RESPECT trial also studied regurgitation by comparing TIF to sham procedure plus PPI for management of regurgitation. The trial randomized 87 patients to the TIF procedure using the EsophyX2 device (Fig. 2.1) plus placebo medication and 42 patients to a sham endoscopy under general anesthesia plus PPI therapy. Inclusion criteria was similar to the TEMPO trial, with patients having persistent symptoms despite PPI therapy for 6 months, abnormal pH testing, and hiatal hernias <2 cm in size. Six-month follow-up demonstrated elimination of regurgitation in 67% (58/87) of the patients in the TIF group and 45% (19/42) in the sham/PPI group ($p = 0.023$). Also, patients undergoing the TIF procedure demonstrated significant decreases in esophageal acid exposure in all parameters measured. DeMeester scores dropped from 33.6 to 23.9 ($p < 0.001$). There were no improvements in pH scores in the sham/PPI group and the DeMeester score increased from 30.9 to 32.7 in this group. In those undergoing TIF who had follow-up endoscopy, 77% had healing of their esophagitis [8].

A similar study by Hakansson et al. randomized patients to TIF versus a sham procedure without PPI. At 6 months, 59% of TIF patients were off PPI medication versus only 18% of sham patients. Additionally, in follow-up pH testing at 6 months, a significant difference in esophageal acid exposure was seen, with 69% of TIF patients having normalized acid exposure, versus only 20% of patients who had the sham procedure [9].

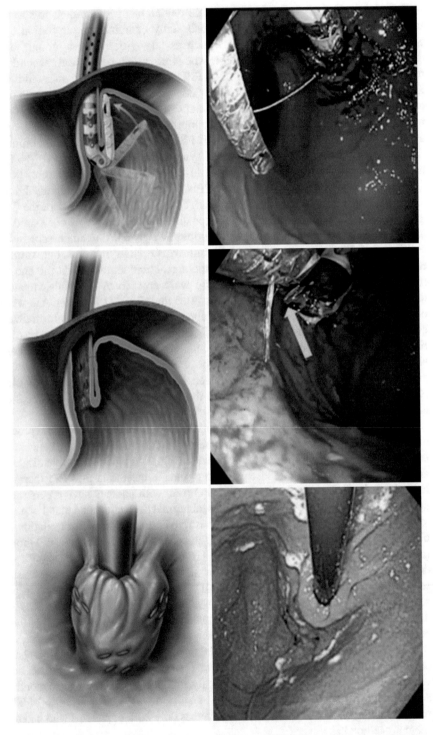

Fig. 2.1 Transoral fundoplication procedure using the EsophyX2 device (Endogastric Solutions, Redmond, WA). (Figure reproduced with permission [8])

Finally, Witteman et al. randomized patients with well-controlled GERD symptoms on PPI to TIF or continuation of PPI treatment, hypothesizing that patients with symptoms controlled with medication would benefit from the endoscopic therapy. At 6 months, 55% (20/37) of patients undergoing TIF saw improvement in GERD-HRQL score of >50%, compared to only 5% (1/20) in the PPI group. Also, 74% of the patients who had TIF were off PPI. However, at 12-month follow-up, only 39% of the patients remained off medication. The study concluded that TIF was successful in the short term but no significant long-term reflux control was obtained [10].

There are several issues that need to be considered when evaluating the literature on TIF. Both the device and technique have evolved since the first reports of this procedure. Additionally, most studies do not report long-term follow-up [11]. With longer-term follow-up, more treatment failures are noted; however, a fairly consistent theme among studies evaluating the TIF device is that the patients who have an initial response are the ones who tend to do well in the long term. An increasing number of studies are now reporting longer-term results with this procedure. At 8 years, Chimukangara et al. demonstrated decreased GERD-HRQL scores as compared to baseline. Notably though, only 23/57 patients were included in the long-term follow-up, and at the long-term follow-up time point, 73% of patients were taking daily anti-acid medications [12]. Testoni et al. reported 6-year follow-up in a cohort of 50 patients. At 6 years (14 patients), only 14.3% of patients were completely off PPI. Most (50%) had reduced their dose by half, and 35.7% of patients were back on full-dose PPI [13]. It is important to recognize that although most patients reduce their doses of PPIs, nearly 40% of patients at longer-term follow-up (4–6 years) will still require PPIs. These data should be interpreted carefully, as it is unknown if these patients have documented objective evidence of recurrent reflux, such as with contrast or pH studies or endoscopic findings [4].

Recently, several groups have published combining traditional hiatal hernia repair (in patients with hiatal hernias >2 cm) with the TIF procedure. The rationale generally provided for this procedure is decreased risk of gas bloat, but, of importance, this is typically in the context of historical data of Nissen fundoplication-associated gas bloat. To date, no study has been completed directly evaluating traditional hiatal hernia repair with TIF as compared to partial (Toupet) fundoplication. A recent retrospective analysis demonstrated improvements in GERD-HRQL scores, reflux symptom index scores, and mean pH scores in patients who underwent laparoscopic hiatal hernia repair with TIF. However, pre- and postoperative follow-up data were obtained in only 29/55 patients; and at a mean follow-up of 296 days, only 76% of patients were noted to have an intact hiatal hernia repair/TIF on endoscopy [14]. It is unclear if improvements in symptom scores and mean pH scores are from restoration of intra-abdominal esophageal length and/or crural closure alone, and whether these preliminary positive results will persist and match the historical long-term follow-up with formal surgical fundoplication.

TIF is an attractive option for patients with endoscopically appropriate anatomy. Advantages of this procedure, similar to most endoscopic procedures for reflux, is a very low rate of severe complications [4], as well as significantly lower rates of gas bloat and dysphagia as compared to traditional laparoscopic Nissen fundoplication. These advantages may be less robust when comparing to partial (Toupet) fundoplication, as recent studies have shown less postoperative gas bloat and dysphagia with partial fundoplication when compared to full Nissen fundoplication [15]. Similar to other endoscopic therapies, the patients who benefit the most are those with no (or very small) hiatal hernias [14, 13], have classic acid reflux symptoms, and respond well to PPI medications. Those with atypical symptoms and PPI non-responders tend to have a less robust response. Increasing number of fasteners utilized also seems to correlate with better long-term response [13]. Repeat TIF for recurrent symptoms after a prior TIF has been described in the literature [16].

Muse

The Medigus Ultrasonic Surgical Endostapler or MUSE (Medigus Ltd., Omer, Israel) procedure is another endoscopic device that can be used to create an endolumenal fundoplication. It differs from EsophyX device in that staples, as opposed to sutures/fasteners, are utilized to create a partial fundoplication. Approved by the FDA in 2015, the procedure similarly is performed under general endotracheal anesthesia in the operating room. MUSE is a single-use endoscopic device that uses a series of five B-shaped, 4.8-mm titanium staples to secure the fundoplication. The shaft of the device houses the staple cartridge and the tip of the endoscope contains the anvil against which to bend the staples during firing. The shaft also houses an ultrasound device to measure tissue thickness and confirm alignment between the cartridge and the anvil. The staples are fired at 3 cm proximal to the gastroesophageal junction and after one fire, the scope is rotated in either direction to perform additional firings to create a partial endoscopic fundoplication (Fig. 2.2). Contraindications to the MUSE procedure are similar to that of TIF, and include BMI <21 or >35 kg/m^2, esophageal stricture/varices, non-reducible hiatal hernia or hiatal hernias >3 cm, and those that do not respond to PPI therapy.

As this is a newer procedure, there is significantly less data available. No randomized trials have been completed on this device to date. The initial pilot study

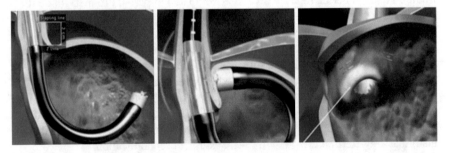

Fig. 2.2 Medigus Ultrasonic Surgical Endostapler or MUSE (Medigus Ltd., Omer, Israel) procedure. (Figure reproduced with permission [17])

consisted of 13 patients on high-dose PPI. Follow-up data at 5 years were available on 11 patients. Five patients were completely off PPIs, three patients had decreased their dose by 50%, and three patients had resumed daily PPIs. Also, 11/13 patients had a greater than 50% reduction in GERD-HRQL scores [17].

A multicenter prospective study was published on 66 patients who underwent the procedure. At 6 months, 64.6% (42/66) were no longer taking PPIs and 56% of the patients who had resumed medication saw a 50% decrease in medication dosage. Additionally, 73% (48/66) had >50% improvement in their GERD-HRQL scores. Esophageal acid exposure was also significantly improved on 6-month pH testing. On follow-up manometry, no significant difference was observed in LES pressure. Serious adverse events were low, and included pneumomediastinum and/or pneumothorax, pleural effusion, esophageal leak, and upper GI bleed (4 patients in the initial 24 patients completed). After the initial 24 patients, there were modifications made to the protocol and device, which resulted in elimination of these particular serious adverse events in the subsequent 48 patients [18].

Kim et al. have reported perhaps the best results in patients undergoing the MUSE procedure. They followed 37 patients for 4 years (from the prospective study) and found 84% and 69% of patients to be off PPIs at 6 months and 4 years, respectively. These patients also had statistically significant improvements in GERD-HRQL scores (off PPI), from mean scores of 29 at baseline to 8.9 at 6 months and 5.3 at 4 years [19].

The most recent results were reported by Lankarani et al. who reported on 71 patients in an international registry undergoing the MUSE procedure. At 1 (47 patients) and 2 (15 patients) years of follow-up, GERD-HRQL scores were improved by >50%. Additionally, 70% and 69% of patients had stopped or decreased their PPI doses by 50% at 1 and 2 years, respectively. There were no new complications present in patients evaluated at 2 years. In patients with pH data available, 4/25 patients had normalization of acid exposure (% time pH ≤ 4) [20].

Stretta

Stretta (Mederi Therapeutics, Greenwich, CN) is an endoscopic device that has been in use the longest of the described procedures, receiving FDA clearance in 2000. It delivers radiofrequency (RF) energy to the muscularis propria to decrease LES compliance and decrease the number of LES relaxations. One benefit of Stretta from the other discussed procedures is that the procedure can be performed under moderate sedation in the outpatient setting. In addition, it does not alter external anatomy as compared to the other transoral fundoplication techniques.

The device consists of a catheter with a balloon at the tip that is inflated with air under pressure control, an irrigation channel, and four needle electrodes that deliver energy to tissue at multiple treatment levels near the Z line and the gastric cardia (Fig. 2.3). The RF generator requires a grounding pad, delivers monopolar current, and gives the operator continuous feedback on tissue temperature, which is

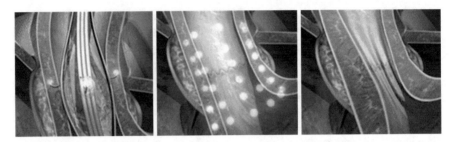

Fig. 2.3 Stretta procedure; schematic demonstrating balloon catheter, treatment areas, and post-treatment appearance. (Figure reproduced with permission [39])

regulated with assistance from irrigation. The device allows maximum heating to 85 °C to the muscularis and 50 °C to the serosa.

The exact mechanism of action is not well understood, but one theory is that the procedure ablates vagal afferent nerve pathways, thereby reducing transient LES relaxations. Another is that LES musculature is altered in response to the heat delivered to the tissue, thus causing a decrease in compliance. Either way, studies have been inconsistent in demonstrating significant change in LES pressures as measured by manometry [21].

Contraindications to Stretta are similar to the other described endoscopic procedures for GERD and include age < 18, pregnancy, hiatal hernias >2 cm, achalasia or incomplete relaxation of the LES in response to swallowing, and American Society of Anesthesiologist (ASA) 4 patients. Relative contraindications include implants near the LES, normal pH studies, PPI non-responders, Barrett's metaplasia, dysphagia, esophageal bleeding, gas bloat, severe esophagitis, coagulation disorders, those who use anticoagulation or antiplatelet therapy, and those with severe medical comorbidities.

Stretta has been studied in several randomized trials and has the benefit of a longer history of use. Corley et al. randomized patients to Stretta ($n = 35$) or sham procedure ($n = 29$). Six-month results favored Stretta, with 61% of those patients off PPI compared to 33% in the sham group. Additionally, GERD-HRQL scores decreased by >50% in 61% of patients undergoing the Stretta procedure. The study did not however demonstrate a difference in esophageal acid exposure between the two arms [22].

Coron et al. studied 43 patients, comparing 23 patients undergoing Stretta to 20 patients remaining on PPI therapy. At 6 months, 78% (18/23) Stretta patients were able to stop or reduce their PPI dose by >50% compared to only 40% in the PPI group ($p = 0.01$). However, these differences did not persist at 12 months. Likewise, there were no differences in GERD-HRQL or other quality of life indexes between the two groups. There were also no differences in esophageal acid exposure at 6 months. Adverse events in the study group included transient abdominal pain, pain with swallowing, and two patients with transient fevers [23].

Abdel Aziz et al. conducted a three-armed trial comparing one or two Stretta procedures to a sham procedure, with 12 patients in each arm. In patients who were randomized to a second procedure, only those without a >75% improvement in GERD-HRQL scores at 4 months went on to a have a second procedure. There were 10/12 patients in this category. At 1 year of follow-up, there was significant improvement in HRQL scores, LES pressures, pH scores, and daily PPI use ($p < 0.01$). Both treatment arms had statistically significant improvement in GERD-HRQL scores compared to the sham procedure. Two of the patients who underwent a second procedure developed gastroparesis as a complication [24].

The most recent systematic review and meta-analysis of Stretta was published by Fass et al. They evaluated 28 studies (2468 patients), including 4 randomized controlled studies. Mean follow-up was approximately 25.4 months. Stretta was associated with significantly improved health-related quality of life (HRQL) scores, heartburn scores, and incidence of erosive esophagitis (decreased by 24%, $p < 0.001$). This meta-analysis also demonstrated reduced esophageal acid exposure ($p < 0.001$) as well as increased mean LES basal pressures (not statistically significant) [25].

It is important to note that these results seem contradictory to another meta-analysis of randomized controlled trials of patients undergoing Stretta therapy [26]. Lipka et al. used normalization of esophageal pH values as a primary endpoint, in which they demonstrated no difference [26]. There are several points that deserve mention. Outcome measures were not uniform in the four randomized trials, therefore the actual number of patients compared with any given endpoint was very low [25]. Normalization of esophageal pH is not seen in most patients undergoing endolumenal anti-reflux therapies (or those taking PPIs). Most studies on Stretta, including in published randomized trials, report improvements in pH exposure. Two of the three studies that reported mean LES pressures demonstrated improvement, as well as improved quality of life scores. Similar to most endolumenal anti-reflux procedures, serious adverse events reported with Stretta are exceptionally low (26 out of >15,000 procedures performed) [27].

Stretta has been described in patients who have undergone laparoscopic Nissen fundoplication with refractory symptoms [28]. It has also been described in patients with reflux after sleeve gastrectomy. However, initial published results in a small cohort of 15 patients demonstrate no changes in pre- and post-procedure quality of life scores and only 20% of patients being able to stop PPI therapy. Also, 66.7% of patients reported not being satisfied at 6 months [29].

Novel Procedures

Two novel procedures are the Anti-Reflux Mucosectomy (ARMS) and Cardia Ligation Anti-Reflux procedure (CLEAR). While little data exist about these procedures, they are described as new, evolving endoscopic treatment options to manage patients with GERD.

Inoue et al. initially described a case report where following endoscopic mucosal resection (EMR) for Barrett's esophagus, GERD symptoms were noted to have been significantly improved. He followed this up with a series of 10 patients having

270-degree circumferential EMR spanning 3 cm in length (1 cm in esophagus and 2 cm in gastric cardia; ARMS procedure). The results showed improvement in DeMeester scores and pH scores and reduction in flap valve grade (Hill grade) from 3.2 to 1.2. Two patients developed stenosis that required balloon dilation. It is thought that the contraction of the cardia during healing after mucosectomy is responsible for the narrowing of the GEJ and contraction of the flap valve, thereby improving GERD symptoms [30].

Another study reported on 19 patients undergoing ARMS for refractory GERD. At 6 months of follow-up, GERD-HRQL scores were significantly improved and 68% (13/19) of patients were off PPI. There were three patients who developed early dysphagia and required balloon dilation and one patient had a muscle injury due to deep resection that was repaired with an endoscopic suturing platform. Three of the six patients who did not respond went on to have formal anti-reflux surgery [31].

The CLEAR procedure is an evolution of the ARMS procedure. The procedure uses multiple sequential band ligations of the cardia (270 degrees), without mucosal resection to cause tissue necrosis and subsequent scarring. The procedure aims to achieve a similar physiologic healing to that of ARMS. The technique has been reported to have been used in two patients with favorable results. One patient underwent repeat subsequent banding for recurrent, although milder, symptoms. The procedure offers the benefit of being technically easier, while limiting the risk of perforation and bleeding that could occur with ARMS [32].

Both of these procedures should be considered investigational and should be performed in the context of well-designed clinical trials.

Conclusion

Endoscopic therapies are an important component in the treatment spectrum of reflux, which also includes lifestyle modification, pharmacotherapy, magnetic sphincter augmentation, and laparoscopic hiatal hernia repair with partial or complete fundoplication, and in patients with morbid obesity and weight loss surgery (Roux-en-Y gastric bypass). As is true for most functional disease, appropriate patient selection is paramount for good outcomes. Both the American Society of Gastrointestinal Endoscopy (ASGE) and the Society of American Gastrointestinal and Endoscopic Surgeons (SAGES) recommend consideration of endolumenal therapies for carefully selected patients with GERD [33, 34].

The patients who tend to do best with endoscopic therapies for GERD include those with favorable endoscopic anatomy (no or very small sliding hiatal hernias of <2 cm), [14, 13], classic symptoms, complete response to PPIs, and normal body mass index [35]. Those with atypical symptoms (particularly regurgitation) may also benefit from endoscopic therapies. In selected cases, endolumenal therapies may be valuable in the patient with recurrent symptoms after formal surgical fundoplication but without evidence of hiatal hernia recurrence. A common theme throughout all endoscopic therapies is that treatment efficacy tends to decrease with time. The longest follow-up has been reported with Stretta, with approximately only ½ of patients remaining completely off anti-acid medications at 10 years [36].

Careful patient workup is important. Endoscopy, including careful endoscopic delineation of esophagogastric junction anatomy including Hill valve grading, upper gastrointestinal series/barium swallow studies, as well as pH probe testing in patients with atypical symptoms or PPI non-responders should be performed. Manometry is not always necessary in patients undergoing endoscopic therapies for GERD, but should be considered in those with a history or imaging that suggests a possible esophageal motility disorder, such as achalasia.

Managing expectations, including discussion of the literature in regard to long-term outcomes, is important when counseling patients who are being considered for endoscopic GERD therapy. Endolumenal therapies do not represent a cure for reflux, but rather an additional tool in the comprehensive management of reflux patients. Endolumenal therapies do not preclude formal laparoscopic, partial or complete, fundoplication for treatment failures [37, 38].

References

1. Rotman SR, Bishop TF. Proton pump inhibitor use in the U.S. ambulatory setting, 2002–2009. PLoS One. 2013;8(2):e56060. https://doi.org/10.1371/journal.pone.0056060.
2. Fass R. Proton pump inhibitor failure–what are the therapeutic options? Am J Gastroenterol. 2009;104 Suppl 2:S33–8. https://doi.org/10.1038/ajg.2009.50.
3. Safety of Long-Term PPI Use. JAMA. 2017;318(12):1177–8. https://doi.org/10.1001/jama.2017.13272.
4. Huang X, Chen S, Zhao H, Zeng X, Lian J, Tseng Y, Chen J. Efficacy of transoral incisionless fundoplication (TIF) for the treatment of GERD: a systematic review with meta-analysis. Surg Endosc. 2017;31(3):1032–44. https://doi.org/10.1007/s00464-016-5111-7.
5. Bell RC, Hufford RJ, Fearon J, Freeman KD. Revision of failed traditional fundoplication using EsophyX transoral fundoplication. Surg Endosc. 2013;27(3):761–7. https://doi.org/10.1007/s00464-012-2542-7.
6. Trad KS, Barnes WE, Simoni G, Shughoury AB, Mavrelis PG, Raza M, Heise JA, Turgeon DG, Fox MA. Transoral incisionless fundoplication effective in eliminating GERD symptoms in partial responders to proton pump inhibitor therapy at 6 months: the TEMPO Randomized Clinical Trial. Surg Innov. 2015;22(1):26–40. https://doi.org/10.1177/1553350614526788.
7. Trad KS, Barnes WE, Prevou ER, Simoni G, Steffen JA, Shughoury AB, Raza M, Heise JA, Fox MA, Mavrelis PG. The TEMPO Trial at 5 years: Transoral Fundoplication (TIF 2.0) is safe, durable, and cost-effective. Surg Innov. 2018;25(2):149–57. https://doi.org/10.1177/1553350618755214.
8. Hunter JG, Kahrilas PJ, Bell RC, Wilson EB, Trad KS, Dolan JP, Perry KA, Oelschlager BK, Soper NJ, Snyder BE, Burch MA, Melvin WS, Reavis KM, Turgeon DG, Hungness ES, Diggs BS. Efficacy of transoral fundoplication vs omeprazole for treatment of regurgitation in a randomized controlled trial. Gastroenterology. 2015;148(2):324–333 e325. https://doi.org/10.1053/j.gastro.2014.10.009.
9. Hakansson B, Montgomery M, Cadiere GB, Rajan A, Bruley des Varannes S, Lerhun M, Coron E, Tack J, Bischops R, Thorell A, Arnelo U, Lundell L. Randomised clinical trial: transoral incisionless fundoplication vs. sham intervention to control chronic GERD. Aliment Pharmacol Ther. 2015;42(11–12):1261–70. https://doi.org/10.1111/apt.13427.
10. Witteman BP, Conchillo JM, Rinsma NF, Betzel B, Peeters A, Koek GH, Stassen LP, Bouvy ND. Randomized controlled trial of transoral incisionless fundoplication vs. pro-

ton pump inhibitors for treatment of gastroesophageal reflux disease. Am J Gastroenterol. 2015;110(4):531–42. https://doi.org/10.1038/ajg.2015.28.

11. Richter JE, Kumar A, Lipka S, Miladinovic B, Velanovich V. Efficacy of laparoscopic nissen fundoplication vs transoral Incisionless fundoplication or proton pump inhibitors in patients with gastroesophageal reflux disease: a systematic review and network meta-analysis. Gastroenterology. 2018;154(5):1298–1308 e1297. https://doi.org/10.1053/j.gastro.2017.12.021.

12. Chimukangara M, Jalilvand AD, Melvin WS, Perry KA. Long-term reported outcomes of transoral incisionless fundoplication: an 8-year cohort study. Surg Endosc. 2019;33(4):1304–9. https://doi.org/10.1007/s00464-018-6403-x.

13. Testoni PA, Testoni S, Mazzoleni G, Vailati C, Passaretti S. Long-term efficacy of transoral incisionless fundoplication with Esophyx (Tif 2.0) and factors affecting outcomes in GERD patients followed for up to 6 years: a prospective single-center study. Surg Endosc. 2015;29(9):2770–80. https://doi.org/10.1007/s00464-014-4008-6.

14. Ihde GM 2nd, Pena C, Scitern C, Brewer S. pH scores in hiatal repair with transoral incisionless fundoplication. JSLS. 2019;23:1. https://doi.org/10.4293/JSLS.2018.00087.

15. Hakanson BS, Lundell L, Bylund A, Thorell A. Comparison of laparoscopic 270 degrees posterior partial fundoplication vs total fundoplication for the treatment of gastroesophageal reflux disease: a randomized clinical trial. JAMA Surg. 2019; https://doi.org/10.1001/jamasurg.2019.0047.

16. Nicolau AE, Lobontiu A. Transoral Incisionless Fundoplication TIF 2.0 with "EsophyX Z(R)" device for GERD: seven years after endo lumenal fundoplication. World's first case report. Chirurgia (Bucur). 2018;113(6):849–56. https://doi.org/10.21614/chirurgia.113.6.849.

17. Roy-Shapira A, Bapaye A, Date S, Pujari R, Dorwat S. Trans-oral anterior fundoplication: 5-year follow-up of pilot study. Surg Endosc. 2015;29(12):3717–21. https://doi.org/10.1007/s00464-015-4142-9.

18. Zacherl J, Roy-Shapira A, Bonavina L, Bapaye A, Kiesslich R, Schoppmann SF, Kessler WR, Selzer DJ, Broderick RC, Lehman GA, Horgan S. Endoscopic anterior fundoplication with the Medigus Ultrasonic Surgical Endostapler (MUSE) for gastroesophageal reflux disease: 6-month results from a multi-center prospective trial. Surg Endosc. 2015;29(1):220–9. https://doi.org/10.1007/s00464-014-3731-3.

19. Kim HJ, Kwon CI, Kessler WR, Selzer DJ, McNulty G, Bapaye A, Bonavina L, Lehman GA. Long-term follow-up results of endoscopic treatment of gastroesophageal reflux disease with the MUSE endoscopic stapling device. Surg Endosc. 2016;30(8):3402–8. https://doi.org/10.1007/s00464-015-4622-y.

20. Lankarani A, Costamagna G, Boskoski I, Nieto J, Lehman GA, Kessler WR, Selzer DJ, Neuhaus H, Beyna T, Mehta S, Shah S, Rey J, Haber GB, Kiesslich R, Starpoli AA, Abu Dayyeh BK, Stavropoulos SN, Caca K, Chang KJ, Fanti L, Testoni PA. Updated results from an international multi-center registry study for endoscopic anterior fundoplication. Gastrointest Endosc. 2018;87(6S):AB282.

21. Franciosa M, Triadafilopoulos G, Mashimo H. Stretta radiofrequency treatment for GERD: a safe and effective modality. Gastroenterol Res Pract. 2013;2013:783815. https://doi.org/10.1155/2013/783815.

22. Corley DA, Katz P, Wo JM, Stefan A, Patti M, Rothstein R, Edmundowicz S, Kline M, Mason R, Wolfe MM. Improvement of gastroesophageal reflux symptoms after radiofrequency energy: a randomized, sham-controlled trial. Gastroenterology. 2003;125(3):668–76.

23. Coron E, Sebille V, Cadiot G, Zerbib F, Ducrotte P, Ducrot F, Pouderoux P, Arts J, Le Rhun M, Piche T, Bruley d, Varannes S, Galmiche JP, Consortium de Recherche Independant sur le Traitement et L'exploration du Reflux Gastro-oesophagien, et al. Clinical trial: radiofrequency energy delivery in proton pump inhibitor-dependent gastro-oesophageal reflux disease patients. Aliment Pharmacol Ther. 2008;28(9):1147–58. https://doi.org/10.1111/j.1365-2036.2008.03790.x.

24. Aziz AM, El-Khayat HR, Sadek A, Mattar SG, McNulty G, Kongkam P, Guda MF, Lehman GA. A prospective randomized trial of sham, single-dose Stretta, and double-dose Stretta for

the treatment of gastroesophageal reflux disease. Surg Endosc. 2010;24(4):818–25. https://doi.org/10.1007/s00464-009-0671-4.

25. Fass R, Cahn F, Scotti DJ, Gregory DA. Systematic review and meta-analysis of controlled and prospective cohort efficacy studies of endoscopic radiofrequency for treatment of gastroesophageal reflux disease. Surg Endosc. 2017;31(12):4865–82. https://doi.org/10.1007/s00464-017-5431-2.

26. Lipka S, Kumar A, Richter JE. No evidence for efficacy of radiofrequency ablation for treatment of gastroesophageal reflux disease: a systematic review and meta-analysis. Clin Gastroenterol Hepatol. 2015;13(6):1058–1067 e1051. https://doi.org/10.1016/j.cgh.2014.10.013.

27. Richardson WS, Stefanidis D, Fanelli RD. Society of American gastrointestinal and endoscopic surgeons response to "no evidence for efficacy of radiofrequency ablation for treatment of gastroesophageal reflux disease: a systematic review and meta-analysis". Clin Gastroenterol Hepatol. 2015;13(9):1700–1. https://doi.org/10.1016/j.cgh.2015.02.007.

28. Noar M, Squires P, Khan S. Radiofrequency energy delivery to the lower esophageal sphincter improves gastroesophageal reflux patient-reported outcomes in failed laparoscopic Nissen fundoplication cohort. Surg Endosc. 2017;31(7):2854–62. https://doi.org/10.1007/s00464-016-5296-9.

29. Khidir N, Angrisani L, Al-Qahtani J, Abayazeed S, Bashah M. Initial experience of endoscopic radiofrequency waves delivery to the lower esophageal sphincter (stretta procedure) on symptomatic gastroesophageal reflux disease post-sleeve gastrectomy. Obes Surg. 2018;28(10):3125–30. https://doi.org/10.1007/s11695-018-3333-6.

30. Inoue H, Ito H, Ikeda H, Sato C, Sato H, Phalanusitthepha C, Hayee B, Eleftheriadis N, Kudo SE. Anti-reflux mucosectomy for gastroesophageal reflux disease in the absence of hiatus hernia: a pilot study. Ann Gastroenterol. 2014;27(4):346–51.

31. Hedberg HM, Kuchta K, Ujiki MB. First experience with banded Anti-reflux Mucosectomy (ARMS) for GERD: feasibility, safety, and technique (with video). J Gastrointest Surg. 2019; https://doi.org/10.1007/s11605-019-04115-1.

32. Chuttani R, De Moura DT, Cohen J. Clear: Cardia ligation anti-reflux procedure for gerd. Gastrointest Endosc. 2017;85(5S):AB110.

33. Committee ASoP, Muthusamy VR, Lightdale JR, Acosta RD, Chandrasekhara V, Chathadi KV, Eloubeidi MA, Fanelli RD, Fonkalsrud L, Faulx AL, Khashab MA, Saltzman JR, Shaukat A, Wang A, Cash B, JM DW. The role of endoscopy in the management of GERD. Gastrointest Endosc. 2015;81(6):1305–10. https://doi.org/10.1016/j.gie.2015.02.021.

34. Dunkin B, Eubanks S, Marks J, Marohn M, Park A, Ponsky J, Rattner D, Rosenthal R, Shah P, Smith CD, Soper N, Swanstrom L, Thaler K. Position statement on endolumenal therapies for gastrointestinal diseases. SAGES. 2009. https://www.sages.org/publications/guidelines/position-statement-on-endolumenal-therapies-for-gastrointestinal-diseases/.

35. Mayor MA, Fernando HC. Endoluminal approaches to gastroesophageal reflux disease. Thorac Surg Clin. 2018;28(4):527–32. https://doi.org/10.1016/j.thorsurg.2018.07.008.

36. Noar M, Squires P, Noar E, Lee M. Long-term maintenance effect of radiofrequency energy delivery for refractory GERD: a decade later. Surg Endosc. 2014;28(8):2323–33. https://doi.org/10.1007/s00464-014-3461-6.

37. Bell RC, Kurian AA, Freeman KD. Laparoscopic anti-reflux revision surgery after transoral incisionless fundoplication is safe and effective. Surg Endosc. 2015;29(7):1746–52. https://doi.org/10.1007/s00464-014-3897-8.

38. Ashfaq A, Rhee HK, Harold KL. Revision of failed transoral incisionless fundoplication by subsequent laparoscopic Nissen fundoplication. World J Gastroenterol. 2014;20(45):17115–9. https://doi.org/10.3748/wjg.v20.i45.17115.

39. Kethman W, Hawn M. New approaches to gastroesophageal reflux disease. J Gastrointest Surg. 2017;21(9):1544–52. https://doi.org/10.1007/s11605-017-3439-5.

Magnetic Sphincter Augmentation

3

Kathleen L. Lak and Jon C. Gould

Introduction

Gastroesophageal reflux disease (GERD) is the most common gastrointestinal disease in the United States with an estimated prevalence of 10–25% [1]. The pathophysiology of GERD is complex and related in part to failure of the antireflux barrier at the esophagogastric (EG) junction [2]. The spectrum of disease that follows may range from troublesome symptoms to esophageal tissue damage [3]. Complications of GERD include reflux esophagitis, esophageal stricture, Barrett's esophagitis, or esophageal adenocarcinoma. Diagnosis, management, and treatment of GERD utilizes over $10 billion in health care expenses with indirect costs of an additional $75 billion per year [4].

Acid-suppression medications are first-line and the predominant treatment for patients with GERD [3]. The mechanism of medical acid suppression is to decrease the acid content and pH of the refluxate with a corresponding improvement in clinical symptoms and reflux esophagitis [3]. Proton pump inhibitors (PPIs) effectively change the character of refluxate but do not always stop reflux entirely. Regurgitation of non-acid refluxate (including bile and other gastric contents) often continues [5]. PPI therapy has been associated with adverse events including *Clostridium difficile* infection, osteoporosis and pathologic bone fractures, dementia, renal insufficiency, myocardial infarction, and B_{12} deficiency [6]. Despite ongoing medical therapy, many patients with GERD remain dissatisfied with their GERD symptom control [7, 8]. Surgical intervention should be offered to patients with medically refractory GERD symptoms, complications as a result of GERD, or to those having a desire to stop acid-suppression therapy due to cost or concern for side effects [2]. Laparoscopic Nissen fundoplication (LNF) is the primary intervention for GERD and has been demonstrated to provide an effective alternative to medical therapy with greater

K. L. Lak · J. C. Gould (✉)
Department of Surgery, Medical College of Wisconsin, Milwaukee, WI, USA
e-mail: jgould@mcw.edu

© Springer Nature Switzerland AG 2021
N. Zundel et al. (eds.), *Benign Esophageal Disease*,
https://doi.org/10.1007/978-3-030-51489-1_3

quality of life in patients with medically refractory symptoms [9]. Despite high estimates on the number of people who qualify for antireflux surgery, it is estimated that less than 1% undergo such a procedure [10]. For many patients, potential side effects of a fundoplication including dysphagia, bloating, and an inability to belch or vomit serve as a major deterrent. In addition, it has been demonstrated that approximately 10% of patients to undergo fundoplication undergo a reoperative procedure, most often secondary to fundoplication failure [11]. Magnetic sphincter augmentation (MSA) is a promising new surgical treatment for GERD with several potential advantages when compared to a fundoplication. The LINX® Reflux Management System (Torax Medical, Inc., Shoreview, MN, USA) is a magnetic sphincter augmentation device for GERD that was approved by the US Food and Drug Administration (FDA) in 2012.

Design and Use

The LINX® MSA device is composed of a ring of titanium beads that slide independently on titanium wires. The beads have neodymium iron boron magnetic cores coated with titanium. The inter-bead attraction provides augmentation of the lower esophageal sphincter (LES) at rest, while having the mobility to expand to accommodate a physiologic bolus such as during swallowing. The device's design utilizes the inter-bead attraction to augment the LES when challenged with low-pressure refluxate; however, higher physiologic challenges, such as with swallowing, vomiting, or belching, are able to overcome the inter-bead attraction.

Surgical placement of the MSA device is performed most often as an outpatient procedure. The device is laparoscopically positioned at the esophagogastric (EG) junction under general anesthesia. Unlike a fundoplication procedure, placement of the MSA device requires less dissection at the hiatus and into the mediastinum, and no mobilization of the fundus or division of the short gastric arteries. A sizing tool is utilized to measure the external circumference of the esophagus at the appropriate location so as to select the appropriately sized device for implantation. A well-positioned device should rest at the EG junction without significant compression of the esophageal tissue. The posterior vagus nerve is typically excluded and the device is placed between the esophagus and the posterior vagus. The surgical technique is simplified compared to a fundoplication and easily reproducible.

Indications and Contraindications

The LINX® MSA device is indicated in patients with refractory GERD despite medical management. Its use is contraindicated in patients with a known or suspected allergy to nickel, stainless steel, titanium, or ferrous materials. The safety and efficacy have not been evaluated by the FDA in patients with a body mass index greater than 35 kg/m², Barrett's esophagus, those with grade C or D (LA Classification) esophagitis, or in patients with significant esophageal motility disorders [10]. The current generation of the LINX® device is compatible with MRI up to 1.5 Tesla.

Early Research and Development

The LINX® device was first approved by the FDA after nearly a decade of development and animal studies [12, 13]. The device was first implanted in a porcine model, which provided preliminary evidence of safety and feasibility. Animals implanted with the device were able to eat normally, gain weight appropriately, and there were no incidents of device erosion. This study was followed by a feasibility clinical trial in humans published in 2008 [14]. In this prospective multicenter trial, 41 patients underwent placement of an MSA device at the esophagogastric junction. Inclusion criteria included patients with clinically significant reflux symptoms at least partially treated with proton pump inhibitors (PPIs), abnormal esophageal acid exposure, and normal esophageal contractility. Notable exclusion criteria included patients with a hiatal hernia >3 cm, esophagitis Grade C or D, or a BMI >35 kg/m^2. All patients in this study had clinical improvement in their symptoms and 80% demonstrated pH normalization.

Post-Market Experience and Long-Term Follow-Up

An update on patients in the pivotal trial was published with 1- and 2-year follow-up. Complete cessation of PPI use was observed in 90% and 86% of patients, respectively [15]. This feasibility trial demonstrated that device implantation was safe with no instances of device migration, erosion, or induced mucosal injury. Initial postoperative dysphagia was reported in 46% of patients and resolved reliably without intervention within 90 days. GERD Health Related Quality of Life (GERD-HRQL) surveys were administered and revealed, respectively, an 85% and 90% reduction in symptom scores at 1 and 2 years postoperatively [15]. At 5 years, no late complications were reported [16]. Bothersome dysphagia was reported by 5% of patients at baseline and by 6% at five 5 postoperatively [16]. Bothersome gas bloating was present in 52% of patients at baseline and this decreased to 8.3% at 5 years. After 5 years of follow-up, the MSA device was determined to provide significant improvement in reflux disease with minimal complications.

The early post-market experience with MSA was chronicled in a number of publications. Lipham et al. described the safety profile of the first 1000 patients implanted with an MSA device [17]. A 0.1% rate of intraoperative/perioperative complications and 3.4% reoperation rate was reported. The most common reason for device removal in this cohort was dysphagia. A different study that focused on device removals included 164 patients, 6.4% of whom underwent explantation (2 for erosions) [18]. The most common reason for explant in this single-center series was recurrent regurgitation or heartburn followed by dysphagia. The authors of this study point out the relative ease with which the MSA device may be removed, even when complicated by an intraluminal erosion.

Bell et al. published the results of a prospective randomized controlled trial designed to evaluate the use of the MSA device in patients with moderate to severe GERD despite once daily PPI therapy [19]. Patients were randomized into two treatment groups—escalation of medical therapy (twice daily PPI dosing) versus surgical placement of an MSA device. At 6 months, 81% of patients in the surgical group experienced a greater than 50% improvement in GERD-HRQL scores compared to 8% in the twice daily PPI group ($p < 0.001$). Regurgitation improved in 89% of patients in the surgical group compared to 10% in the medical treatment group. Six months following MSA implantation, 91% of patients in the surgical group were off PPI therapy.

While a randomized comparative study of medical therapy versus MSA has been conducted and published as described, no such comparison between MSA and laparoscopic fundoplication has been conducted. The closest comparative study was published by Reynolds et al. and utilized matching via propensity scores in order to compare patients with a similar disease severity prior to surgery [20]. Symptomatic outcomes up to 1 year following surgery were compared in matched patients to undergo both laparoscopic Nissen fundoplication and laparoscopic MSA implantation. For both fundoplication and MSA implantation, similar rates of GERD symptom improvement, dysphagia, and patient satisfaction were achieved. There was a significant difference in the ability to belch or vomit favoring MSA. The MSA patients experienced an 8.5% rate of inability to belch and 4.3% rate of inability to vomit compared to 25.5% and 21.3% in the LNF group ($p = 0.004$). There was no significant difference in the need for endoscopic dilations in the first postoperative year between treatment groups.

Implantation of an MSA device inherently involves a sunk cost for the device itself not applicable to laparoscopic fundoplication. In general, most MSA patients are discharged on the day of their procedure and the majority of fundoplication patients spend a night in the hospital. Operating room time is typically greater for fundoplication when compared to MSA. To compare costs associated with a surgical encounter to perform a fundoplication versus implanting an MSA device, Reynolds et al. published another study where they determined that in their experience there was no significant difference in mean charges between procedure types (laparoscopic MSA $48,491 versus laparoscopic fundoplication $50,111; $p = 0.506$) [21]. The authors of this study concluded that the MSA provides a similar efficacy and safety to fundoplication with lower hospital charges.

As the post-market experience with MSA has steadily increased, surgeons have expanded their indications and have started to implant devices in patients with conditions not studied in the FDA premarket research. Publications regarding the outcomes in patients with conditions listed as precautions are appearing in the literature with good reported outcomes. Outcomes in patients with hiatal hernia and even Barrett's esophagus have been published [22–24]. Whereas the initial post-market technique for implanting an MSA device involved minimal dissection at the hiatus and an emphasis on preserving the phrenoesophageal ligament, the technique has evolved to include a complete hiatal dissection. Tatum et al. compared outcomes in the "minimal dissection" era to outcomes in patients to undergo a full hiatal dissection with division of the phrenoesophageal membranes and ligament [24]. Recurrent reflux and lower reoperation rates were observed in those to undergo a full dissection. Rona et al. retrospectively reviewed 192 patients who underwent MSA, 27.1% of whom had a hiatal hernia ≥3 cm. Those patients with hiatal hernias ≥3 cm were found to have decreased PPI requirements and lower GERD-HRQL scores at a median follow-up of 12 months compared to those with a hernia <3 cm in size or no hernia [23]. In this study, there was no difference in the ability to achieve symptom resolution nor the need for intervention for dysphagia. These authors suggest that short-term outcomes are similar for those patients with and without a large hiatal hernia managed with MSA.

Conclusion

GERD is the most common gastrointestinal condition in the United States. Medical therapy with acid suppression is not completely effective in many patients, and concerns about long-term medical therapy are progressively increasing. Despite these facts, antireflux surgery is utilized in a very small portion of patients who would otherwise qualify or benefit. This is largely due to the invasiveness, side effects, and failure rate associated with laparoscopic fundoplication. MSA is a novel and promising new option with a side-effect profile that has several advantages when compared to fundoplication. MSA implantation is safe and effective, and a viable as well as important option for patients with GERD.

References

1. Dent J, El-Serag HB, Wallander MA, Johansson S. Epidemiology of gastro-oesophageal reflux disease: a systematic review. Gut. 2005;54(5):710–7.
2. Stefanidis D, Hope WW, Kohn GP, et al. Guidelines for surgical treatment of gastroesophageal reflux disease. Surg Endosc. 2010;24(11):2647–69.
3. Kahrilas PJ, Shaheen NJ, Vaezi MF, Institute AGA, Committee CPaQM. American Gastroenterological Association Institute technical review on the management of gastroesophageal reflux disease. Gastroenterology. 2008;135(4):1392–413, 1413.e1391–95.
4. El-Serag HB. Time trends of gastroesophageal reflux disease: a systematic review. Clin Gastroenterol Hepatol. 2007;5(1):17–26.
5. Vela MF, Camacho-Lobato L, Srinivasan R, Tutuian R, Katz PO, Castell DO. Simultaneous intraesophageal impedance and pH measurement of acid and nonacid gastroesophageal reflux: effect of omeprazole. Gastroenterology. 2001;120(7):1599–606.
6. Maes ML, Fixen DR, Linnebur SA. Adverse effects of proton-pump inhibitor use in older adults: a review of the evidence. Ther Adv Drug Saf. 2017;8(9):273–97.
7. Dean BB, Gano AD, Knight K, Ofman JJ, Fass R. Effectiveness of proton pump inhibitors in nonerosive reflux disease. Clin Gastroenterol Hepatol. 2004;2(8):656–64.
8. Sharma N, Agrawal A, Freeman J, Vela MF, Castell D. An analysis of persistent symptoms in acid-suppressed patients undergoing impedance-pH monitoring. Clin Gastroenterol Hepatol. 2008;6(5):521–4.
9. Anvari M, Allen C, Marshall J, et al. A randomized controlled trial of laparoscopic Nissen fundoplication versus proton pump inhibitors for the treatment of patients with chronic gastro-esophageal reflux disease (GERD): 3-year outcomes. Surg Endosc. 2011;25(8):2547–54.
10. Telem DA, Wright AS, Shah PC, Hutter MM. SAGES technology and value assessment committee (TAVAC) safety and effectiveness analysis: LINX. Surg Endosc. 2017;31(10):3811–26.
11. Zhou T, Harnsberger C, Broderick R, et al. Reoperation rates after laparoscopic fundoplication. Surg Endosc. 2015;29(3):510–4.

12. Ganz RA, Gostout CJ, Grudem J, Swanson W, Berg T, DeMeester TR. Use of a magnetic sphincter for the treatment of GERD: a feasibility study. Gastrointest Endosc. 2008;67(2):287–94.
13. committee. GaUDPottMDa. LINX Reflux Management PMA briefing. 2012. Accessed 25 Jan 2019.
14. Bonavina L, Saino GI, Bona D, et al. Magnetic augmentation of the lower esophageal sphincter: results of a feasibility clinical trial. J Gastrointest Surg. 2008;12(12):2133–40.
15. Bonavina L, DeMeester T, Fockens P, et al. Laparoscopic sphincter augmentation device eliminates reflux symptoms and normalizes esophageal acid exposure: one- and 2-year results of a feasibility trial. Ann Surg. 2010;252(5):857–62.
16. Saino G, Bonavina L, Lipham JC, Dunn D, Ganz RA. Magnetic sphincter augmentation for gastroesophageal reflux at 5 years: final results of a pilot study show long-term acid reduction and symptom improvement. J Laparoendosc Adv Surg Tech A. 2015;25(10):787–92.
17. Lipham JC, Taiganides PA, Louie BE, Ganz RA, DeMeester TR. Safety analysis of first 1000 patients treated with magnetic sphincter augmentation for gastroesophageal reflux disease. Dis Esophagus. 2015;28(4):305–11.
18. Asti E, Siboni S, Lazzari V, Bonitta G, Sironi A, Bonavina L. Removal of the magnetic sphincter augmentation device: surgical technique and results of a single-center cohort study. Ann Surg. 2017;265(5):941–5.
19. Bell R, Lipham J, Louie B, et al. Laparoscopic magnetic sphincter augmentation versus double-dose proton pump inhibitors for management of moderate-to-severe regurgitation in GERD: a randomized controlled trial. Gastrointest Endosc. 2019;89(1):14–22.e11.
20. Reynolds JL, Zehetner J, Wu P, Shah S, Bildzukewicz N, Lipham JC. Laparoscopic magnetic sphincter augmentation vs laparoscopic Nissen fundoplication: a matched-pair analysis of 100 patients. J Am Coll Surg. 2015;221(1):123–8.
21. Reynolds JL, Zehetner J, Nieh A, et al. Charges, outcomes, and complications: a comparison of magnetic sphincter augmentation versus laparoscopic Nissen fundoplication for the treatment of GERD. Surg Endosc. 2016;30(8):3225–30.
22. Alicuben ET, Tatum JM, Bildzukewicz N, et al. Regression of intestinal metaplasia following magnetic sphincter augmentation device placement. Surg Endosc. 2019;33(2):576–9.
23. Rona KA, Reynolds J, Schwameis K, et al. Efficacy of magnetic sphincter augmentation in patients with large hiatal hernias. Surg Endosc. 2017;31(5):2096–102.
24. Tatum JM, Alicuben E, Bildzukewicz N, Samakar K, Houghton CC, Lipham JC. Minimal versus obligatory dissection of the diaphragmatic hiatus during magnetic sphincter augmentation surgery. Surg Endosc. 2019;33(3):782–8.

Surgical Therapy for GERD

4

Ariel Shuchleib, Elias Chousleb, and Natan Zundel

Introduction

Anti-reflux surgery has a long history. It was in 1936 when Rudolph Nissen performed the first fundoplication. However, this was not done to prevent reflux but to "protect" an anastomosis from a distal esophagectomy. In 1951, Allison described for the first time a surgery with the intent to prevent reflux and the Nissen fundoplication for reflux was done a few years later, in 1955 [1].

However, the popularity of anti-reflux surgery did not pick up until the 1990s, with the creation of laparoscopic surgery. During that decade, there was a steady increase in the procedures performed in the USA According to data from the Nationwide Inpatient Sample (NIS), 31,695 cases were done in 1999, and since then a steady decrease in fundoplications has been noticed. The reason for this decline could be the increased efficacy on medication, newer endoscopic and surgical procedures, or the concern for long-term results [2].

In this chapter, we review the physiopathology of reflux, preoperative evaluation, the current surgical therapies, and their results.

A. Shuchleib (✉)
Department of General Surgery, ABC Medical Center, Mexico City, Mexico

E. Chousleb
Department of General Surgery, The Bariatric and Sleeve Gastrectomy Center at Jackson North, Miami, FL, USA

N. Zundel
Department of Surgery, University at Buffalo, Miami, FL, USA

© Springer Nature Switzerland AG 2021
N. Zundel et al. (eds.), *Benign Esophageal Disease*,
https://doi.org/10.1007/978-3-030-51489-1_4

Symptomatology and Pathophysiology

The most common manifestations of gastroesophageal reflux disease (GERD) are the typical symptoms such as heartburn, regurgitation, dysphagia, or sleep disturbances. However, multiple atypical symptoms on different systems such as ENT, pulmonary, cardiac, or dental can be related to GERD. Some of the most common atypical symptoms are laryngitis, hoarseness, sore throat, sinusitis, otitis, asthma, chronic cough, bronchitis/pneumonia, chest pain, dental problems, and halitosis, among others. It is estimated that 60% of the asthmatic population in the USA could have a component related to reflux [3].

Gastroesophageal Junction (GEJ) Incompetence

This junction is a complex with different anti-reflux mechanisms; the dysfunction of any of those leads to reflux disease.

- Transient lower esophageal sphincter relaxations (TLESRs)
  - The TLESR is a mechanism that allows clearing air from the stomach and belching. When it happens, the LES relaxes, the stimuli to the diaphragmatic crura gets inhibited, and the longitudinal muscular layer of the esophagus contracts.
  - When this occurs, acid also refluxes in up to 93% of the events.
- Hypotensive lower esophageal sphincter (LES)
  - This is defined as LES pressure <10 mmHg.
  - It is an uncommon etiology for reflux, reflux occurs while straining or if severely hypotensive, could happen freely.
- Anatomic disruption of the GEJ
  - If the LES is not aligned with the diaphragmatic crura, the efficiency of the anti-reflux mechanism decreases significantly, which leads to GERD.
  - Most commonly after a hiatal hernia. Patients with large hiatal hernias also have weaker LES pressures and esophageal peristalsis [4].

Increased Acid Production

In most patients with GERD, the acid production is normal; however, in certain populations with a hypersecretory state such as patients with Zollinger-Ellison, the increased levels of acid overcome the protective mechanisms and lead to severe reflux.

When acid, bile, and the digestive enzymes come in contact with the esophagus, it can lead to some complications such as Barret's or even esophageal cancer [5].

Impaired Esophageal Motility and Acid Clearance

Following exposure to gastric acid, esophageal clearance is required to limit the symptoms and the damage. A prolonged contact with fluid with a pH <4 can lead to severe mucosal injury.

Failed or hypotensive esophageal motility (<30 mmHg) can be a contributing factor to GERD; however, reflux itself can lead to worsening of the motility. When reflux is corrected and the vicious cycle is broken, some improvement can be seen in the esophageal motility, particularly in patients with severe esophagitis [4, 6].

Obesity

Obesity is an important risk factor for developing GERD. Obesity is not a single mechanism, but a combination of multiple factors previously explained. Central obesity leads to an increase in intraabdominal pressure. That increase in pressure diminishes the threshold required to defeat the natural anti-reflux mechanisms. Obesity also increases the susceptibility of the patients to develop a hiatal hernia.

On top of the previously stated, obese people have an increased prevalence of esophageal motor disorders, a decreased resting LES tone, a decreased esophageal peristalsis, and an increased number of TLESR [7].

Jacobson et al. did a study in >10,000 women in which they found an almost linear correlation between BMI and reflux symptoms [8].

Sleeve Gastrectomy

Obesity continues to rise around the world, and nowadays sleeve gastrectomy is the procedure most commonly performed. It is estimated that it accounts for nearly 60% of all the bariatric procedures.

One of the most important concerns regarding this surgery is the potential for reflux. There are many papers that have been written about the relation between sleeve and de novo or worsening reflux and the development of Barret's [9].

Some of the proposed mechanisms for GERD after sleeve are lack of gastric compliance, increased intraluminal pressure, removal of the fundus, decreased LES pressure, and further increase in pressure if there is a partial obstruction due to a technical problem such as a twist or narrowing on the sleeve [10].

Preoperative Workup

In order to be able to talk about the possible surgical therapies, it is important to have a precise diagnosis of GERD because symptoms alone can have a specificity as low as 30% [11]. Endoscopy is a mandatory test that should be done in all patients; it can not only give us the diagnosis when we find mucosal breaks but also allows us to find associated pathology such as Barret's, *H. pylori*, eosinophilic esophagitis, or even adenocarcinoma. Another benefit of the procedure is that biopsies can be taken for additional diagnoses [12].

- Barium swallow: It delineates the anatomy very clearly; this study can identify hiatal hernias or specific situations such as a short esophagus. On top of that, the extent of the reflux can be seen in fluoroscopy [13], as well as estimates of esophageal motility.
- 24-hour pH-monitoring: This remains the gold standard for the diagnosis of GERD; however, in our practice we do not perform this study routinely unless we have doubts about the diagnosis [12].
- Manometry +/− impedance: This study allows us to evaluate the esophageal motility, which we believe is important. So we perform it routinely; however, some evidence exists that there is no benefit in a tailored approach to the fundoplication [14, 15].

Surgical Interventions

Fundoplication

The procedure most commonly performed for GERD is fundoplication. Many technical variations regarding the procedure exist, but the most common techniques are the posterior partial fundoplication (Toupet) and the total or 360° (Nissen).

Multiple prospective studies have been done throughout the years comparing surgical and medical treatment for GERD with good follow-up, and it has been shown that surgical therapy is a good alternative and, in many cases, more efficient than the medical therapy. Prospective trials favor surgery with objective and subjective findings on manometry, pH-metry, and questionnaires, especially on patients who had a partial response to proton pump inhibitors (PPIs) [16–18].

When talking about surgeries for a chronic disease, it is important to see the long-term results and follow-up. Marandani randomized 137 patients to either open Nissen or Toupet fundoplication and followed them for 18 years. Symptoms were controlled in 80–90% of the patients [19]. Similarly, Campanello followed his patients in Sweden for 5, 10, and 20 years after a laparoscopic fundoplication and found that 87% of the patients were satisfied with the results after the surgery, and 84% would recommend the surgery to their loved ones [20].

Multiple studies have compared partial to total fundoplication; however, a definitive consensus regarding which procedure is better has not been achieved.

Some authors advocate for a tailored approach, which means doing a total fundoplication on patients who have good esophageal motility and a partial on patients with motility issues, but this has also been a subject of controversy [21–25].

In order to compare these two procedures Hajibandeh et al. [21] did a metanalysis that included three randomized controlled trials (RCT) with a total of 220 patients who had either a Nissen or a Toupet fundoplication. Dysphagia was significantly higher on the Nissen group OR = 10.32 (95% CI = 3.47–30.67, $P < 0.0001$) compared to the Toupet one, despite the latter group having a higher incidence of preoperative esophageal dysmotility/dysphagia. The study did not provide data regarding heartburn or regurgitation, or objective reflux data.

Wang randomized 80 consecutive patients to either a Nissen or a Toupet. The patients were fully worked up with EGD, manometry, and pH-metry. The last two studies were repeated in the postoperative period. On their last follow-up, the DeMeester score decreased from 43.0 ± 42.1 to 10.37 ± 3.10 in the Nissen group and 42.58 ± 39.38 to 12.03 ± 2.18 in the Toupet ($P < 0.05$ in both groups). In both groups, a significant increase on the LES tone was seen between 7 and 18 mmHg, as well as a great improvement in the esophageal function. In their study, despite there being a statistically significant difference on the DeMeester score favoring the Nissen group, clinical symptoms were similar, and the only thing that had a clinical relevance was an increased rate of dysphagia in total fundoplication group [26].

On a different metanalysis with systematic review from seven RCT (three were used in the study from Hajibandeh), Broeders [23] found no difference in acid exposure, esophagitis, symptomatic recurrence, or satisfaction between the two groups. However, the rates of dysphagia (R.R 1.6), surgical reintervention (R.R 2.1), esophageal dilation (R.R 2.4), and inability to belch (R.R 2.0) were higher on the Nissen group. In their opinion, Toupet should be the treatment of choice.

Conversely, Patti [22] did a retrospective study of 357 patients who were followed for 70 months. The first 235 receive a tailored approach depending on the manometric results. Patients who had esophageal dysmotility had a partial fundoplication and patients with normal motility a total fundoplication. Postoperatively, patients who received a partial fundoplication had a DeMeester score of 46 +/− 56 compared with 24 +/−33 in the patients who had a Nissen. Reflux symptoms were also higher in the first group; 33% vs. 15%. Lastly, dysphagia was only marginally higher on the Nissen group, 11% vs 8%.

In the following 122 patients, they did a Nissen regardless of the manometric scores and, at the end, they did a comparison between patients with weak motility who had a partial vs. patients with weak motility who had a total. The DeMeester score postoperatively on the partial fundoplication arm was 46 +/− 56 vs 10 +/− 8 on the total, reflux was 33% vs 13%, and dysphagia was 8% vs 9%. Due to their results, the authors recommend a 360° procedure regardless of the preoperative manometry.

A recent metanalysis compared an anterior 180° with a total fundoplication; the study reviewed six RCT with 531 patients. Their findings were similar DeMeester scores and symptomatic relief with a tendency favoring the Nissen group in both groups. Dysphagia rates were similar in patients with a follow-up shorter than 60 months, and in the patients with a longer follow-up less dysphagia was seen in the first group (RR = 0.67, 95% CI, 0.49–0.90, $P = 0.009$). However, the number of endoscopic dilations required, gas bloating symptoms, and inability to belch were similar in both groups. The main difference between the two groups was the need for a reoperation due to recurrent symptoms in the group with the anterior approach (RR = 3.58, 95% CI, 1.30–9.88, $P = 0.01$) [27].

Hopkins randomized 191 patients to either a 90° anterior fundoplication or to a posterior 360°; he followed them for 10 years with questionnaires. He saw similar overall satisfaction in both groups, yet heartburn scores and the need to take PPIs was higher in the anterior group, whereas dysphagia was higher in the Nissen one [28].

While comparing an anterior fundoplication with a Toupet, SAGES guidelines found a statistically significant higher use of PPIs, increased esophageal acid exposure, more reoperations, and less satisfaction with the anterior fundoplication without any benefit on dysphagia. For that reason, they concluded that an anterior repair should not be recommended for GERD [13].

Although it is a safe procedure, complications can occur, gastric or esophageal injuries are more frequent after redo operations and its incidence is around 1% [29, 30].

Capnothorax can happen if the pleura is violated (around 2% of the time) and sometimes is noted by the anesthesia team by a sudden rise in CO_2. It usually does not have a significant clinical repercussion and resolves by hyperventilation, giving positive pressure before extubation and observation. Supplemental O_2 and a chest X-ray can be done in the postoperative course, but is not routinely necessary.

The spleen is the most commonly injured solid organ during a fundoplication, and it happens as a result of a direct injury or by excessive traction while mobilizing the gastric fundus. Those injuries present in 2.4% of the cases and their consequences vary from inconsequential small tears to splenic hematomas and lacerations, or to significant bleeding requiring conversion to open and/or a splenectomy [5].

A transthoracic approach was used frequently before the creation of laparoscopic Nissen fundoplication; however, its popularity has been decreasing significantly and nowadays we seldom see any publications regarding this approach. Since morbidity is higher with the Belsey Mark IV for reflux or small hiatal hernias, that procedure is almost exclusively done for large hiatal/paraoesophageal hernias, significant previous abdominal surgery, redo surgery, esophageal dysmotility, and extreme esophageal shortening [31].

Not much evidence exists comparing the laparoscopic Nissen fundoplication (LNF) with the Belsey Mark IV, but there is a role for it in certain cases with pinpoint indications. A group at Mayo Clinic published recently their experience of 118 patients with large paraoesophageal hernias (>50% of the stomach) that were operated between 2002 and 2011. They matched those patients with patients who had a laparoscopic Nissen fundoplication (LNF) around the same time. Recurrence rates were similar between both groups with reference to the quality of life scores; nonetheless, esophageal leak was higher on the LNF group (6.8% vs 0%) as well as reoperations (9.3% vs 2.5%) [32].

Esophageal Lengthening Procedures

Collis gastroplasty is not an anti-reflux procedure itself, but more of an adjunct therapy while doing a fundoplication. Its use has been debated significantly; the first point of debate is its indication. This procedure is used when not enough esophagus can be brought intraabdominally. The existence of a short esophagus by itself has been challenged by some authors [33]. Some of the concerns that linger around this procedure are leaving an amotile segment of stomach that could hinder the esophageal emptying and generating dysphagia [34], leaving parietal cells in the neoesophagus that could lead to increased reflux, and lastly the concern from complications of the staple line.

Making a comparison between a fundoplication in a patient who required a Collis and one that did not can be inaccurate, since patients that require it already have an advanced disease that leads to the short esophagus in the first place. On top of that, in some series, the Collis group have greater revisional rates [35].

In the Zehetner series, the rate of dysphagia decreased from 58% to 16% after the Collis had only two new cases of dysphagia [34]. Weltz et al. did a retrospective study in which they compared the results of 149 patients who had an anti-reflux procedure with a Collis gastroplasty and 331 patients that only had the anti-reflux procedure. As expected, the time of surgery was greater in the Collis group; however, 30-day readmissions, complications, and quality of life were equivalent in both groups at 12 months [35].

Laparoscopic Magnetic Sphincter Augmentation

The lower esophageal sphincter has two mechanisms to prevent reflux, the pinch by both diaphragmatic crura and the intrinsic muscular sphincter, a magnetic device was created and approved by the FDA in 2012 to increase the pressure of the LES and decrease reflux when the previously stated mechanisms fail.

The LINX® Reflux Management System (Torax Medical, Inc., Shoreview, MN, USA) is a magnetic chain of titanium beads linked together around the esophagus that increases the pressure of the LES. The magnets separate when the food bolus passes through but prevent reflux since the back pressure is lower. When back pressure increases even further, the device opens to allowing belching or vomiting.

Currently, this device is targeted for patients with pathologic reflux with normal esophageal motility without esophagitis or a significant hiatal hernia.

Ganz reported 100 consecutive patients with a 3-year follow-up. He showed that 94% of the patients were satisfied with the procedure, and 84% were off PPIs. After 5 years, he did a follow-up study that still showed good results without major complications [36].

The most commonly reported adverse event after placement of the device is dysphagia in 45–68% of the patients. However, for most cases, it resolves on its own with time but pulse steroids or, in some cases, esophageal dilations are required. The prevalence of dysphagia in the USA at 5 years decreased to 6%. The removal rate goes from 3% to 6% and the reasons are persistent dysphagia, odynophagia, and chest pain, and the most worrisome ones are migration and erosion [37].

According to Alicuben, there have only been 29 reported cases of erosions worldwide, which represent 0.3% of the devices placed. If the device erodes into the stomach, this could be removed with either an endoscopic or laparoscopic procedure in most cases [38].

Gastric Bypass

The gastric bypass is one of the oldest procedures that could be done for GERD. It was first described by Dr. Mason in 1967 [39]. In the following decades, the relation between the bypass and reflux was extensively studied.

One of the main reasons for which a fundoplication is not performed on obese patients is because the recurrence rate is close to 30% in that population [40] on top of not having any significant impact on the weight, and potentially making the revisional surgery either for weight loss or recurrence of symptoms significantly harder and with higher morbidity. SAGES guidelines recommend avoiding a fundoplication and performing a bariatric surgery on patients with a BMI >35 kg/m^2 and recommend further studying performing bariatric surgery on patients with a BMI between 30 kg/m^2 and 35 kg/m^2 [13].

Multiple mechanisms are related to the correction of reflux with the gastric bypass. First, as previously mentioned in this chapter, obesity is a significant risk factor for GERD, so when patients lose weight, reflux diminishes. Also, due to the size of the gastric pouch, the number of parietal cells on it significantly decreases and by extension the acid production. Lastly, with a standard bypass technique, in order for the acid or bile to reach the pouch or the esophagus, it would have to travel backwards on the alimentary limb for 100 cm or more.

On a series of 152 patients, a statistical and clinically significant improvement in heartburn, water brash, laryngitis, wheezing and aspiration was seen after the bypass. Their consumption of PPI went from 44% to 9% and the occasional use of H2 blockers from 60% to 10% [40].

On a recent randomized controlled trial 217, patients with obesity were assigned to either a gastric bypass or a sleeve and were followed for 5 years. Weight loss was the same between the two groups; however, reflux resolution was seen in 60% of the bypass group against 25% of the sleeve gastrectomy patients [41].

Mortality rates after a bypass on expert hands now approaches 0.16% and it is primarily due to a pulmonary embolism, leaks rates 1% and bleeding 0.4%. Long-term complications such as internal hernias could be as high as 16%; however, if the mesenteric defects are closed with non-absorbable sutures, the rate decreases significantly. Lastly, marginal ulcerations can occur in 4.5%, especially in patients who smoke or have a gastro-gastric fistula [42].

Electrical Lower Sphincter Augmentation (EndoStim)

LES stimulation with electricity can increase the tone of the sphincter without affecting the esophageal peristalsis. In 2012, Rodriguez et al. did the first studies in humans in which he proved that by implanting a device that stimulates the LES, the resting tone can increase and reflux diminishes [43].

The way the LES stimulator device (by EndoStim St Louis. MO) works is by placing laparoscopically two electrodes on the anterior wall of the GEJ 1.5 cm apart from each other and those electrodes are connected to an implantable impulse generator that gets placed on a subcutaneous pocket. The generator can be interrogated and programed wirelessly [44]. The device delivers up to 12 thirty-minute sessions of electrical stimulation during the day and those sessions can be programed before or after meals or when patients are symptomatic.

So far, small series have been published with a follow-up of 3 years with promising results, improving reflux and with low morbidity [45]; however, case numbers are still too small with a relatively short follow-up to be able to recommend this therapy for the general population.

Reflux After Sleeve Gastrectomy

As previously stated in this chapter, sleeve gastrectomy is the most common bariatric procedure performed worldwide and it has been linked to GERD, management of reflux after sleeve can be complicated. Here is an algorithm on how it could be managed Fig. 4.1.

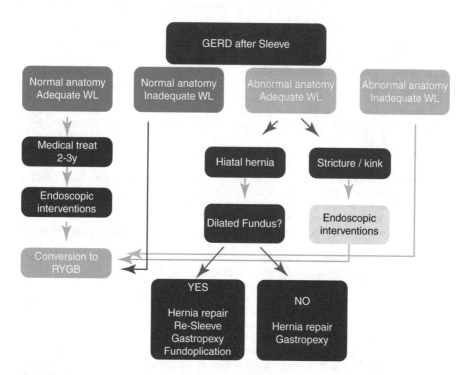

Fig. 4.1 Obtained from: Chousleb et al. Gastroesophageal Reflux Disease (GERD) post Sleeve Gastrectomy. Review of the literature and proposal of a management algorithm. (On: the perfect sleeve. 2020 with permission by the authors)

References

1. Stylopoulos N, Rattner DW. The history of hiatal hernia surgery: from Bowditch to laparoscopy. Ann Surg. 2005;241(1):185–93.
2. Finks J, Wei Y, et al. The rise and fall of antireflux surgery in the United States. Surg Endosc. 2006;20:1698–701.
3. Vaezi MF. Atypical manifestations of gastroesophageal reflux disease. MedGenMed. 2005;7(4):25.
4. Kahrilas PJ. Pathophysiology of reflux esophagitis. In: Grover S, editor. UpToDate. Waltham, MA: UpToDate Inc. https://www.uptodate.com. Accessed on 25 Dec 2019.
5. Flores L, Krause C, et al. Novel therapies for gastroesophageal reflux disease. Curr Probl Surg. 2019;56(12):100692.
6. Katada N, Moriya H, et al. Laparoscopic antireflux surgery improves esophageal body motility in patients with severe reflux esophagitis. Surg Today. 2014;44(4):740–7.
7. Chang P, Friedenberg F. Obesity & GERD. Gastroenterol Clin North Am. 2014;43(1):161–73.
8. Jacobson B, Somers SC, et al. Body-mass index and symptoms of gastroesophageal reflux in women. N Engl J Med. 2006;354(22):2340–8.
9. Chousleb E, Zundel N, et al. Gastroesophageal Reflux Disease (GERD) post Sleeve Gastrectomy. Review of the literature and proposal of a management algorithm. On: the perfect sleeve 2020.
10. Stenard F, Iannelli A. Laparoscopic sleeve gastrectomy and gastroesophageal reflux. World J Gastroenterol. 2015;21(36):10348–57.
11. Csendes A, Rencoret G, et al. Relationship between gastroesophageal reflux symptoms and 24 h esophageal pH measurements in patients with normal or minimally abnormal upper endoscopies. Rev Med Chil. 2004;132:19–25. (in Spanish).
12. Melillo R, Herbella F. Preoperative workup, patient selection, surgical technique and follow-up for a successful laparoscopic Nissen fundoplication. Mini-invasive Surg. 2017;1:6–11.
13. SAGES Guidelines for surgical treatment of gastroesophageal reflux disease (GERD). 2010.
14. Fibbe C, Layer P, et al. Esophageal motility in reflux disease before and after fundoplication: a prospective, randomized, clinical, and manometric study. Gastroenterology. 2001;121:5–14.
15. Yang H, Watson DI, et al. Esophageal manometry and clinical outcome after laparoscopic Nissen fundoplication. J Gastrointest Surg. 2007;11:1126–33.
16. Anvari M, Allen C, et al. A randomized controlled trial of laparoscopic Nissen fundoplication versus proton pump inhibitors for treatment of patients with chronic gastroesophageal reflux disease: One-year follow-up. Surg Innov. 2006;13:238–49.
17. Mahon D, Rhodes M, et al. Randomized clinical trial of laparoscopic Nissen fundoplication compared with proton-pump inhibitors for treatment of chronic gastro-oesophageal reflux. Br J Surg. 2005;92:695–9.
18. Mehta S, Bennett J, et al. Prospective trial of laparoscopic Nissen fundoplication versus proton pump inhibitor therapy for gastroesophageal reflux disease: seven-year follow-up. J Gastrointest Surg. 2006;10:1312–6; discussion 1316–1317.
19. Maradani J, Lundell L, et al. Total or posterior partial fundoplication in the treatment of GERD: results of a randomized trial after 2 decades of follow-up. Ann Surg. 2011;253:875–8.
20. Campanello M, Westin E, et al. Quality of life and gastric acid-suppression medication 20 years after laparoscopic fundoplication. ANZ J Surg. 2020;90(1–2):76–80.
21. Hajibandeh S, Hajibandeh S, et al. Impact of Toupet versus Nissen fundoplication on dysphagia in patients with gastroesophageal reflux disease and associated preoperative esophageal dysmotility: a systematic review and meta-analysis. Surg Innov. 2018; [epub ahead of print]
22. Patti MG, Fisichella PM, et al. Impact of minimally invasive surgery on the treatment of esophageal achalasia: a decade of change. J Am Coll Surg. 2003;196(5):698–703.
23. Broeders J, Mauritz F, et al. Systematic review and meta-analysis of laparoscopic Nissen (posterior total) versus Toupet (posterior partial) fundoplication for gastro-oesophageal reflux disease. Br J Surg. 2010;97:1318–30.

24. Fernando HC, Luketich JD, et al. Outcomes of laparoscopic Toupet compared to laparoscopic Nissen fundoplication. Surg Endosc. 2002;16:905–8.
25. Håkanson BS, Lundell L, et al. Comparison of laparoscopic 270° posterior partial fundoplication vs total fundoplication for the treatment of gastroesophageal reflux disease: a randomized clinical trial. JAMA Surg. 2019;154(6):479–86.
26. Wang B, Zhang W, et al. A Chinese randomized prospective trial of floppy Nissen and Toupet fundoplication for gastroesophageal disease. Int J Surg. 2015;23:35e40.
27. Du X, Wu JM, et al. Laparoscopic Nissen (total) versus anterior 180° fundoplication for gastroesophageal reflux Disease A meta-analysis and systematic review. Medicine (Baltimore). 2017;96(37):e8085.
28. Hopkins RJ, Irvine T, et al. Long-term follow-up of two randomized trials comparing laparoscopic Nissen 360◦ with anterior 90◦ partial fundoplication. Br J Surg. 2020 Jan;107(1):56–63.
29. Hunter JG, Smith CD, et al. Laparoscopic fundoplication failures: Patterns of failure and response to fundoplication revision. Ann Surg. 1999;230(4):595–604; discussion 604–6.
30. Watson DI, de Beaux AC. Complications of laparoscopic antireflux surgery. Surg Endosc. 2001;15(4):344–52.
31. Coosemans W, De Leyn P, Deneffe G, Van Raemdonck D, Lerut T. Laparoscopic antireflux surgery and the thoracic surgeon: what now? Eur J Cardiothorac Surg. 1997;12(5):683–8.
32. Laan DV, Agzarian J, et al. A comparison between Belsey Mark IV and laparoscopic Nissen fundoplication in patients with large paraesophageal hernia. J Thorac Cardiovasc Surg. 2018;156(1):418–28.
33. Madan AK, Frantzides CT, et al. The myth of the short esophagus. Surg Endosc. 2004;18(1):31–4.
34. Zehetner J, DeMeester S, et al. Laparoscopic wedge fundectomy for Collis gastroplasty creation in patients with a foreshortened esophagus. Ann Surg. 2014;260(6):1030–3.
35. Weltz AS, Zahiri HR, et al. Patients are well served by Collis gastroplasty when indicated. Surgery. 2017;162(3):568–76.
36. Ganz RA, Edmundowicz SA, et al. Long-term outcomes of patients receiving a magnetic sphincter augmentation device for gastroesophageal reflux. Clin Gastroenterol Hepatol. 2016;14:671–7.
37. Richter JE. Laparoscopic magnetic sphincter augmentation: potential applications and safety are becoming more clear-but the story is not over. Clin Gastroenterol Hepatol. 2020;18(8):1685–7.
38. Alicuben ET, Bell RCW, et al. Worldwide experience with Erosion of the magnetic sphincter augmentation device. J Gastrointest Surg. 2018;22(8):1442–7.
39. Mason EE, Ito C. Gastric bypass in obesity. Surg Clin N Am. 1967;47:1345–51.
40. Frezza EE, Ikramuddin S, et al. Symptomatic improvement in gastroesophageal reflux disease (GERD) following laparoscopic Roux-en-Y gastric bypass. Surg Endosc. 2002;16:1027–31.
41. Peterli R, Wölnerhanssen BK, et al. Effect of laparoscopic sleeve gastrectomy vs laparoscopic roux-en-Y gastric bypass on weight loss in patients with morbid obesity the SM-BOSS randomized clinical trial. JAMA. 2018;319(3):255–65.
42. Higa KD, Ho T, et al. Laparoscopic Roux-en-Y gastric bypass: 10-year follow-up. Surg Obes Relat Dis. 2011;7:516–25.
43. Rodriguez L, Rodriguez P, et al. Short-term electrical stimulation of the lower esophageal sphincter increases sphincter pressure in patients with gastroesophageal reflux disease. Neurogastroenterol Motil. 2012;24:446–50.
44. Paireder M, Kristo I. Electrical lower esophageal sphincter augmentation in patients with GERD and severe ineffective esophageal motility—a safety and efficacy study. Surg Endosc. 2019;33:3623–8.
45. Rodríguez L, Rodriguez PA. Electrical stimulation therapy of the lower esophageal sphincter is successful in treating GERD: long-term 3-year results. Surg Endosc. 2016;30(7):2666–72.

Recurrence of Symptoms After Surgical Therapies

5

Sammy Ho and Sara Welinsky

Gastroesophageal reflux disease (GERD) is a common problem in the outpatient setting with increasing prevalence in the Western world, affecting 18.1–27.8% of patients in North America [1]. Although GERD is most commonly managed with medical therapy including proton pump inhibitors (PPI) or histamine antagonists, invasive techniques including surgical Laparoscopic Nissen Fundoplication or endoscopic Transoral Incisionless Fundoplication (TIF) provide treatment alternatives for difficult-to-control GERD symptoms. There is no consensus on which of the different treatment options is best.

Laparoscopic Nissen Fundoplication is the gold standard for surgical management of GERD. Multiple studies have compared the efficacy of medical therapy with Laparoscopic Fundoplication to determine reflux recurrence. Various outcomes have been emphasized in the literature, with studies showing excellent short-term results for surgical management but with varying outcomes for long-term efficacy [2]. One randomized control trial compared total Laparoscopic Nissen Fundoplication with PPI therapy by measuring time to treatment failure and found that medical and surgical interventions had similar 3-year remission rates at 90% for surgical patients and 93% for medically treated patients ($p = 0.25$) [3]. In another randomized control trial, surgery showed more heartburn free days in the surgical group with a treatment failure of 11.8% in the surgical group and 16% treatment failure in the medically managed group [1].

In contrast, multiple large cohort studies have shown a high risk of recurrence after Laparoscopic Fundoplication [4]. One cohort study with a mean follow-up of 5.9 years showed that of the 37% of patients taking acid-reducing medications

S. Ho
Montefiore Medical Center, Bronx, NY, USA

S. Welinsky (✉)
Columbia University Medical Center, New York, NY, USA

© Springer Nature Switzerland AG 2021
N. Zundel et al. (eds.), *Benign Esophageal Disease*,
https://doi.org/10.1007/978-3-030-51489-1_5

post-operatively, 17% never stopped taking the medications after surgery and 83% restarted the medication at a mean of 2.5 years [5]. Another large cohort study using nationwide Swedish registries investigated 2655 post-surgical patients and showed 17.7% had recurrent gastroesophageal reflux disease requiring long-term medication use or secondary antireflux surgery [4]. Some risk factors that were associated with recurrent symptoms included older age and female sex.

Although Laparoscopic Nissen Fundoplication is thought to be a successful treatment modality for GERD, recurrence of symptoms is not uncommon and between 3% and 6% of patients will undergo a second procedure [6]. In most cases, Laparoscopic Fundoplication failure can be attributed to one of the following explanations: (1) wrong indications for the operation; (2) wrong preoperative workup; or (3) failure to execute the proper technical steps [6]. If heartburn symptoms can be controlled with medications, a repeat procedure can often be avoided, but if symptoms persist and an obvious anatomic issue exists, then a second operation is often considered [6]. Long-term results for surgical re-intervention are limited. One literature review found that re-operation was associated with higher morbidity and mortality when compared to primary anti-reflux surgery and had a lower success rate at 81% for subjective symptom improvement [7].

TIF has become increasingly popular in helping to bridge the gap between medical therapy and surgical intervention due to its minimally invasive approach. Given the novelty of this procedure, long-term efficacy is unknown. Studies comparing TIF to PPI therapy have demonstrated a beneficial effect. One study showed significant symptom improvement in the TIF group compared with the PPI group, with pH normalization for the TIF group of 50% compared with 63% ($p < 0.001$) for the PPI group immediately after the procedure [8]. However, the same study looked at esophageal acid exposure at 12 months and found that although the quality of life showed sustained improvement, there was no long-term improvement in esophageal acid exposure [8].

There have been no head-to-head comparisons of TIF and surgical Nissen Fundoplication, but one study performed a systematic review and meta-analysis to compare the relative efficacies of TIF versus Laparoscopic Nissen Fundoplication and showed that TIF had the highest probability of increasing health-related quality of life (0.96), followed by Nissen Fundoplication (0.66), followed by PPI therapy (0.042) [9].

With increasing prevalence of GERD in the Western world, understanding the effectiveness of different treatment modalities is essential. Although medical management is often the primary treatment, invasive techniques with surgical Laparoscopic Nissen Fundoplication or endoscopic TIF are being utilized with increasing frequency. Comparison of PPI therapy and surgical Laparoscopic Nissen Fundoplication has been well-studied with variable outcomes. Treatment failure for Laparoscopic Nissen Fundoplication has been reported as low as 11.8% [1], while other studies have shown the need to restart acid-reflux medications after surgery in as high as 37% [5]. Further head-to-head comparison is needed to contrast the effectiveness of Laparoscopic Nissen Fundoplication and TIF.

References

1. Anvari M, Allen C, Marshall J, et al. A randomized controlled trial of laparoscopic Nissen fundoplication versus proton pump inhibitors for the treatment of patients with chronic gastro-esophageal reflux disease (GERD): 3-year outcomes. Surg Endosc. 2011;25(8):2547–54.
2. Castelijns PS, Ponten JE, Poll MC, Bouvy ND, Mulders JF. Quality of life after Nissen fun-doplication in patients with gastroesophageal reflux disease: Comparison between long- and short-term follow-up. J Mimim Access Surg. 2018;14(3):213–20.
3. Lundell L, Attwood S, Ell C, et al. Comparing laparoscopic antireflux surgery with esomepra-zole in the management of patients with chronic gastro-oesophageal reflux disease: a 3-year interim analysis of the LOTUS trial. Gut. 2008;57(9):1207–13.
4. Maret-Ouda J, Wahlin K, El-Serag HB, et al. Association between laparoscopic antireflux sur-gery and recurrence of gastroesophageal reflux. JAMA. 2017;318:939–46.
5. Wijnhoven BP, Lally CJ, Kelly JJ, Myers JC, Watson DI. Use of antireflux medication after antireflux surgery. J Gastrointest Surg. 2008;12(3):510–7.
6. Patti MG, Allaix ME, Fisichella PM. Analysis of the causes of failed antireflux surgery and the principles of treatment: a review. JAMA Surg. 2015;150(6):585–90.
7. Furnée EJ, Draaisma WA, Broeders IA, Gooszen HG. Surgical reintervention after failed anti-reflux surgery: a systematic review of the literature. J Gastrointest Surg. 2009;13(8):1539–49.
8. Witteman BP, Conchillo JM, Rinsma NF, Betzel B, Peeters A, Koek GH, Stassen LP, Bouvy ND. Randomised controlled trial of Transoral incisionless Fundoplication vs proton pump inhib-itor for treatment of gastroesophageal reflux disease. Am J Gastroenterol. 2015;110(4):531–42.
9. Richter JE, Kumar A, Lipka S, Miladinovic B, Velanovich V. Efficacy of Laparoscopic Nissen fundoplication vs transoral incisionless fundoplication or proton pump inhibitors in patients with gastroesophageal reflux disease: a systematic review and network meta-analysis. Gastroenterology. 2018;154(5):1298–1308.e7.

Short Esophagus: Its Relationship with Fundoplication Failure and Postoperative Recurrence of the Hiatal Hernia

6

Italo Braghetto and Owen Korn

Since the 1950s, the discussion about the acquired shortened esophagus has continued. It is a very controversial issue because some surgeons recognize the existence of a real short esophagus, while others do not recognize it at all. Both have experimental and clinical arguments, based on anatomical studies, radiologic manometrics, and findings during surgical exploration that support the existence or inexistence of an acquired short esophagus. On the other hand, the relation between the short esophagus and antireflux surgery has been a topic of keen interest in the esophageal literature of the past 40 years.

History

The history of the short esophagus is long and full of misunderstandings. In 1950, Barrett established the concept of congenital short esophagus by arbitrarily considering that the organs are defined by their epithelia. Thus, when the columnar epithelium was found at the distal end of the esophagus, it was estimated that it was the stomach and therefore the esophagus was short. In 1953, Allison demonstrated the presence of esophageal submucosal glands under the columnar epithelium and showed that what was believed to be the stomach was in fact esophagus. Barrett took 4 years to acknowledge his mistake.

In 1957, Lortat Jacob was the first to describe the phenomenon of acquired esophageal shortening. He described the pathophysiology of reflux esophagitis leading to stenosis, in some cases to acquired esophageal shortening, and named it "endobrachiesophagus." During the same period, Leigh Collis described his combined technique of gastroplasty with hiatal hernia repair.

I. Braghetto (✉) · O. Korn
Department of Surgery, Hospital "Dr. José J. Aguirre", University of Chile,
Santiago, RM, Chile
e-mail: ibraghet@hcuch.cl

© Springer Nature Switzerland AG 2021
N. Zundel et al. (eds.), *Benign Esophageal Disease*,
https://doi.org/10.1007/978-3-030-51489-1_6

Some important dates:

1950	Barrett defines congenital short esophagus
1953	Allison/Johnstone identified esophagus instead of stomach
1957	Barrett recognized the confusion and error
1957	Collis published his technique
1970/1980	Pearson, Orringer, and Sloan use the Collis-Nissen Collis-Belsey technique
1995–2001	Swanstrom, DeMeester, Hunter, Richardson: laparoscopic approach

Pathophysiology

Physiologically, an intrinsic shortening of the esophagus would result, most commonly, from the chronic inflammation that accompanies gastroesophageal reflux disease. An inflammatory response ensues, with the inevitable stages of edema, inflammatory cell infiltration, subsequent healing, and eventual fibrosis. This process eventually involves the deeper muscular layers of the esophageal wall and may even extend transmurally into the periesophageal tissues of the mediastinum. With repeated cycles of injury and repair over time, functional and irreversible damage occurs to the involved esophagus. Contraction of the collagen in the transmural fibrous scar can occur circumferentially, producing a peptic stricture, or longitudinally, resulting in a short esophagus [1–3]. Manometric, radiologic, and experimental studies support the existence of short esophagus.

Although this pathophysiological process is undoubted, it does not necessarily lead to an anatomical shortening of the esophagus. Some authors have suggested to separate two different presentations, one that is true short esophagus but susceptible to be elongated, and one that cannot be elongated. For the unbelievers, the esophagus will be longer or shorter depending on the adequate intra-mediastinal dissection of the esophagus and, therefore, these authors definitely do not recognize this entity. Most of the authors in their clinical practice have found a short esophagus situation only in highly exceptional cases, and in our experience, after working for many years in esophageal surgery, the presence of a "true" short esophagus has been uncommon to say the least.

Why Yes, Why No

As mentioned, the reason for esophageal anatomical shortening is due to a chronic inflammatory process secondary to long-standing gastroesophageal reflux that first produces severe mucosal (ulceration) and then transmural compromise that results in damage to the muscle fibers. The healing process leads to stenosis and eventual esophageal shortening.

Some older studies would support this hypothesis. In a study performed on opossum, it was demonstrated that the infusion of acid into the esophagus to produce inflammation caused esophageal shortening with manometric displacement of the inferior esophageal sphincter toward the proximal and consequently, a hiatal hernia would appear [2]. It is a convenient theory but the studies were very unconvincing due to the great mobility and physiological displacement of the sphincter. Does a couple of centimeters of retraction really determine a short esophagus? On the other hand, it can be seen that the acid can induce a contractile response of the muscle fiber without there being a histological fibrotic scar substrate that causes the permanent shortening.

Renowned esophageal surgeons such as Griffith Pearson, Karen Horvath, Tom DeMeester, Jeffrey Peters, Lee Swanstrom, Sandro Mattioli, and others accept and promote the existence of a short esophagus, especially in patients with hiatal hernia, peptic stenosis of the esophagus with Barrett's esophagus, and recurrence after Nissen fundoplication [3]. On the other hand, other well-known surgeons such as Ronald Hinder, Attila Csendes, and Lucius Hill himself have never recognized a short esophagus in practice.

Evaluation and Diagnosis

Much has been written about the preoperative diagnosis and predictive factors of a short esophagus. Some authors base their literature on manometric, endoscopic, or radiological studies, and others on the presence of esophageal stenosis, Barrett's esophagus, or large hiatal hernias. None of these studies can assure the existence of a short esophagus without intraoperative confirmation of its true existence [3]. It is accepted that the gold standard for diagnosing a supposed short esophagus is during the surgical procedure.

Anatomy

For years, it was thought that the scarring process secondary to reflux esophagitis that caused the shortening of the esophagus had as a direct consequence on the appearance of hiatal hernia, and some studies suggested a relationship between the severity of esophagitis and the appearance of hiatal hernia in different sizes. However, it has been observed in children with hiatal hernia in whom no esophagitis has been found [1]. Hence, the explanation could be the other way around, that is, a large hiatal hernia could be the cause of esophagitis and not esophagitis the cause of the appearance of the hernia. The possibility of esophagitis itself contributing to the appearance of a hiatal hernia has been ignored by many authors [2].

So far in the literature, there has not been a clear anatomical demonstration of the shortening of the esophagus and many descriptions do not go beyond being impressions that are based on the external appearance of the gastroesophageal junction.

A short anatomical esophagus means that a segment several centimeters in length of the distal esophageal tube disappears and the union of the esophageal tube with the gastric pouch ascends. The sphincter and gastroesophageal vestibule also ascend and the short vessels would lengthen just like the artery and left gastric veins

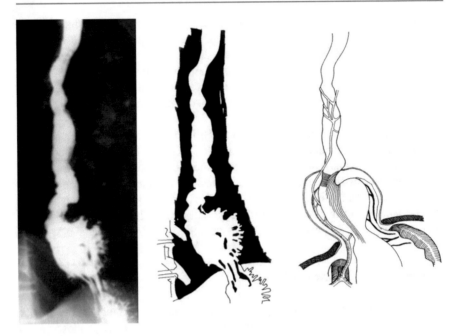

Fig. 6.1 Hiatal Hernia with "accordionated" esophagus

following the stomach. The vagal trunks, which do not shorten with the esophagus, would be redundant. The esophagus does not fall back under the hiatus, and the stomach, its serosa and its accompanying vessels permanently remain in the thorax because they cannot be lowered. Some believe that this description is found in at least 15% or 20% of patients with GERD.

A true hiatal or paraesophageal hernia (Type II, III or IV) has a dilated hiatus with a large peritoneal sac and an "accordioned" esophagus because it has to accommodate itself if the stomach rises, and the vessels and vagus follow the organs without losing their relations (Fig. 6.1).

Endoscopy

Endoscopic study has been suggested as a preoperative predictor of short esophagus, measuring the distance from the dental incisura to the gastroesophageal junction in relation to height. This method can very clearly determine the limit of squamous-columnar mucosa change but does not determine the exact location of the gastroesophageal sphincter, especially in patients with hiatus hernia or Barrett's esophagus in whom it is not possible to identify the exact point of the gastroesophageal junction due to dilation of the cardia and loss of Hiss angle. The endoscopic landmarks present great variation and there is a lot of misunderstanding regarding the location of peptic esophageal stenosis in relation to the change of mucous membranes and the exact location of the esophagogastric junction. This, in turn, results in the mistaken concept of the existence of a short esophagus. A study was made with the measurement of the length of the esophagus taken from the incisors to the gastroesophageal junction in patients undergoing Nissen or Toupet fundoplication. The study also included another group in whom Collis gastroplasty had to be performed and the length relationship of the patients was calculated using their height. It was concluded that there was a difference of 3.8 cm between both groups, but a great dispersion of the values was observed in both groups, with a specificity of 95% and a negative predictive value of 83%. The study by the Nebraska group that compared the length of the esophagus in patients subjected to a Collis gastroplasty versus a control group in which there was no need for esophageal elongation lacks scientific rigor since it does not consider the esophageal dissection factor. According to other opinions, this endoscopic measurement is absolutely reliable [4]. On the other hand, correlating these measurements with the intraoperative confirmation of a short esophagus will depend, as we have already mentioned, on the type of mediastinal dissection performed.

Manometry

The best way to determine the length of the esophagus is the manometric method, determining the limits of the cricopharyngeal sphincter and the distance to the LES and correlating it with the height of the patients. However, it has been seen that there is a low correlation between these parameters and there is also a large dispersion of values between normal subjects and patients with gastroesophageal reflux.

In 1971, our Surgical Department simultaneously performed radiological and manometric studies demonstrating that below the stricture area motility existed that corresponded to the esophagus and not the stomach and therefore it was not a true short esophagus [5] (Fig. 6.2).

Peters and DeMeester [6] found progressive shortening of the esophagus according to the severity of the esophagitis with up to 2 cm of difference, coinciding with Korn's studies in our group. The measured shortening is in the range of 2 cm and could be explained by the shortening of the sphincter pressure area. No significant differences were found between patients with esophagitis or complicated Barrett's esophagus [7]. In Fig. 6.3, the findings in the two studies are shown. On the other hand, Gastal describes the manometric length of the esophagus in patients undergoing Collis gastroplasty, after esophageal mobilization with laparoscopic approach. When compared to a normal one, 28% short esophagus, 6% definitive short esophagus and 12% short esophagus catalogued as apparent were found, but the differences are also no more than 2cms. [8].

The positive predictive value of the manometric study is only 36%. In Fig. 6.4, we show our results studying esophageal length in control subjects and patients with reflux esophagitis, non-complicated and complicated Barrett's esophagus. [6] Based on this study, for us, the so-called true short esophagus does not exist and is not relevant between different degrees of severity of the disease nor does it have an

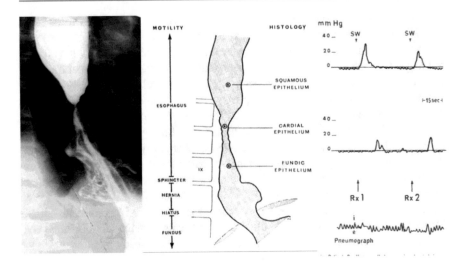

Fig. 6.2 Simultaneous radiologic and manometric study demonstrating that the segment below the stricture corresponds to esophagus and not the stomach

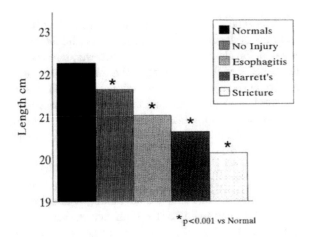

Fig. 6.3 Manometric length of esophagus according to severity of esophagitis. (Refs. [6, 7])

Subject's height	Control subjects (n)	Reflux esophagitis (n)	Long-segment Barrett's (n)	Long-segment complicated Barrett's (n)
≥180	30.3 ± 3.1 (6)	28.2 ± 2.4 (5)	28.2 ± 2.6 (5)	28.0 (1)
170-179	28.2 ± 2.5 (43)	26.0 ± 2.1 (13)	26.7 ± 2.4 (17)	26.6 ± 3.1 (12)
160-169	27.2 ± 2.9 (82)	25.6 ± 2.3 (34)	26.1 ± 2.4 (33)	25.1 ± 3.3 (7)
≤159	26.1 ± 2.3 (59)	25.5 ± 2.8 (25)	25.4 ± 2.5 (19)	26.4 ± 2.8 (9)

*There were not statistically significant differences among the different groups compared by range of height. All values are represented as cm ± SD.

Fig. 6.4 Manometric length of esophagus (cm) according to height in controls and patients with reflux esophagitis and Barrett's esophagus

important role in the choice of the surgical technique to be used. The minimum differences of 1–2 cm between patients with different degrees of esophagitis can be explained by the decrease in the length of the sphincter or by the dilation of the gastroesophageal junction and not by an anatomical shortening of the esophagus. [9].

Radiology

It has been suggested that if it is observed that the gastroesophageal junction is located more than 5 cm above the diaphragmatic crura or hiatal hernia and it cannot be reduced in a standing position; a short esophagus may be present. Radiological studies are inaccurate because they do not precisely determine the location of the LES. When the barium column is swallowed, the LES relaxes and ascends proximally. The classic image for those who think of a short esophagus is presented in Fig. 6.5. The segment below the esophageal narrowing (a) would correspond to a gastric segment pulled proximally by the esophageal shortening; however, it was found that this segment corresponds anatomically and histologically to the esophagus with a dilated gastroesophageal junction (point b).

The positive predictive value of the preoperative barium esophagram was only 50%.

In a study comparing the preoperative radiological image and the intraoperative findings in which a short esophagus was found and subjected to Collis gastroplasty, the positive predictive value of the preoperative barium esophagram was only 50%.

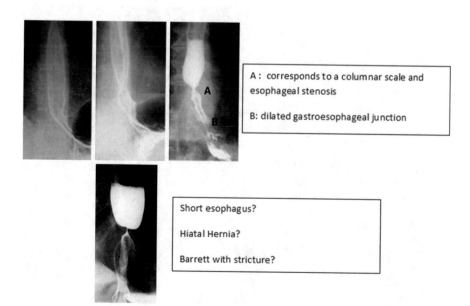

A : corresponds to a columnar scale and esophageal stenosis

B: dilated gastroesophageal junction

Short esophagus?

Hiatal Hernia?

Barrett with stricture?

Fig. 6.5 Preoperative evaluation with barium swallow

However, once again, the question arises of how the measurement was made and how meticulous the intra-mediastinal dissection to adequately mobilize the esophagus was. [10].

When these three methods of evaluation are jointly used for the diagnosis of the supposed short esophagus, the specificity is 100% but the sensitivity is only 28%. [10].

Intraoperative Measurement

Despite all the preoperative diagnostic considerations, the definitive diagnosis of a short esophagus is confirmed during a surgical procedure after extended esophageal mediastinal dissection. In some cases, identification of EGJ can be difficult even with intraoperative endoscopy in patients with hiatal hernia or Barrett's esophagus. Mattioli et al. have conducted a very elegant method for measuring the length of the intraabdominal segment of esophagus after a 6–8 cm dissection of the mediastinal esophagus. The distance between EGJ and the apex of the hiatus was determined. When the sub-diaphragmatic segment of esophagus is less than 1.5 cm, it was categorized as a short esophagus. [11] In this study, after preoperative barium swallow, short esophagus was found in 1.2%, while during surgery, 37% presented an intra-abdominal esophagus shorter than 1.5 cm. Collis gastroplasty was performed in 14.5% and Collis-Nissen procedure in 3.8%. These results are very inconsistent. In our experience, after esophageal dissection, we always obtained the intra-abdominal segment of distal esophagus more than 2–3 cm, even in patients with hiatal hernia or complicated Barrett's esophagus (Fig. 6.6).

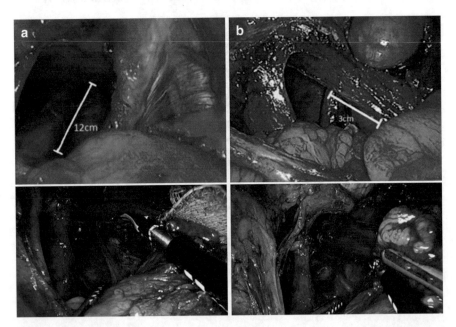

Fig. 6.6 Intraoperative measurement of mediastinal dissection of distal esophagus (**a**) and intra-abdominal esophageal segment after dissection (**b**)

Reported Incidence

The precise incidence of the truly shortened esophagus is unknown. In a review of the open and laparoscopic literature, the frequency of esophageal shortening ranges widely from the 60% reported by Pearson and Todd to 0% reported by Hill and some laparoscopic series [12–14]. In the laparoscopic literature, the incidences of esophageal shortening requiring a Collis gastroplasty are 3–5%. This enormous variation is due, in part, to the magnitude and type of intra-medastinic dissection of the esophagus. An extensive review carried out by Herbella [14] establishes that the true existence depends on the extension of the esophageal dissection of the surgical approach and of the basic pathology. These criteria are fundamental to determining the exact incidence of the existence of a true short esophagus. According to Dallemagne, the esophagus should be mobilized up to 5–7 cm above the hiatus, and Swanstrom suggested continuing dissection to the level of the lower pulmonary vein. This high mobilization of the esophagus enables the reconstruction of a sufficiently long abdominal esophageal segment which is possible to obtain in a high proportion of cases. For us, in agreement with the majority of authors, a true short esophagus is very rare. For Hinder, the true short esophagus is less than 1% [12–15].

In Table 6.1, we show a summary of the reported incidence of a short esophagus.

In our surgical experience, after 40 years of work in esophageal surgery, we have only seen three cases of short esophagus in difficult dissection situations, in which, when attempting to descend, there was a transversal tear in a scar area that forced esophageal resuturing and gastroplasty repair.

Post-fundoplication Failure: Technical Failure or Short Esophagus?

In a study by Swanstrom's group, it was clearly established that a good intramediastinal dissection reduces the failure rate of Nissen fundoplication without the need for a Collis gastroplasty, which otherwise does not guarantee good

Table 6.1 Reported incidence of short esophagus

	Incidence Short Esophagus
Patients with GERD	1.53%
Laparotomy approach	0.08%
Laparoscopic approach	0.84%
Thoracotomic approach	57.4%
Thoracoscopic approach	5.4%
Paraesophageal hernia	11.9%
Barrett's esophagus	0.95%
Reoperation after fundoplication	2.9%

results, aside from its complexity as a process. Poor results have been described with a high rate of postoperative complications, persistence of abnormal acid reflux in more than 50% of cases determined by 24 h pH monitoring, and poor long-term results such as dysphagia, esophageal peristalsis, and recurrence. Therefore, a good intra-mediastinal mobilization of the esophagus, of at least 7 cm (Type II intra-mediastinal dissection), should be chosen, which results in an adequate length of the abdominal esophagus to perform a fundoplication [16–17].

Recurrence of Postoperative Hiatal Hernia: Is the Short Esophagus the Cause? Failure in the Dissection of the Sac and Mobilization of the Esophagus?

It is widely accepted that in order to avoid a post-repair recurrence of a hiatal hernia, a fundoplication should be performed on the free abdominal esophagus, for which at least 2–3 cm of the intra-abdominal esophagus should be obtained. If this is not obtained, one could think of the existence of a short esophagus. It has been perceived by those who recognize it that a short esophagus contributes to a recurrence in 15–35% of the patients, but as we have already mentioned, with a wide dissection of the intra-mediastinal hernia sac, sectioning all the fibrous tracts that keep traction toward proximal hernia content and good dissection (Type II), it is possible to obtain an optimal length of intra-abdominal esophagus, which has been corroborated in many reported experience [10–17].

Collis Gastroplasty: When to Indicate?

Therefore, given the low incidence of the true short esophagus and accepting that there are exceptional situations, the question is when to perform a Collis Nissen gastroplasty and how often should it be performed? Here, there is great bias due to the partiality with which patients are handled. In some centers prone to accepting the existence of a short esophagus, the Collis gastroplasty or Collis-Nissen technique is more openly performed. For some, the short esophagus simply does not exist and they have never performed a Collis gastroplasty [14–16], and others have performed it in up to 14% of the patients operated on for GERD [17–22].

Figure 6.7 shows the algorithm for the treatment of GERD suggested more recently; however, it has not been accepted at all [23].

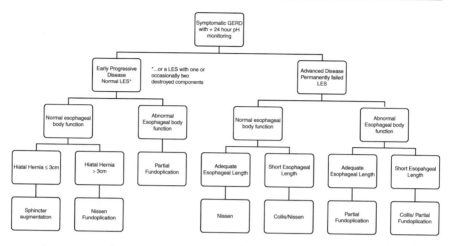

Fig. 6.7 Algorithm for treatment of gastroesophageal reflux disease according to the preoperative evaluation and intraoperative findings

References

1. Stephens HB. The problem of the acquired short esophagus. Calif Med. 1949;71:385–90.
2. Paterson WG, Kolyn DM. Esophageal shortening induced by short term intraluminal acid perfusion in opossum: a cause for hiatus hernia. Gastroenterology. 1994;107:1736–40.
3. Puri V, Jacobsen K, Bell JM, Crabtree TD, Kreisel D, Krupnick AS, Patterson GA, Meyers BF. Hiatal hernia repair with or without esophageal lengthening: is there a difference. Innovations. 2013;8:341–7.
4. Yano F, Stadlhuber RJ, Tsuboi K, Garg N, FilipiCh J, Mittal SK. Preoperative predictability of the short esophagus: endoscopic criteria. Surg Endosc. 2009;23:1308–12.
5. Heitmann P, Csendes A, Strauszer T. The myth of short esophagus. Dig Dis. 1971;16:307–20.
6. Korn O, Csendes A, Burdiles P, et al. Length of the esophagus in patients with gastroesophageal reflux disease and Barrett's esophagus compared to controls. Surgery. 2003;133:358–63.
7. Peters JH, Kauer WKH, DeMeester TR. Tailored antireflux surgery. In: Bremner CG, DeMeester TR, Peracchia A, editors. Modern approach to benign esophageal disease. St Louis, MO: Quality Medical Publishing, Inc; 1995. p. 57–68.
8. Gastal OL, Hagen JA, Peters JH, et al. Short esophagus: analysis of predictors and clinical implications. Arch Surg. 1999;134:633–6.. [discussion: 637–8]
9. Kunio NR, Dolan JP, Hunter JG. Short Esophagus. Surg Clin N Am. 2015;95:641–52.
10. Awad ZT, Mittal SK, Roth TA, et al. Esophageal shortening during the era of laparoscopic surgery. Worl J Surg. 2001;25:558–61.
11. Mattioli S, Lugaresi M, Costantini M, et al. The short esophagus: intraoperative assessment of esophageal length. J Thorac Cardiovasc Surg. 2008;136:834–41.
12. Bochkarev V, Lee YK, Vitamvas M, Oleinikov D. Short esophagus: how much length can we get? Surg Endosc. 2008;22:2123–7.
13. Migaczewski M, Zub-Pokrowiecka A, Grzesiak-Kulk A, Pedziwiatr M, Major P, Rubinkiewicz M, Winiarski M, Natkaniec M, Budzynski A. Incidence of true short esophagus among patients submitted to laparoscopic Nisen fundoplication. Videosurgery Mininv. 2015;10:10–4.
14. Herbella FAM, Del Grande JC, Colleoni R. Short esophagus: literature incidence. Dis Esoph. 2002;15:125–31.

15. Swanstrom LL, Marcus DR, Galloway GQ. Laparoscopic Collis gastroplasty is the treatment of choice for the shortened esophagus. Am J Surg. 1996;171:477–81.
16. Madan AK, Frantzides CT, Patsavas KL. The myth of short esophagus. Surg Endosc. 2004;18:31–4.
17. Hill LD, Gelfand M, Bauermeister D. Simplified management of reflux esophagitis with stricture. Ann Surg. 1970;172:638–51.
18. Larrain A, Csendes A, Strauszer T. The short esophagus: a surgical myth. Actagastroenterologca Latinoam. 1971;3:125–33.
19. Demeester SR, Demeeser TR. The short esophagus: going, going, gone? Surgery. 2003;133:364–7.
20. Pearson FG, Cooper JD, Patterson GA, et al. Gastroplasty and fundoplication for complex reflux problems. Long-term results. Ann Surg. 1987;206:473–81.
21. Kauer WK, Peters JH, DeMeester TR, et al. A tailored approach to antireflux surgery. J Thorac Cardiovasc Surg. 1995;110:141–7.
22. Durand L, De Anton R, Caracoche M, Covian E, Gimenez M, Ferraina P, Swanstrom L. Short esophagus: selection of patients for surgery and long term results. Surg Endosc. 2012;26:704–13.
23. Worrell SG, Greene CL, DeMeesterTR. The state of surgical treatment of gastroesophageal reflux disease after five decades. J. Am Coll Surg. 2014;219:819.

Hiatal Hernia

7

Kamil Nurczyk, Marco Di Corpo, and Marco G. Patti

Hiatal hernia (HH) is a common finding in the general population, and given the aging and the prevalence of obesity of the population in the United States, these numbers will increase in the future [1]. It is a condition in which the stomach, in some cases together with other structures, herniates through the esophageal hiatus into the mediastinum. HH is a frequent finding in patients with gastroesophageal reflux disease (GERD) eliminating a key component of the antireflux mechanism as it interrupts the synergistic action between the lower esophageal sphincter (LES) and the diaphragmatic crura [2]. HH has a distinct connection with obesity due to increased intra-abdominal pressure [3, 4], which also increases the risk of recurrence [5].

Classification

The HH are divided into four groups [6]:

- *Type I HH,* so called sliding HH, is the most common, and it is responsible for more than 95% of the cases. The gastroesophageal junction (GEJ) herniates upward into the posterior mediastinum through the esophageal hiatus [7] (Fig. 7.1).
- *Type II HH* is the pure paraesophageal hernia (PEH). There is no displacement of the GEJ, which is located below the diaphragm, but there is herniation of the gastric fundus above the GEJ and lateral to the esophagus. Type II is the least common among the PEH.

K. Nurczyk · M. G. Patti (✉)
Departments of Surgery and Medicine, University of North Carolina, Chapel Hill, NC, USA
e-mail: marco_patti@med.unc.edu

M. Di Corpo
Department of Surgery, University of North Carolina, Chapel Hill, NC, USA

© Springer Nature Switzerland AG 2021
N. Zundel et al. (eds.), *Benign Esophageal Disease*,
https://doi.org/10.1007/978-3-030-51489-1_7

Fig. 7.1 Hiatal
hernia type I

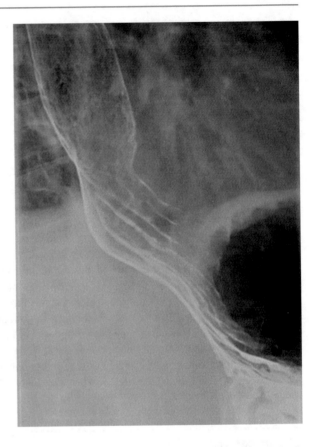

- *Type III PEH* is the combination of types I and II as the GEJ and fundus are both herniated into the mediastinum [6]. More than 90% of PEH are Type III (Fig. 7.2).
- *Type IV PEH* is characterized by the presence of other structures, such as the omentum, colon, small bowel, spleen, and/or pancreas within the hernia sac in mediastinum (Fig. 7.3).

Symptoms and Complications

Although many patients with HH are asymptomatic, each type of HH may present with different symptoms. Complaints related to GERD, such as heartburn, regurgitation, chronic cough, laryngitis, and asthma, are the consequence of the antireflux mechanism disruption and are typical for type I HH. This may lead to GERD complications such as esophagitis, Barrett esophagus, and strictures. Respiratory complications vary from chronic cough to asthma, aspiration pneumonia, and even pulmonary fibrosis. According to Schlottmann et al. patients with larger HH have more frequent episodes of coughing and wheezing, decreased pressure of the lower esophageal sphincter, weaker peristalsis, more acid reflux (as documented by pH

Fig. 7.2 Hiatal hernia
type III

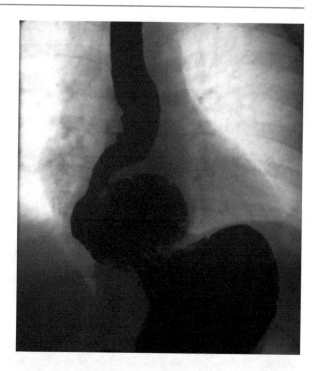

Fig. 7.3 Hiatal
hernia type IV

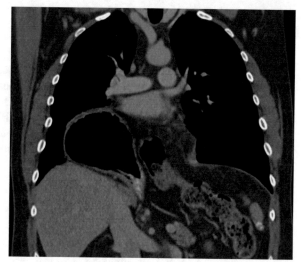

monitoring), and more severe esophagitis [8]. While in type I HH dysphagia is usually secondary to abnormal peristalsis, in PEH it may be caused by compression of
the distal esophagus by the hernia. Large PEH may lead to respiratory and cardiac
impairment caused by direct compression of the thoracic organs [9]. Another complication is anemia secondary to bleeding from venous stasis of the gastric wall or

Cameron lesions [10]. Acute symptoms are more common for PEH. Volvulus, strangulation, obstruction, ischemia, necrosis, and perforation are potentially lethal complications [11].

Evaluation

Most patients require an esophagogastroduodenoscopy, barium swallow examination, high resolution manometry, and pH monitoring. A chest and abdomen CT is key for the diagnosis of a type IV hernia, which can be suspected in a chest X-ray.

Endoscopy

Endoscopy gives information about the presence of esophagitis or Barrett's esophagus and rules out other gastric or duodenal pathology.

Barium Swallow

It determines the size and type of HH. While this test is important to delineate the anatomy, it should not be considered diagnostic for GERD.

Esophageal Manometry

High-resolution manometry (HRM) determines the level of the crura, the respiratory inversion point, and the location of the lower esophageal sphincter (LES). It may also give information regarding the size of sliding HH, the pressure of the LES, and the quality of esophageal peristalsis. In addition, HRM enables a pH probe to be properly positioned 5 cm above the upper border of the LES. The manometry and pH monitoring are often omitted in elderly patients with type III HH.

pH Monitoring

Ambulatory pH monitoring is used to determine the presence of abnormal reflux, and the correlation between symptoms experienced by the patient and episodes of reflux. This is key before planning surgical treatment of GERD with a fundoplication.

Computed Tomography

CT scan is recommended when a type IV HH is suspected or in case of acute complications.

Surgical Treatment

Asymptomatic HH do not need surgery. However, patients with large PEH should have regular follow-up as the annual probability of developing acute symptoms is around 1% [12]. The surgical approach and the indications for surgery differ depending on the type of HH.

Type I Most patients with GERD are treated with acid reducing medications. The indications for surgery are intolerance to medical therapy or inadequate symptom control despite optimal medical management, patient preference for surgery despite successful medical management, complications of GERD, such as stricture while taking PPI, and/or persistence of extra-esophageal symptoms despite medical therapy. The technique will be described in the chapter that treats GERD.

Types II, III, and IV Surgery is indicated when the patient is symptomatic. It is usually elective surgery. When ischemia is present, urgent repair is needed [13]. Surgical techniques for HH evolved over time [14]. Previous studies have shown that laparoscopic HH repair, as compared to open, was associated with significantly better postoperative outcomes in terms of morbidity, mortality, length of hospital stay, and costs [15]. The following describes the technical steps of the repair of a type III hiatal hernia. In most cases, the type IV hiatal hernia can also be treated laparoscopically as it is possible to reduce all the organs. However, when severe adhesions are present, a left thoracotomy might be necessary.

Patient Positioning

Laparoscopic HH repair is performed under general anesthesia. During the procedure, patient lies in supine position. The beanbag mattress is useful especially when using the reverse Trendelenburg position. Patient's legs are positioned on stirrups with knees flexed at 30 degrees. After inducing anesthesia, the anesthesiologist inserts an oro-gastric tube to decompress the stomach. During the operation, the surgeon's position is between the patient's legs with assistants on both sides of the operating table (Fig. 7.4).

Trocar Placement

The operation is performed using 5 trocars. After abdominal cavity insufflation using a Verres needle, trocar 1 is placed 14 cm below the xiphoid process in the midline or slightly to the left. Trocar 2 is placed in the left midclavicular line at the level of trocar 1. Trocar 3 for the liver retractor is placed in the right midclavicular line at the level of trocar 1. Trocars 4 and 5 are placed under the costal margins on the left and right side, and are used for the dissecting and suturing instruments (Fig. 7.5).

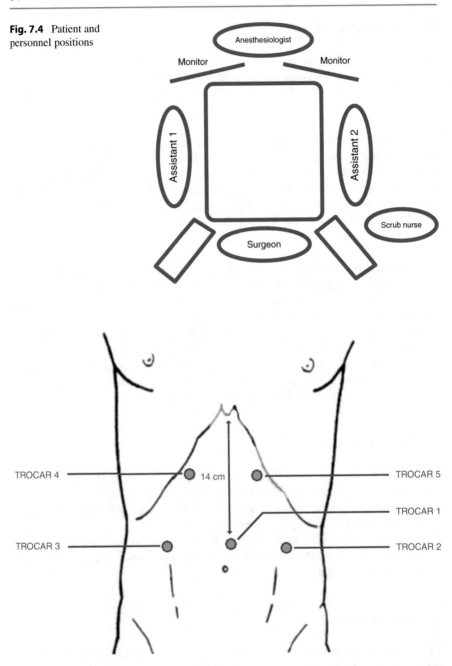

Fig. 7.4 Patient and personnel positions

Fig. 7.5 Trocar positioning

Dissection of the Hernia Sac and Mobilization of the Esophagus

Traction is applied to the herniated stomach to reduce it below the diaphragm as much as possible (Fig. 7.6).

The short gastric vessels are divided and the left pillar of the crus is reached. The left crus approach reduces the risk of injury to an accessory left hepatic artery that can occur if the dissection is started over the gastrohepatic ligament, with resultant bleeding difficult to control (Fig. 7.7). The hernia sac is incised at the junction with the left crus and an anterior and lateral mobilization of the esophagus is performed (Fig. 7.8). Next the gastrohepatic ligament is divided at the pars flaccida above the caudate lobe of the liver toward the right pillar of the crus, and the esophagus is further dissected in the posterior mediastinum paying attention not to damage the parietal pleura and the vagus nerves. A posterior window behind the esophagus is then created, and a Penrose drain is placed around the esophagus, incorporating both the anterior and the posterior vagus nerves. This maneuver facilitates exposure to complete the dissection (Fig. 7.9). Dissection is continued in the posterior mediastinum circumferentially around the esophagus. During this part of the dissection, it is important to avoid injury to the pleura and the vagus nerves. If proper dissection

Fig. 7.6 Paraesophageal hernia

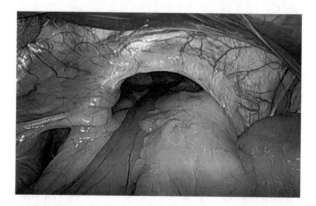

Fig. 7.7 Dividing short gastric vessels

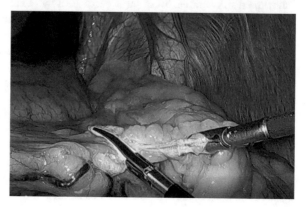

Fig. 7.8 Hernia sac
dissection

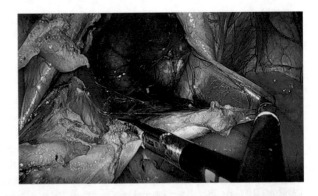

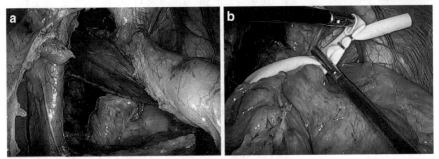

Fig. 7.9 Posterior window (**a**) and Penrose drain placement (**b**)

is performed, it is usually possible to have about 3 cm of esophagus below the diaphragm without tension. In our experience, a lengthening procedure is rarely necessary.

Closure of the Diaphragmatic Crura

The right and left pillar of the crus are approximated behind the esophagus using interrupted silk sutures. Suturing is performed by placing stitches at 1 cm intervals. In some cases, when the hiatal defect is large, some stitches can be placed anterior to the esophagus. The recurrence rate after laparoscopic PEH with cruroplasty is significant [16–22]; however, in the majority of cases the recurrent hernia is asymptomatic and small [22–24]. Some studies have demonstrated lower recurrence rates after nonabsorbable mesh PEH repair compared with cruroplasty [25, 26]. At the same time, the use of synthetic mesh has been associated with severe complications, such as erosions through the esophageal wall, esophageal stenosis, and infections [27, 28]. To avoid these complications, the use of biological materials has been investigated [24, 29–32]. While a significant lower early recurrence rate 6 months after the surgery was reported in the group of patients treated with mesh repair compared to the group of patients who underwent cruroplasty (9% vs. 23%) [24], at 5-year follow-up the recurrence rate was similar in the two groups of patients (54%

vs. 59%) [33]. Interestingly, both group of patients reported similar symptom improvement and a reoperation was necessary in only 3% of cases regardless of the technique used to close the hiatal defect. As literature shows that using mesh does not reduce the recurrence rate, it is associated with long-term complications, and implies high costs for the healthcare system, surgeons should not routinely use mesh at the hiatus and consider its use only for a very selected group of patients. Most likely patients with a giant PEH, redo operations, or cases where the tension-free cruroplasty cannot be achieved are mostly benefited by the use of mesh (Fig. 7.10).

Fundoplication

Fundoplication is the last step of the procedure. It both prevents gastroesophageal reflux and works as a gastropexy. If the quality of peristalsis has been assessed and found to be normal, a 360 degree fundoplication is performed over a 56–60 French bougie [34]. But in elderly patients and when the manometry has not been performed, a partial posterior fundoplication is the procedure of choice. Failure of the closure of the crura and an anatomically incorrect wrap are the main reasons for failure of antireflux surgery [35–37] (Fig. 7.11).

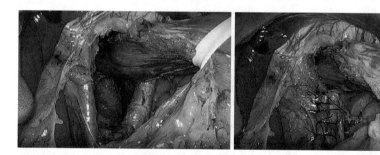

Fig. 7.10 Closure of the esophageal hiatus

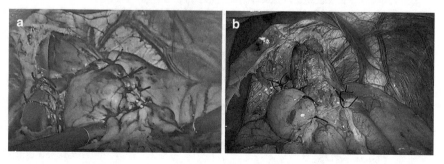

Fig. 7.11 Nissen fundoplication (**a**) and partial posterior fundoplication (**b**)

References

1. Davis SS Jr. Current controversies in paraesophageal hernia repair. Surg Clin North Am. 2008;88(5):959–78.
2. Gordon C, Kang JY, Neild PJ, et al. The role of the hiatus hernia in gastro-oesophageal reflux disease. Aliment Pharmacol Ther. 2004;20:719–32.
3. Wilson LJ, Ma W, Hirschowitz BI. Association of obesity with hiatal hernia and esophagitis. Am J Gastroenterol. 1999;94(10):2840–4.
4. Pandolfino JE, El-Serag HB, Zhang Q, Shah N, Ghosh SK, Kahrilas PJ. Obesity: a challenge to esophagogastric junction integrity. Gastroenterology. 2006;130(3):639–49.
5. Perez AR, Moncure AC, Rattner DW. Obesity adversely affects the outcome of antireflux operations. Surg Endosc. 2001;15(9):986–9.
6. Kahrilas PJ, Kim HC, Pandolfino JE. Approaches to the diagnosis and grading of hiatal hernia. Best Pract Res Clin Gastroenterol. 2008;22(4):601–16.
7. Curci JA, Melman LM, Thompson RW, Soper NJ, Matthews BD. Elastic fiber depletion in the supporting ligaments of the gastroesophageal junction: a structural basis for the development of hiatal hernia. J Am Coll Surg. 2008;207(2):191–6.
8. Schlottmann F, Andolfi C, Herbella FA, Rebecchi F, Allaix ME, Patti MG. GERD: presence and size of hiatal hernia influence clinical presentation, esophageal function, reflux profile, and degree of mucosal injury. Am Surg. 2018;84(6):978–82.
9. Khanna A, Finch G. Paraesophageal herniation: a review. Surgeon. 2011;9(2):104–11.
10. El Khoury R, Ramirez M, Hungness ES, Soper NJ, Patti MG. Symptom relief after laparoscopic Paraesophageal hernia repair without mesh. J Gastrointest Surg. 2015;19(11):1938–42.
11. Roman S, Kahrilas PJ. The diagnosis and management of hiatus hernia. BMJ. 2014;349:g6154.
12. Stylopoulos N, Gazelle GS, Rattner DW. Paraesophageal hernias: operations or observation? Ann Surg. 2002;236(4):492–500; discussion 500–1
13. Peters JH. SAGES guidelines for the management of hiatal hernia. Surg Endosc. 2013;27(12):4407–8.
14. Stylopoulos N, Rattner DW. The history of hiatal hernia surgery: from Bowditch to laparoscopy. Ann Surg. 2005;241(1):185–93.
15. Schlottmann F, Strassle PD, Farrell TM, Patti MG. Minimally invasive surgery should be the standard of care for paraesophageal hernia repair. J Gastrointest Surg. 2017;21(5):778–84.
16. Luketich JD, Nason KS, Christie NA, et al. Outcomes after a decade of laparoscopic giant paraesophageal hernia repair. J Thorac Cardiovasc Surg. 2010;139:395–404.
17. Hashemi M, Peters JH, DeMeester TR, et al. Laparoscopic repair of large type III hiatal hernia: objective follow-up reveals high recurrence rate. J Am Coll Surg. 2000;190:553–61.
18. Mattar SG, Bowers SP, Galloway KD, et al. Long-term outcome of laparoscopic repair of paraesophageal hernia. Surg Endosc. 2002;16:745–9.
19. Pierre AF, Luketich JD, Fernando HC, et al. Results of laparoscopic repair of giant paraesophageal hernias: 200 consecutive patients. Ann Thor Surg. 2002;74:1909–15.
20. Smith GS, Isaacson JR, Draganic BD, et al. Symptomatic and radiological follow-up after para-esophageal hernia repair. Dis Esophagus. 2004;17:279–84.
21. Zaninotto G, Portale G, Costantini M, et al. Objective followup after laparoscopic repair of large type III hiatal hernia. Assessment of safety and durability. World J Surg. 2007;31:2177–83.
22. Dallemagne B, Kohnen L, Perretta S, Weerts J, Markiewicz S, Jehaes C. Laparoscopic repair of paraesophageal hernia. Long-term follow-up reveals good clinical outcome despite high radiological recurrence rate. Ann Surg. 2011;253(2):291–6.
23. Aly A, Munt J, Jamieson GG, et al. Laparoscopic repair of large hiatal hernias. Br J Surg. 2005;92:648–53.
24. Oelschlager BK, Pellegrini CA, Hunter J, et al. Biologic prosthesis reduces recurrence after laparoscopic paraesophageal hernia repair. A multicenter, prospective, randomized trial. Ann Surg. 2006;244:481–90.

25. Frantzides CT, Madam AK, Carlson MA, et al. A prospective, randomized trial of laparoscopic polytetrafluoroethylene (PTFE) patch repair vs simple cruroplasty for large hiatal hernia. Arch Surg. 2002;137:649–52.
26. Johnson JM, Carbonell AM, Carmody BJ, et al. Laparoscopic mesh hiatoplasty for paraesophageal hernias and fundoplications. A critical analysis of the available literature. Surg Endosc. 2006;20:362–6.
27. Carlson MA, Condon RE, Ludwig KA, et al. Management of intrathoracic stomach with polypropylene mesh prosthesis reinforced transabdominal hiatus hernia repair. J Am Coll Surg. 1998;187:227–30.
28. Tatum RP, Shalhub S, Oelschlager BK, et al. Complications of PTFE mesh at the diaphragmatic hiatus. J Gastrointest Surg. 2007;12:953–7.
29. Lee YK, James E, Bochkarev V, et al. Long-term outcome of cruroplasty reinforcement with human acellular dermal matrix in large paraesophageal hiatal hernia. J Gastrointest Surg. 2008;12:811–5.
30. Tatum RP, Shalhub S, Oelschlager BK, Pellegrini CA. Complications of PTFE mesh at the diaphragmatic hiatus. J Gastrointest Surg. 2008;12(5):953–7.
31. Stadlhuber RJ, Sherif AE, Mittal SK, Fitzgibbons RJ Jr, Michael Brunt L, Hunter JG, Demeester TR, Swanstrom LL, Daniel Smith C, Filipi CJ. Mesh complications after prosthetic reinforcement of hiatal closure: a 28-case series. Surg Endosc. 2009;23(6):1219–26.
32. Parker M, Bowers SP, Bray JM, Harris AS, Belli EV, Pfluke JM, Preissler S, Asbun HJ, Smith CD. Hiatal mesh is associated with major resection at revisional operation. Surg Endosc. 2010;24(12):3095–101.
33. Oelschlager BK, Pellegrini CA, Hunter JG, Brunt ML, Soper NJ, Sheppard BC, Polissar NL, Neradilek MB, Mitsumori LM, Rohrmann CA, Swanstrom LL. Biologic prosthesis to prevent recurrence after laparoscopic paraesophageal hernia repair:long-term follow-up from a multicenter, prospective, randomized trial. J Am Coll Surg. 2011;213(4):461–8.
34. Patterson EJ, Herron DM, Hansen PD, Ramzi N, Standage BA, Swanström LL. Effect of an esophageal bougie on the incidence of dysphagia following Nissen fundoplication: a prospective, blinded, randomized clinical trial. Arch Surg. 2000;135(9):1055–61.
35. Horgan S, Pohl D, Bogetti D, et al. Failed antireflux surgery: what have we learned from reoperations? Arch Surg. 1999;134:809–15.
36. Hunter JG, Smith CD, Branum GD, et al. Laparoscopic fundoplication failures: patterns of failure and response to fundoplication revision. Ann Surg. 1999;230:595–604.
37. van Beek DB, Auyang ED, Soper NJ. A comprehensive review of laparoscopic redo fundoplication. Surg Endosc. 2011;25:706–12.

Redo Antireflux Surgery

8

Brett Parker and Kevin Reavis

Introduction

Laparoscopic antireflux surgery (ARS) has become the gold standard for medically refractory gastroesophageal reflux disease (GERD) since it was first introduced by Dallemagne et al. in 1991 [1]. ARS also aids in eliminating the need for life-long antisecretory medications, such as proton pump inhibitors (PPIs), and therefore avoiding side effects such as osteoporosis, clostridium difficile infections, gastric polyposis, and aspiration pneumonia. Though primary ARS has excellent safety and outcomes, up to 10% of patients undergoing laparoscopic fundoplication will eventually require laparoscopic reoperative antireflux surgery (redo-ARS) [2]. A recent study demonstrated this rate can be reduced to 4.5% at 15-year follow-up, in the expert hands of an experienced foregut surgeon [3]. This is a testament to the fact that primary ARS should become standardized, with careful deliberation given to the appropriate operative approach for each individual patient population. Table 8.1 highlights the multitude of antireflux operations a foregut surgeon may choose to perform, as well as the complexity of the decision-making process. Proper patient and procedure selection can be a complex endeavor, with the lowest, most predictable outcomes generated by high-volume centers.

Reoperative gastroesophageal surgery after failed ARS can be one of the most challenging procedures a surgeon will face. Redo-ARS is notoriously difficult with higher complication rates and worse outcomes when compared to the primary operation, and requires a high level of laparoscopic surgical skills [4–7]. It is crucial for the surgeon and the patient to come to an agreement on postoperative expectations prior to embarking on revisional surgery, with a clear understanding that outcomes

B. Parker (✉)
Providence Portland Medical Center, The Oregon Clinic GMIS, Portland, OR, USA

K. Reavis
Division of Minimally Invasive Surgery, The Oregon Clinic, Portland, OR, USA

© Springer Nature Switzerland AG 2021
N. Zundel et al. (eds.), *Benign Esophageal Disease*,
https://doi.org/10.1007/978-3-030-51489-1_8

Table 8.1 Surgical options for primary antireflux, along with some notable complexities of the decision-making process

Procedure	Adjuncts and considerations	Approach
Complete 360° fundoplication (Nissen)	Bougie size, length, number of sutures, configuration (greater curvature to greater curvature, or anterior-posterior), adequate motility, viable fundus	Open, laparoscopic, robotic
Partial posterior 180° fundoplication (Toupet)	Bougie size, crural or diaphragmatic pexy, inadequate motility	Open, laparoscopic, robotic
Partial anterior 270° fundoplication (Dor)	Bougie size, concurrent esophageal myotomy for pseudoachalasia	Open, laparoscopic, robotic
Posterior gastropexy (Hill)	Cardia calibration, avoid injury to aorta and celiac axis	Open, laparoscopic, robotic
Posterior plication (Belsey-Mark IV)	Frozen abdomen, avoid injury to pericardium or pulmonary vasculature	Open transthoracic, thoracoscopic
Roux-en-Y reconstruction	Bypass vs. gastrectomy, total vs. subtotal, limb length, pouch size	Open, laparoscopic, robotic
Magnetic sphincter augmentation (LINX®)	Minimal dissection technique vs. complete circumferential hiatal dissection, hiatal hernia size	Laparoscopic
Transoral incisionless fundoplication (TIF)	Concomitant laparoscopic hiatal hernia repair	Endoscopic
Radiofrequency therapy (Stretta®)	Low risk, no impact on future interventions	Endoscopic
Minimally invasive esophagectomy (MIE)	Conduit type and viability	Abdominal, thoracic, cervical

are generally worse after redo-ARS than after the already-failed primary ARS. Despite the technical challenges redo-ARS presents, more than 80% of patients report satisfaction with their revision [7].

Causes of Fundoplication Failure

There are a multitude of reasons a primary ARS may have failed. Recognizing these patterns of failure is crucial for the reoperative surgeon to produce a favorable outcome. Patients' demographics and risk factors associated with failure include morbid obesity, female gender, advanced age, chronic cough, hiatal hernia, concurrent esophageal dysmotility, initial atypical reflux symptoms, lack of response to medications, and postoperative retching or dry heaving [8–13]. Surgeon technical errors that may contribute to failure of initial ARS involve loose crural closure, low placement of the fundoplication, failure to gain adequate intra-abdominal esophageal length, and configuring an extremely loose or tight fundoplication [7]. Typical intraoperative findings during revisional surgery include, in order of likelihood, intrathoracic wrap migration, disruption of the fundoplication, slipped fundoplication, and malpositioned or mis-calibrated wrap [7]. Less commonly, patients with ongoing postoperative reflux can develop a gastroesophageal stricture warranting revisional surgery. Awais, Luketich, and colleagues reported recurrent hiatal hernia to be the most common cause of failure (64%) in a series of 275 redo-ARS, followed by short esophagus (43%), misplaced wrap (16%), wrap being too loose or tight (14%), and wrap breakdown (4%) [14] (Figs. 8.1 and 8.2).

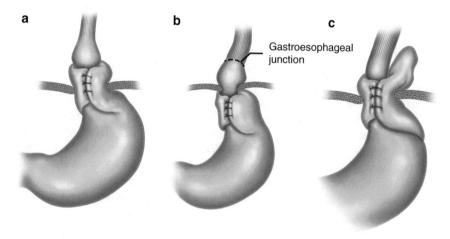

Fig. 8.1 Patterns of fundoplication herniation. (**a**) GEJ and wrap herniate together above the diaphragm. (**b**) GEJ only is herniated above the diaphragm, while fundoplication remains intraabdominal. (**c**) Paraesophageal hernia

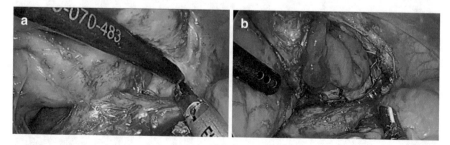

Fig. 8.2 (**a, b**) Intraoperative images of a perforated herniated fundoplication. The surgeons left-handed suction device is retracting the fundus. The right-handed ultrasonic shear is pointing to the left crus. A recurrent hiatal hernia with dense inflammatory tissue extending into the mediastinum can be seen in the center of the image. (Image courtesy of Christy Dunst)

Early Failure

Whether the primary antireflux operation failed early or late can be a valuable clue in determining the underlying cause of the failure. Identifying the underlying cause is important so that the same mistake is not made again during the revisional surgery. Early failure is typically secondary to an unexpected stress applied to the repair. Immediate nausea, retching, dry heaving, and coughing should be aggressively controlled in the recovery room and continued to be treated prophylactically during the immediate postoperative period. Patients should have assistance during ambulation to prevent traumatic falls, and heavy lifting and straining should be avoided to minimize intra-abdominal pressures. Patients should also be warned against the risks of over-zealous oral intake in the immediate postoperative period. Technical error is not a common cause of early failure at high-volume centers but should always be considered part of the differential.

Dysphagia is a common complaint after ARS. If the patient is stable, it is wise to allow several days for the postoperative edema to resolve. Intravenous steroids may assist in this process. If the patient cannot manage their own secretions, the surgeon should assume the fundoplication or hiatus is too tight, a hiatal hernia has recurred, or that the patient's esophageal motility is too weak to overcome the newly increased distal esophageal pressure. An initial chest X-ray in the recovery room is sometimes all that is needed to make the diagnosis (Fig. 8.3), though a contrast esophagram is most helpful in making the diagnosis. If the anatomy appears normal, then physiologic dysphagia can typically be improved with endoscopic balloon dilation.

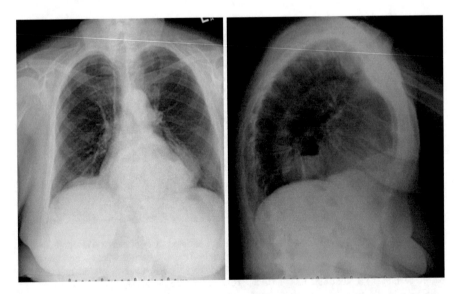

Fig. 8.3 An A-P and Lateral chest Xray obtained in the immediate postoperative period showing an acute recurrence of the hiatal hernia. Note the air fluid level above the diaphragm. The patient was taken back to surgery for immediate repair

If an anatomic derangement is discovered on immediate postoperative imaging, the patient should return to the operating room for repair of the recurrent hiatal hernia or revision of the fundoplication. If this is discovered several days postoperatively, it is best theoretically to wait approximately 3 months to undergo redo-ARS to avoid the dense adhesions and inflammatory response seen during this portion of the healing process. Should the surgeon unfortunately be forced to operate during this period, a tedious dissection should be expected, with an increased risk of intraoperative complications.

Late Failure

Late failure is generally defined as a patient who initially experienced good postoperative results having return of symptoms more than 90 days after surgery. Late failure is much more common than early failure. Reflux symptoms are typically due to an anatomic breakdown of the hiatal repair or disruption of the fundoplication, while dysphagia is usually secondary to scarring or twisting at the hiatus. The average length of time between primary and redo-ARD has recently been shown to be approximately 42 months [15]. Morgenthal et al. report that despite a recurrence rate of approximately 32% at 10 years, most of these patients are asymptomatic, and 93.3% of all patients state they would have the procedure again [16, 17].

Presentation

The most common symptoms leading to reoperative antireflux surgery are recurrent reflux, dysphagia, and regurgitation [7]. Return of reflux and heartburn, or atypical symptoms of reflux such as chronic couch, hoarseness, or aspiration are the prevailing symptoms when there has been a wrap disruption. Improvement of symptoms after re-initiation of antisecretory medication can be a key clinical clue during the patient interview. Dysphagia, noncardiac chest pain, and regurgitation occur more frequently after recurrent hiatal hernia or crural stenosis. This can be seen also in patients with complications from prior hiatal mesh placement. Good response to endoscopic balloon dilation can be an important clinical indicator. Postprandial bloating, early satiety, and irregular bowel movements should raise suspicion for iatrogenic vagal nerve injury resulting in gastroparesis.

Approximately two-thirds of failure patients report recurrent or persistent reflux. When analyzing this data, it is important to define failure, as it is widely accepted that subjective symptoms often do not correlate with objective testing. In fact, studies show that abnormal pH-studies are found in only 23–39% of patients reporting postoperative reflux symptoms [18]. Conversely, pathologic esophageal acid exposure after fundoplication may not always be symptomatic. Hunter et al. reported that 13% of patients had abnormal routine pH-studies 12 weeks after laparoscopic fundoplication, but none of these patients reported reflux symptoms [19].

Dysphagia occurs is approximately one-third of patients with failed ARS. Dysphagia is more common after a complete 360 degree fundoplication when compared to partial fundoplication [9, 20]. Oftentimes, patients who complain primarily of dysphagia have no obvious cause on preoperative workup or intraoperative exploration. For patients with ongoing symptoms with no underlying cause after a complete physiologic and anatomic foregut workup, consider a psychological evaluation to rule out psychosomatic disorders. For the above reasons, it is crucial to establish regularly scheduled 24-hr pH monitoring as part of all patients' postoperative follow-up protocol, with the addition of a more extensive foregut workup for symptomatic patients, including endoscopy, barium esophagram, and high-resolution esophageal manometry.

Workup

The complexity of redo-ARS requires a comprehensive evaluation of the patient to determine the exact etiology of their symptoms and to determine candidacy for certain revisional techniques. It is of utmost importance to obtain the operative note from the primary surgery, with attention focused on the extent of dissection, status of the vagus nerves, possible mesh placement, and configuration of the wrap. The first diagnostic step in working up a symptomatic patient with prior ARS presenting to your office is typically a contrast esophagram to outline the patient's anatomy and give some indication to the physiology of bolus transit.

Repeat esophagogastroduodenoscopy should be performed, ideally by the operative surgeon, to identify the location of the gastroesophageal junction (GEJ) and assess for hiatal hernia or esophagitis (Fig. 8.4). The

Fig. 8.4 Contrast esophagram showing recurrent hiatal hernia in a patient with prior Nissen fundoplication who presented with nausea and epigastric discomfort. Note the presence of the fundoplication above the diaphragm. (Image courtesy of Christy Dunst)

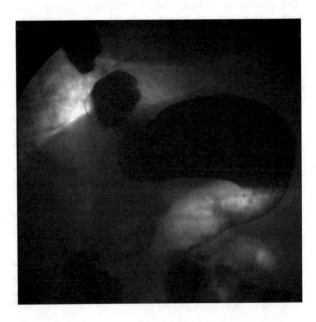

Fig. 8.5 Endoscopic retroflexed view of a herniated wrap. The image depicts an intact fundoplication, tightly adherent to the shaft of the scope, which has migrated above the diaphragm. The crus is seen in the left lower corner of the picture. (Image courtesy of Christy Dunst)

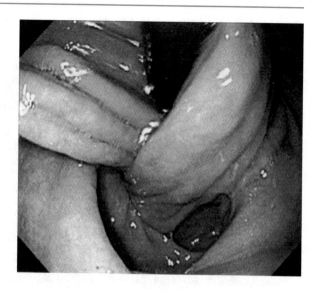

squamocolumnar junction (SCJ) should be characterized and biopsied. If the patient had a previously placed mesh, it is imperative to assess for erosion, which can be managed with endoscopic resection and expectant extrusion prior to the redo-ARS (Fig. 8.5).

A 48-hour Bravo™ pH capsule or Restech™ Dx-pH sensor can be inserted during this same endoscopic procedure to objectively test for pathologic esophageal acid exposure and establish a baseline esophageal DeMeester or oropharyngeal RYAN Score for postoperative follow-up pH testing. Alternatively, the patient can undergo catheter-based 24-hr pH monitoring. It is imperative to ensure the patient is not actively taking antisecretory medications that may mask the results. High-resolution esophageal manometry (HRM) is essential, as patients with esophageal motility disorders such as achalasia who present with regurgitation are unfortunately still misdiagnosed with GERD. HRM can also help guide the surgeon's decision as to what type of fundoplication to perform. If the patient has evidence of ineffective esophageal motility, a partial fundoplication may prevent postoperative dysphagia. Patients who present with large paraesophageal hernias may not be able to have manometry successfully performed, and if completed, the results may be difficult to interpret. Figure 8.6 depicts the topography of a patient with prior fundoplication, who has manometric evidence of a recurrent hiatal hernia.

If postprandial abdominal bloating is present, a nuclear medicine gastric emptying study is helpful to assess for gastroparesis, which can occur after iatrogenic injury of the vagus nerves during the primary procedure. If delayed gastric emptying is discovered, the patient would likely benefit from a concurrent pyloroplasty or decompressive gastrostomy tube.

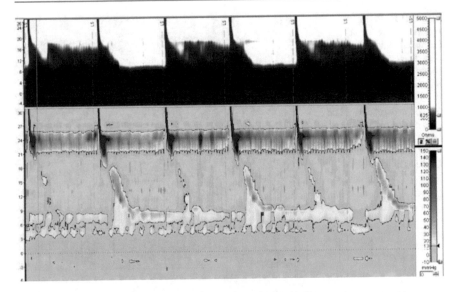

Fig. 8.6 High resolution manometry of a patient with prior Nissen fundoplication, showing recurrent hiatal hernia. Note the presence of normal peristalsis, but two distal esophageal high-pressure zones. (Image courtesy of Christy Dunst)

Surgical Options and Techniques

As previously mentioned, there are several techniques available for patients with failure of ARS. Many of these options can be approached via the abdomen or transthoracic, either open or laparoscopic, depending on surgeon preference. Robotic assistance is also becoming part of many surgeons' armamentarium. The most common surgical options include redo-fundoplication with the addition of a Collis gastroplasty or hiatal hernia repair as needed, conversion to Roux-en-Y (RNY) gastrojejunostomy, or minimally invasive esophagectomy (MIE). With the advent of newer antireflux procedures, such as the transoral incisionless fundoplication (TIF) and the magnetic sphincter augmentation (MSA) device, revisional techniques have also been established, and will be described later.

Redo-Fundoplication

Revisional fundoplication is the preferred surgical technique at many advanced foregut centers for patients with prior failed ARS. Redo fundoplication is known to be technically challenging and laborious, and for this reason, has historically required a laparotomy or thoracotomy. As today's surgeons have gained more expertise in advanced laparoscopy, redo-fundoplication is now primarily completed via a laparoscopic approach, which offers superior visualization of the upper abdomen and mediastinum. The conversion rate from laparoscopy to open is approximately 1–2.5% [21, 22].

Technique

The patient isss placed supine or in lithotomy position with steep reverse Trendelenburg. After careful access to the abdomen is gained, the pneumoperitoneum is established. Perihepatic adhesiolysis is performed and a liver retractor is placed. An energy device is used to transect the pars flaccida and the gastrohepatic ligament, using the caudate lobe of the liver as a reliable landmark to begin the dissection. Dissection is carried toward the right crus taking care not to injure the celiac artery pedicle or inferior vena cava, as there are often wrap adhesions in this area and distorted tissue planes can mislead the surgeon. A previously placed mesh can also produce a challenge in the dissection of the retro-esophageal window. If the approach from the right crus seems too difficult, moving to the left crus is recommended, using the greater curvature of the stomach as a reliable landmark to begin dissection. The esophagus is circumferentially freed from all surrounding adhesions, with special attention toward identifying and protecting the anterior and posterior vagus nerves, if present. A Penrose drain placed around the GEJ can assist with retraction. If a hiatal hernia is found, the recurrent hernia sac, if one has reformed, is reduced and excised. Extensive mediastinal dissection is performed, freeing the intrathoracic esophagus at least 5 cm above the hiatus, ensuring ligation of any penetrating arterial branches from the aorta. The previously created wrap is taken down by cutting the gastro-gastric sutures with an ultrasonic shear or laparoscopic scissors. The epiphrenic fat pad is then excised. Adequate intra-abdominal esophagus is then ensured to be at least 2–3 cm in length without applying traction. At this juncture, the need for an esophageal lengthening procedure via wedge fundectomy is assessed.

Crural repair is then completed with permanent suture in a sequential horizontal mattress fashion, with the option of adding an onlay mesh for reinforcement to the cruroplasty. If undue tension is present, a diaphragmatic relaxing incision with inlay permanent mesh patch closure may be required. Lowering the pneumoperitoneum during hiatal closure can also be a useful adjunct. The short gastric vessels are then ensured to be properly ligated, and the new fundoplication is created. Intraoperative impedance planimetry with EndoFLIP® can also be useful to act as a "smart" bougie during the formation of the fundoplication to measure the length and distensibility of the wrap (Fig. 8.7) [23]. Whether a complete or partial fundoplication is performed should be dependent on each patient's clinical scenario, symptoms, and preoperative high-resolution manometry. In general, complete fundoplication is performed for reflux and hiatal hernias, while partial fundoplication is chosen for patients with preoperative dysphagia. Many surgeons perform intraoperative upper endoscopy to rule out underlying mucosal injury or perforation via an air insufflation test, as well as to inspect the quality and configuration or the wrap. A transhiatal closed suction drain is typically left at the end of the procedure.

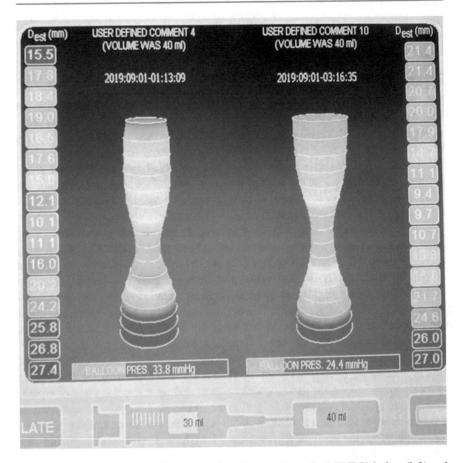

Fig. 8.7 The functional lumen imaging probe balloon catheter (EndoFLIP®) before (left) and after (right) fundoplication. Sixteen impedance planimetry sensors measure a distensibility index to help guide the creation of the wrap. An elongated hourglass appearance depicts a properly formed fundoplication. Note the absence of overt stenosis or high pressurization. (Image courtesy of Christy Dunst)

Hiatal Hernia Repair with Mesh Reinforcement

It is the author's practice to always use an onlay bilayered fully resorbable mesh for complex hiatal closures (Fig. 8.8). This can be secured to the crura with either laparoscopic sutures or laparoscopic tacks. If tacks are used, care is taken to avoid injury to the IVC, aorta, or pericardium. A study of 26 patients with previous mesh cruroplasty, undergoing redo-ARS, reported a recurrent hiatal hernia rate of 70% [15]. It should be noted that nearly half of these patients had biologic mesh placed during the primary operation, which is known to have high recurrence rates.

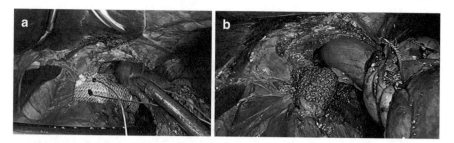

Fig. 8.8 (**a, b**) Placement of an absorbable onlay mesh, incorporated into the cruroplasty closure with permanent suture. The final hiatal suture is secured after Bougie is removed. (Image courtesy of Christy Dunst)

Fig. 8.9 Collis gastroplasty completed with an articulating linear cutting stapler, to obtain >3 cm intra-abdominal neo-esophageal length. The stapler is placed tightly alongside a bougie dilator to prevent a proximal dog ear, which can lead to the formation of a postoperative epiphrenic diverticulum. (Image courtesy of Christy Dunst)

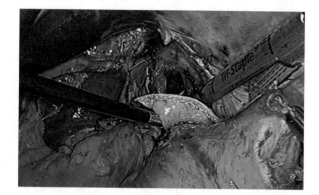

Collis Gastroplasty for the Short Esophagus

Axial tension is a major contributor to recurrent hiatal hernia, the leading cause of failed primary ARS. Short esophagus has been estimated to be present in 21–43% of patients undergoing redo-ARS [14, 24]. Due to the prevalence of the short esophagus and the high rate of recurrent hiatal hernias, it is necessary for the reoperative surgeon to have a low threshold to tubularize the stomach and create a neoesophagus in order to gain adequate intra-abdominal length. One study showed that patients with a short esophagus and prior failed ARS reported better subjective symptoms resolution and satisfaction scores after Roux-en-Y reconstruction versus redo-fundoplication with Collis gastroplasty (Fig. 8.9). It should be noted that this study actually reported no difference in objective outcomes and a lower complication rate in the subset of patients undergoing redo-fundoplication and Collis gastroplasty [25].

Diaphragmatic Relaxing Incision

Radial tension is also a major component of recurrent hiatal hernia and failure of antireflux operations. Redo-ARS notoriously have scarred, fibrotic crura that will not easily oppose one another. If the cruroplasty seems to have undue tension, the best way to control this is via a diaphragm-relaxing incision. Covering a tight repair with an onlay mesh will not offload the radial tension on the crus, and therefore large defects with high radial tension should not be considered an indication for mesh placement. The right diaphragm should be the first option for making a relaxing incision, as this is easier to perform. If full-thickness incision of the right diaphragm between the IVC and right crus does not gain adequate relief, then a left-diaphragm relaxing incision should be made. Diaphragmatic defects are then patched with a permanent inlay mesh. It is important to leave an adequate cuff a diaphragm along the IVC for successful patch closure (Fig. 8.10).

Roux-en-Y Gastrojejunostomy

Morbid obesity has been shown in most studies to be an independent risk factor for the development of GERD, as well as for failure of ARS [26–28]. However, there is some evidence to also support equivalent outcomes between obese and nonobese patients undergoing primary ARS, raising concern for publication bias [29]. There is clear evidence in the bariatric literature to show that GERD improves after RNY gastric bypass [28, 30]. Knowing this, there has been an increasing trend to convert prior failed fundoplications to a Roux-en-Y gastrojejunostomy (RNY), particularly in patients with morbid obesity, as the procedure not only improves reflux by bypassing or eliminating gastric-acid-producing cells, but also offers additional health benefits seen with weight loss. Additionally, RNY is gaining traction as the preferred technique for patients with prior failed ARS and concomitant gastroparesis, esophageal dysmotility, intraoperative gastroesophageal injury during redo-ARS, or many previous foregut procedures. In cases of extremely distorted

Fig. 8.10 Full thickness right diaphragmatic relaxing incision to offload radial tension on the cruroplasty. Care is taken to avoid injury to the IVC, which is behind the surgeons left-handed grasper in this image. (Image courtesy of Christy Dunst)

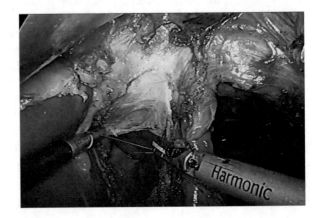

postprocedural anatomy, or in the event of gastric cardia or distal esophageal injury, a total gastrectomy with RNY esophagojejunostomy is offered. Interestingly, Kent et al. demonstrated improved outcomes with RNY as the primary surgery for patients with scleroderma and severe esophageal dysmotility [31]. In general, if patients with two or three prior failed ARS present with severe recurrent foregut symptoms not amenable to endoscopic therapy, an RNY or total gastrectomy should be offered [32, 33].

Converting to an RNY has shown to be effective in nearly 93% of patients, with high subjective patient satisfaction scores [2]. There is also great objective evidence to support this technique in the morbidly obese, with DeMeester scores demonstrated to decrease from approximately 57–12.5 after revisional RNY [3]. One concern with RNY becoming the procedure of choice is the high complication rate published in the literature, ranging from 21% to 46% [7]. The anastomotic stricture rate can approach 28%, and this is likely due to the relatively small pouch created during RNY, and the resultant ischemia from the many prior foregut surgeries this patient population undergoes. Luckily, most of these strictures can be successfully managed with endoscopic dilation [34]. Mittal et al. concluded that despite the higher postoperative complication rate, patients with more complex foregut pathology benefit more from conversion to an RNY reconstruction rather than redo-fundoplication, as evidenced by higher one-year postoperative satisfaction scores [25]. However, one must remember that with this technique comes the accepted long-term risk of dumping syndrome, nutritional deficiencies, internal hernia, marginal ulcer, afferent limb syndrome, and bacterial overgrowth, which are not typically seen after redo-fundoplication.

Technique

After gaining abdominal access and establishing pneumoperitoneum, the right crus is identified, and dissection is carried out in a clockwise direction until the left crus is identified. The previous fundoplication is circumferentially freed from the hiatus and any adhesions. If the vagus nerves are still intact, these are identified and protected. If any remaining short gastric vessels are present, these are then ligated with a bipolar device or an ultrasonic scalpel. The previous wrap is completely deconstructed and the GEJ is identified. Alternatively, the previous fundoplication can be left in place and the stomach can be transected just distal to this. The short gastric vessels are ensured to be adequately transected. An endo-GIA linear cutting stapler is used to create a gastric pouch, ensuring to preserve the left gastric artery. Creating a small 5–10 cm pouch is extremely important to ensure no acid-producing parietal cells remain in direct communication with the esophagus. There is debate whether to leave to remnant stomach in place or perform a subtotal gastrectomy. Leaving it in place offers the benefit of a simpler procedure and reserving a gastric conduit in the event an esophagectomy is required in the future. The omentum is divided with an energy device to decrease tension on the anastomosis. The RNY reconstruction is then created with a >50 cm biliopancreatic limb to minimize the risk of bile reflux and a >100 cm alimentary limb in an ante-colic fashion. The antimesenteric gastrojejunal anastomosis and jejunojejunostomy are created with an endo-GIA stapler, and the common enterotomies are closed with intracorporeal suturing. Stapling of the common enterotomy between the jejunojejunostomy can also be used.

Minimally Invasive Esophagectomy

Minimally invasive esophagectomy (MIE) is typically considered the last resort for patients with severe esophageal dysmotility and previously failed ARS, or in patients who develop esophageal pathology following several previously failed ARS such as a long esophageal stricture not amenable to dilation or pseudoachalasia with massive esophageal dilation. It is also a bail-out strategy in the event that the GEJ cannot be reconstructed. Reoperative intervention in patients with mesh at the hiatus is associated with a higher need for esophageal resection [15]. Managing the anatomic and physiologic complexities in these patients can be quite challenging, and indications for up-front esophagectomy are still debated. An alternative rescue procedure, known as the Meredino procedure, as recently been proposed for patients with many prior failed fundoplications. It involves resection of the gastroesophageal junction with jejunal interposition. A 2018 series of 12 patients undergoing this alternative technique found high postoperative complication rates (67%), with 25% of patients ultimately requiring conversion to an RNY within 12 months [35]. At this time, the Merendino procedure does not appear to be a viable surgical strategy for redo-ARS for the majority of patients.

Technique

There are many MIE techniques, each with its own advantages and disadvantages. This procedure is technically demanding, requires a significant learning curve, and should be performed only by experienced surgeons at high-volume centers. MIE can be done with a combination of laparoscopic, thoracoscopic, or robotic approaches. Each technique is safe and efficacious, and the preferred approach depends on surgeon or institutional preference. The two most popular approaches for benign foregut disease are the transhiatal approach and the Ivor-Lewis technique. The transhiatal approach involves an abdominal and left cervical incision with the anastomosis placed in the left neck. This technique does not require single-lung ventilation and only supine positioning. The placement of the anastomosis outside of the chest has a theoretical advantage of decreasing the morbidity of anastomotic leaks. It is a great option for benign disease of the GEJ and patients with poor pulmonary function. The transthoracic Ivor Lewis technique involves an abdominal and right thoracic approach with a right chest anastomosis. Patients require single-lung ventilation and typically require both supine and left lateral positioning. Avoiding a neck incision leads to decreased recurrent laryngeal nerve injury compared to other techniques. This approach also allows for better lymph node harvest in achalasia patients who have developed squamous cell carcinoma. Lastly, the three-incision McKeown technique requires right thoracic, abdominal, and left cervical incisions with a left cervical anastomosis. This approach allows for greater length of proximal resection and is typically reserved for proximal malignant disease.

Reoperative Antireflux Surgery After Prior Transoral Incisionless Fundoplication

The transoral incisionless fundoplication (TIF) procedure is a popular technique for the endoscopic treatment of GERD and is generally very well tolerated with minimal side effects. TIF uses the EsophyX device (EndoGastric Solutions, Inc., Redmond, WA, USA) to create a full-thickness partial fundoplication with permanent T-fasteners between the stomach and the esophagus. If the wrap becomes disrupted, the patient develops a hiatal hernia, or the patient experiences post-procedural reflux, redo-ARS is often necessary.

A systematic review of 559 patients undergoing both early (TIF1) and newer (TIF2) versions of the TIF procedure demonstrated that 7.2% of these patients underwent laparoscopic revision to a fundoplication at median 9.5-month follow-up [36]. A subsequent single institutional prospective study of 165 patients undergoing TIF reported that 15% of patients required redo-ARS [37]. Out of this patient population, 28 patients underwent revision of TIF to laparoscopic fundoplication, with no reported intraoperative or postoperative complications at median 14 month follow-up. This evidence suggests that the laparoscopic dissection and reconfiguration of the gastric fundus can be performed safely after TIF, as only 14% of the revised patients had dense adhesions [37]. It is still unknown how revisional fundoplication after TIF affects GERD long term, as postoperative pH testing was not reported in these patients. One study did report that after 15 patients with failed TIF underwent successful redo-ARS, 33% did report troublesome postoperative dysphagia. It should be noted that these authors did not use a bougie to calibrate the fundoplication [38].

During revisional surgery, it is important to note that the left crus can oftentimes be included in the T-fasteners, and this should be considered when performing revisional surgery to ensure the surgeon is operating in the right dissection plane. The T-fasteners should not be pulled out to avoid injuring the mural tissue; rather they should be cut and left to fall into the lumen. This is of supreme importance to decrease the risk of perforation or postoperative abscess formation. There is also a theoretical risk of the T-fasteners leading to traction diverticulum of the distal esophagus. The surgeon should be aware of this potential during hiatal dissection to avoid esophageal injury. Additionally, if during dissection, the fundus is found to be fused with the esophageal wall, it may be best to leave this intact and simply roll the wall of the stomach over the fused portion and incorporate it into the fundoplication [37]. Whether to perform a partial or complete fundoplication should be guided by the severity of the disease, as severe reflux is best treated with complete fundoplication, though patients with mild to moderate disease may do better with partial fundoplication to prevent dysphagia.

Reoperation After Failed Magnetic Sphincter Augmentation

Laparoscopic insertion of a magnetic sphincter augmentation (MSA) device, commonly known as the LINX® Reflux Management System (Torax® Medical, Inc. Shoreview, MN), has become a popular alternative to laparoscopic fundoplication. Although the placement of this circumferential foreign body at the gastroesophageal junction (GEJ) was initially met with concern for erosion similar to the bariatric gastric band, it has since been shown to be safe and effective [39–41]. Despite good evidence supporting its use, some MSA devices will inevitably require removal.

Most patients who require explantation experience dysphagia, followed by objective persistent or recurrent reflux, or food impaction. If a concurrent hiatal hernia repair was performed during the initial operation, it is plausible that a patient's dysphagia may be due to a tight crural closure rather than a constricting device, and this can often be improved with serial endoscopic balloon dilations. Recurrent or persistent reflux could be due to progressive or recurrent hiatal hernia, or due to the device being placed low on the stomach. These differentials should be evaluated with preoperative imaging prior to offering a patient LINX removal surgery.

Studies thus far report the rate of MRS device removal to range between 1.1% and 6.7% [42–44]. Erosions occur in 0.15–1.2% of patients [42, 43]. If a patient develops intraluminal erosion, they should be offered LINX removal. Patients who experience erosion can have the device removed endoscopically, due to the fibrotic capsule formed around the device after placement. This is done by cutting the wire with endoscopic scissors and pulling back on the wire with endoscopic forceps. Alternatively, laparoscopic removal is accomplished by using monopolar energy to open the fibrotic capsule, cutting the wire with laparoscopic scissors, and gently applying upward traction on the beads while continuing to free the capsule (Fig. 8.11). If the patient is having the MSA device removed for ongoing reflux, then a subsequent fundoplication is beneficial. For hiatal hernias, it is at the surgeon's discretion whether to repair the hiatal hernia and replace the

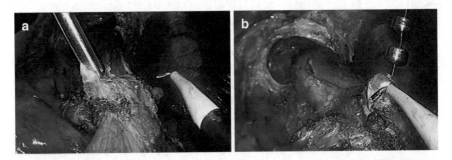

Fig. 8.11 (a, b) Laparoscopic removal of a LINX® device. Monopolar energy is used to free the beads from the surrounding fibrotic capsule, taking care not to injure the underlying esophagus. An enlarged hiatal defect can also be seen in the background. (Image courtesy of Christy Dunst)

MSA device or perform a fundoplication. If the indication is dysphagia, some surgeons contend that no further ARS is required, due to the inflammatory response caused by the foreign body. For perforations, Graham patch closure only is typically indicated [45].

Outcomes

In general, intraoperative complications are higher during laparoscopic surgery, and postoperative complications are higher after open surgery. Redo-ARS carries an overall complication rate ranging from 9.7% to 24% [46]. Furnee et al. demonstrated the intraoperative complication rate from redo-ARS to be approximately 21.4%. The most common intraoperative complications were iatrogenic perforation (13.1%) and lacerations of the liver or spleen resulting in significant bleeding (1.9%), though the postoperative leak rate was just 1.5% [47]. A 2015 analysis of several studies monitoring objective outcomes after redo-ARS reported over 80% of patients to have normal acid exposure on pH monitoring or lack of esophagitis on endoscopy [7]. A recent prospective study of 46 patients showed a significantly improved Gastroesophageal Reflux Symptom Scale (GERSS) and Gastroesophageal Reflux Disease Health-Related Quality of Life (GERD-HRQL) scores at median 16.5 months after redo-LARS. Additionally, 82% of these patients reported satisfaction with their operation, and 96% stated that they would undergo the redo-ARS again if given the choice [46].

Studies suggest the rate of a second failed ARS necessitating a third operation to be approximately 11% at median 3.3 years follow-up [14]. It has been suggested that while revisional third and even fourth time ARS is possible, positive outcomes decrease by approximately 20% after each redo surgery [46]. Signhal et al. grouped 940 patients into four groups including primary ARS, first reoperative, second reoperative, and greater than three reoperative ARS groups. In their study, conversion to laparotomy, conversion to RNY, operative time, blood loss, visceral perforation, postoperative leak, and vagal injury all significantly increased with each subsequent revisional surgery [48]. This study also reported a progressive decline in patient-reported satisfaction with each redo intervention. These conclusions certainly reflect the increased risk and surgical difficulty encountered by the surgeon with each subsequent redo and are excellent data to consider when weighing surgical options for patients who present in your office with failed ARS.

References

1. Dallemagne B, et al. Laparoscopic Nissen fundoplication: preliminary report. Surg Laparosc Endosc. 1991;1(3):138e143.
2. Zorrilla L, et al. Standardized steps for conversion of anti-reflux surgery operation to Roux-en-Y gastric bypass. Surg Obes Relat Dis. 2017;13(10)
3. Obeid NR, et al. Patterns of reoperation after failed fundoplication: an analysis of 9462 patients. Surg Endosc. 2017;32(1):345–50.

4. Byrne JP, et al. Symptomatic and functional outcome after laparoscopic reoperation for failed antireflux surgery. Br J Surg. 2005;92(8):996e1001.
5. Dutta S, et al. Outcome of laparoscopic redo fundoplication. Surg Endosc. 2004;18(3):440e443.
6. Pessaux P, et al. Laparoscopic antireflux surgery: five-year results and beyond in 1340 patients. Archiv Surg (Chicago, Ill. 1960). 2005;140(10):946e951.
7. Grover BT, Kothari SN. Reoperative antireflux surgery. Surg Clin N Am. 2015;95(3):629–40.
8. Morgenthal CB, Lin E, Shane MD, et al. Who will fail laparoscopic Nissen fundoplication? Preoperative prediction of long-term outcomes. Surg Endosc. 2007;21(11):1978–84.
9. Broeders JA, Roks DJ, Draaisma WA, et al. Predictors of objectively identified recurrent reflux after primary Nissen fundoplication. Br J Surg. 2011;98(5):673–9.
10. Power C, Maguire D, McAnena O. Factors contributing to failure of laparoscopic Nissen fundoplication and the predictive value of preoperative assessment. Am J Surg. 2004;187(4):457–63.
11. Soper NJ, Dunnegan D. Anatomic fundoplication failure after laparoscopic antireflux surgery. Ann Surg. 1999;229(5):669–76.
12. O'Boyle CJ, Watson DI, DeBeaux AC, et al. Preoperative prediction of long-term outcome following laparoscopic fundoplication. ANZ J Surg. 2002;72(7):471–5.
13. Jackson PG, Gleiber MA, Askari R, et al. Predictors of outcome in 100 consecutive laparoscopic antireflux procedures. Am J Surg. 2001;181(3):231–5.
14. Awais O, Luketich JD, Schuchert MJ, et al. Reoperative antireflux surgery for failed fundoplication: an analysis of outcomes in 275 patients. Ann Thorac Surg. 2011;92(3):1083–9.
15. Nandipati K, Bye M, Yamamoto SR, Pallati P, Lee T, Mittal SK. Reoperative intervention in patients with mesh at the Hiatus is associated with high incidence of esophageal resection—a single-center experience. J Gastrointest Surg. 2013;17(12):2039–44.
16. Morgenthal CB, et al. The durability of laparoscopic Nissen fundoplication: 11-year outcomes. J Gastrointest Surg. 2007;11(6):693–700. https://doi.org/10.1007/s11605-007-0161-8.
17. White BC, et al. Do recurrences after paraesophageal hernia repair matter? Surg Endosc. 2007;22(4):1107–11. https://doi.org/10.1007/s00464-007-9649-2.
18. Oor JE, et al. Outcome for patients with pathological esophageal acid exposure after laparoscopic fundoplication. Ann Surg. 2018;267(6):1105–11.
19. Hunter JG, Trus TL, Branum GD, et al. A physiologic approach to laparoscopic fundoplication for gastroesophageal reflux disease. Ann Surg. 1996;223:673–85. discussion 685–7
20. Broeders JA, Mauritz FA, Ahmed Ali U, et al. Systematic review and meta-analysis of laparoscopic Nissen (posterior total) versus Toupet (posterior partial) fundoplication for gastrooesophageal reflux disease. Br J Surg. 2010;97:1318–30.
21. Khajanchee YS, O'Rourke R, Cassera MA, et al. Laparoscopic reintervention for failed antireflux surgery: subjective and objective outcomes in 176 consecutive patients. Arch Surg. 2007;142(8):785–901.
22. Pennathur A, Awais O, Luketich JD. Minimally invasive redo antireflux surgery: lessons learned. Ann Thorac Surg. 2010;89(6):S2174–9.
23. Su B, Novak S, Callahan Z, Kuchta K, Carbray J, Ujiki M. Using impedance planimetry (EndoFLIP™) in the operating room to assess gastroesophageal junction distensibility and predict patient outcomes following fundoplication. Surg Endosc. 2020;34:1761–8.
24. Iqbal A, Awad Z, Simkins J, Shah R, Haider M, Salinas V, et al. Repair of 104 failed anti-reflux operations. Ann Surg. 2006;244(1):42–51.
25. Mittal, Sumeet K., et al. "Roux-En-Y reconstruction is superior to redo fundoplication in a subset of patients with failed antireflux surgery." Surg Endosc, vol. 27, no. 3, June 2012, pp. 927–935.
26. Zainabadi K, Courcoulas AP, Awais O, et al. Laparoscopic revision of Nissen fundoplication to Roux-en-Y gastric bypass in morbidly obese patients. Surg Endosc. 2008;22(12):2737–40.
27. Frezza EE, Ikramuddin S, Gourash W, et al. Symptomatic improvement in gastroesophageal reflux disease (GERD) following laparoscopic Roux-en-Y gastric bypass. Surg Endosc. 2002;16(7):1027–31.
28. Patterson EJ, Davis DG, Khajanchee Y, et al. Comparison of objective outcomes following laparoscopic Nissen fundoplication versus laparoscopic gastric bypass in the morbidly obese with heartburn. Surg Endosc. 2003;17(10):1561–5.

29. Telem DA, Altieri M, Gracia G, Pryor AD. Perioperative outcome of esophageal fundoplication for gastroesophageal reflux disease in obese and morbidly obese patients. Am J Surg. 2014;208:163–8.
30. Nelson LG, Gonzalez R, Haines K, Gallagher SF, Murr MM. Amelioration of gastroesophageal reflux symptoms following Roux-en-Y gastric bypass for clinically significant obesity. Am Surg. 2005;71(11):950–3.
31. Kent MS, Luketich JD, Irshad K, Awais O, Alvelo-Rivera M, Churilla P, Fernando HC, Landreneau RJ. Comparison of surgical approaches to recalcitrant gastroesophageal reflux disease in the patient with scleroderma. Ann Thorac Surg. 2007;84(5):1710–5.
32. Makris KI, Lee T, Mittal SK. Roux-en-Y reconstruction for failed fundoplication. J Gastrointest Surg. 2009;13:2226–32.
33. Awais O, Luketich JD, Tam J, et al. Roux-en-Y near esophagojejunostomy for intractable gastroesophageal reflux after antireflux surgery. Ann Thorac Surg. 2008;85:1954–9.
34. Yamamoto SR, Hoshino M, Nandipati KC, Lee TH, Mittal SK. Long-term outcomes of reintervention for failed fundoplication: redo fundoplication versus Roux-en-Y reconstruction. Surg Endosc. 2013;28(1):42–8.
35. Analatos A, Lindblad M, Rouvelas I, Elbe P, Lundell L, Nilsson M, et al. Evaluation of resection of the gastroesophageal junction and jejunal interposition (Merendino procedure) as a rescue procedure in patients with a failed redo antireflux procedure. A single-center experience. BMC Surg. 2018;18(1)
36. Wendling MR, Melvin WS, Perry KA. Impact of transoral incisionless fundoplication (TIF) on subjective and objective GERD indices: a systematic review of the published literature. Surg Endosc. 2013;27:3754–61.
37. Bell, Reginald C. W., et al. "Laparoscopic anti-reflux revision surgery after transoral incisionless fundoplication is safe and effective." Surg Endosc, vol. 29, no. 7, Aug. 2014, pp. 1746–1752., doi:https://doi.org/10.1007/s00464-014-3897-8.
38. Witteman BP, Kessing BF, Snijders G, Koek GH, Conchillo JM, Bouvy ND. Revisional laparoscopic antireflux surgery after unsuccessful endoscopic fundoplication. Surg Endosc. 2013;27:2231–6.
39. Bonavina L, DeMeester T, Fockens P, et al. Laparoscopic sphincter augmentation device eliminates reflux symptoms and normalizes esophageal acid exposure: one- and 2-year results of a feasibility trial. Ann Surg. 2010;252:857–62.
40. Ganz RA, Peters JH, Horgan S, et al. Esophageal sphincter device for gastroesophageal reflux disease. N Engl J Med. 2013;368:719–27.
41. Reynolds JL, Zehetner J, Wu P, Shah S, Bildzukewicz N, Lipham JC. Laparoscopic magnetic sphincter augmentation vs. laparoscopic nissen fundoplication: a matched-pair analysis of 100 patients. J Am Coll Surg. 2015;221:123–8.
42. Asti E, Siboni S, Lazzari V, Bonitta G, Sironi A, Bonavina L. Removal of the magnetic sphincter augmentation device: surgical technique and results of a single-center cohort study. Ann Surg. 2017;265:941–5.
43. Smith CD, Ganz RA, Lipham JC, Bell RC, Rattner DW. Lower esophageal sphincter augmentation for gastroesophageal reflux disease: the safety of a modern implant. J Laparoendosc Adv Surg Tech A. 2017;27:586–91.
44. Lipham JC, Taiganides PA, Louie BE, Ganz RA, DeMeester TR. Safety analysis of the first 1000 patients treated with magnetic sphincter augmentation for gastroesophageal reflux. Dis Esophagus. 2015;28:305–11.
45. Tatum JM, et al. Removing the magnetic sphincter augmentation device: operative management and outcomes. Surg Endosc. 2018;33(8):2663–9.
46. Campo, Sara E. Martin Del, et al. "Laparoscopic redo fundoplication improves disease-specific and global quality of life following failed laparoscopic or open fundoplication." Surg Endosc, vol. 31, no. 11, July 2017, pp. 4649–4655.
47. Furnee EJ, et al. Surgical intervention after failed antire flux surgery: a systematic review of the literature. J Gastrointest Surg. 2009;13(8):1539e1549.
48. Singhal S, et al. Primary and redo antireflux surgery: outcomes and lessons learned. J Gastrointest Surg. 2017;22(2):177–86.

Motility Disorders: Workup and Evaluation

9

Samuel Szomstein, Alejandro Cracco, and Jose Melendez-Rosado

Introduction

The esophagus is tubular muscular structure composed of striated and smooth muscle, which propels food from the mouth to the stomach through an orchestrated combination of peristaltic contractions and muscle relaxation [1]. It can be divided anatomically into the upper esophageal sphincter, esophageal body, and lower esophageal sphincter (LES). Motility disorders of the esophagus usually affect the body and LES. The main function of the LES is the prevention of reflux of gastric contents to the esophagus. In its resting state, the LES is in a tonic contraction, and when swallowing occurs, it relaxes to allow passage of the food bolus into the stomach. This complex coordination of muscles is driven by the innervation of the vagus nerve that arises from the dorsal motor nucleus and nucleus ambiguous in the brain stem communicating directly with the myenteric plexus within the esophagus [2]. Excitatory and inhibitory neurotransmitters such as acetylcholine and nitric oxide, respectively, are released into the neuromuscular junction causing either muscle contraction or relaxation, stimulating peristaltic contraction [3, 4]. Failure of any of these components can result in ineffective propulsion of the food bolus and consequently patient will present with a variety of symptoms, predominantly dysphagia.

Although radiographic and endoscopic information is important as part of the workup for esophageal motility disorder, the gold standard test is the use of high-resolution manometry (HRM). HRM consists of a probe that is introduced through the nostril down the gastroesophageal junction (GEJ). This probe contains multiple sensors that measure pressures, from the upper esophageal sphincter to the

S. Szomstein (✉) · A. Cracco
Cleveland Clinic Florida – Weston, Weston, FL, USA
e-mail: szomsts@ccf.org

J. Melendez-Rosado
Eisenman & Eisenman M.D., Advanced Gastro Consultants, Lake Worth, FL, USA

© Springer Nature Switzerland AG 2021
N. Zundel et al. (eds.), *Benign Esophageal Disease*,
https://doi.org/10.1007/978-3-030-51489-1_9

Fig. 9.1 Normal color pressure topography on high-resolution manometry

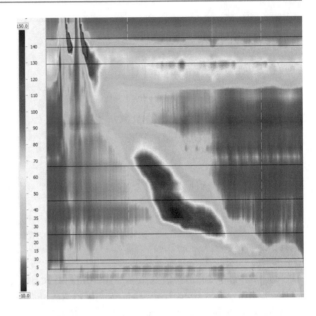

GEJ. Once in position, the patient is asked to swallow 5 mL of water in 10 different swallows. The coordination and degree of pressure throughout esophagus give rise to a color pressure topography plot that allows physicians to distinguish different types of esophageal motility disorder (Fig. 9.1). The color pressure topography is further breakdown to measure different manometric parameters such as integrated relaxation pressure (IRP) that measures relaxation of LES, distal latency (DL), and contractile front velocity (CFV) that measures peristaltic propagation, and distal contractile integral (DCI) that measures the contractile force. In 2015, the International HRM Working Group releases The Chicago Classification v3.0 (CC), which is the most updated version to classify esophageal motility disorders [5]. It utilizes a hierarchical diagnostic approach, categorizing disorder into (1) disorders of esophagogastric junction (EGJ) outflow that includes achalasia and EGJ outflow obstruction; (2) major disorders of peristalsis, which include diffuse esophageal spasms (DES), Jackhammer esophagus (JHE), and absent contractility; (3) minor disorders of peristalsis, which include ineffective motility and fragmented peristalsis (FP). The findings of some of the different esophageal motility disorders will be explained in this chapter.

Achalasia

Achalasia is a disease that results from destruction of myenteric neurons and aganglionosis in the esophagus [4]. Currently, the evidence points to an autoimmune phenomenon causing inflammation in the esophageal myenteric plexus, and although viral infections have been suggested as possible triggers, evidence is still mixed in this regards [6, 7]. This neuronal damage causes an imbalance between the inhibitory and excitatory hormones; however, in achalasia the predominant pathophysiologic mechanism is an absent or abnormal inhibitory innervation of the LES, which causes a failure of the LES to relax appropriately in the process of deglutition [8]. Over time patient will have progressive dilation of the esophagus and abnormal peristalsis. Over time chronic changes such as megaesophagus, tortuous esophagus, and angulation may be seen. Overall, the disease is rare; however, recent studies have noticed an increase in incidence with rates as high as of 1.6/100,000 per year [9]. The peak incidence is between 30 and 60 years of age. It is unclear if this increase in incidence is because of more awareness of the disease, better access to health care, and diagnostic tools.

Symptoms

The most common symptom achalasia patient present with is dysphagia. This is typically to solids and liquids, which distinguish a motility disorder from an anatomical cause, where dysphagia to solids is more predominant [10]. Another predominant symptom that may mimic gastroesophageal reflux disease (GERD) and that occurs in up to 75% of patients is heartburn [11, 12]. Heartburn in achalasia patients is not associated with the typical GERD, but from bacterial fermentation of retained food in the esophagus due to poor esophageal clearance [13]. Noncardiac chest pain, which can also be seen in GERD, is reported in about 60% of patients with achalasia particularly in young patients [14].

Given that achalasia can be misdiagnosed because of these overlapping symptoms, and if chest pain is encountered, a full cardiac evaluation should be considered in elderly patients and those with risk factor for coronary artery disease [15]. If heartburn is a presenting symptom, particularly in those patients who have failed a trial of proton pump inhibitors and have had a negative endoscopic evaluation, HRM should be considered [16].

Diagnosis

The diagnosis of achalasia is suspected on the basis of symptoms and is further confirmed by imaging and manometric studies. The first diagnostic evaluations in patients with suspected achalasia should be an esophagogastroduodenoscopy (EGD). EGD with detailed inspection of the esophageal mucosa and gastric cardia on retroflexion is essential to rule out other obstructive processes that may cause dysphagia such as esophageal strictures, severe esophagitis, eosinophilic esophagitis, or malignancy. On EGD, patients with achalasia will have a dilated and often tortuous esophagus with mild resistance in the LES. They may also have retained saliva, liquid or undigested food in the esophagus, and candida esophagitis because of food stasis. In cases where there is an increase in risk for aspiration pneumonia, endotracheal intubation to protect the airway may be needed prior to EGD.

Fig. 9.2 Bird beak sign on barium esophagogram

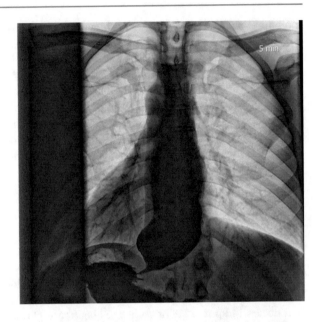

Barium will demonstrate the classic radiologic finding of a dilated esophagus and a smooth tapering of the LES that gives the classic appearance of a "Bird's beak" representing impair relaxation of LES [17] (Fig. 9.2). Although this is very characteristic for achalasia, another possibility can be pseudoachalasia from esophageal cancer or gastric cardia tumor. This should be suspected when patients have advanced age, short duration of symptoms, considerable weight loss, and difficulties to pass EGD through the GEJ [18]. In these cases, any abnormal mucosa in the lower esophagus should be biopsy and cross-sectional imaging such as computed tomography scan of the abdomen and/or endoscopic ultrasound should be considered. Other rare cause of pseudoachalasia is the use of laparoscopic adjustable gastric band for the treatment of obesity and a tight Nissen fundoplication [19, 20].

Timed barium esophagogram is an imaging technique to asses esophageal clearance of barium after therapy for achalasia [21]. It involves measuring the width and height of barium column at 1, 2, and 5 minutes after ingestion of barium before and after therapy. A <50% improvement on barium height has been associated with lack of symptomatic improvement [22].

HRM is the gold standard test to confirm the diagnosis of achalasia. This technology is able to distinguish three different subtypes of achalasia, type I, II, and III [5] (Fig. 9.3). Although the subtypes have different characteristics on HRM, they all share a fundamental abnormality, which is failure of LES relaxation and esophageal body dysmotility. Failure of LES relaxation gives an IRP >15 mmHg on HRM. Type I is characterized by aperistalsis of the body of esophagus, type II by pressurization of the body of the esophagus, and type III by a rapidly propagated esophageal pressurization attributable to spastic contractions. It is essential to differentiate the three subtypes of achalasia as they may have different outcomes depending on the treatment [23, 24].

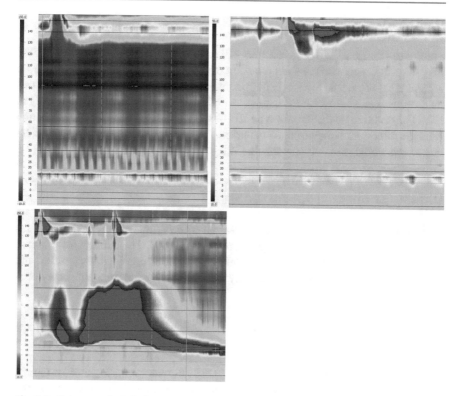

Fig. 9.3 Subtypes of achalasia

Esophagogastric Junction Outflow Obstruction (EGJO)

This disorder describes a subgroup of patients in which HRM noticed to have incomplete relaxation of the LES, with preserved peristalsis, therefore not meeting the criteria for achalasia [25]. Previously this disorder was also known as LES disrelaxation or functional obstruction and it has been suggested to be caused by infiltrative diseases, or a variant or incomplete onset of achalasia [26, 27].

Symptoms

Clinically, this disorder may present with similar symptoms as achalasia. However, it has been noted that some patients with symptoms responded to achalasia treatment, whether in others their symptoms disappeared spontaneously or were not related to outflow obstruction [26, 27]. Therefore, subsequent diagnostics tests should be used to identify true EGJO obstruction from incidental elevated IRP pressures [28].

Diagnosis

Similar to achalasia, EGJO obstruction will have an IRP >15 mmHg; however, they may have sufficient peristalsis in the body of the esophagus to not meet criteria for achalasia based on HRM [5]. It is important to perform the HRM off opioids as this medications can cause a LES dysfunction and have a similar manometric finding to EGJO obstruction and achalasia type III [29]. If opioids-induced LES dysfunction is on the differential diagnosis, then a priority should be to discontinue the medication as this findings may be reversible [30].

Diffuse Esophageal Spasm (DES)

DES is a hypermotility disorder characterized by repetitive and simultaneous premature contractions of the esophageal musculature [31]. The etiology of this rare disorder is unclear, but appears to be related to a defective inhibitory reflex and spontaneous contractions generated by independent discharges of acetylcholine [32].

Symptoms

Chest pain is a characteristic symptom of DES. In many occasions, chest pain is confused as pain of cardiac origin as it also may radiate to the jaw, and upper extremities. It is also frequently associated with dysphagia and regurgitation [33].

Diagnosis

Barium esophagogram can be suggestive of DES with the classic finding of simultaneous, lumen obliterating contractions of the circular muscle giving the appearance of "corkscrew" esophagus [34]. Despite this classic finding, these contractions can be intermittent and not always present at the time of evaluation. The gold standard diagnostic evaluation is HRM. Given that premature contraction can be seen in normal subjects, the CC has established that this abnormality has to be present ≥20% (DL <4.5) to make a diagnosis [5, 35].

Jackhammer Esophagus (JHE)

JHE is a rare hypercontractile condition of the esophagus with unclear etiology.

Fig. 9.4 Jackhammer
esophagus

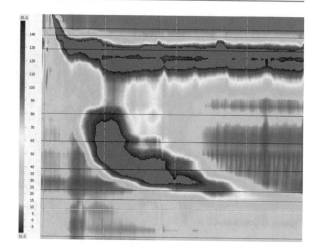

Diagnosis

The hallmark of this condition is a DCI ≥8000 mmHg/cm/sec in ≥20% swallows on HRM [5] (Fig. 9.4). Isolated increased wave amplitude contractions was not always associated with symptoms, and could also be found in healthy asymptomatic patients [36]. This led to the introduction of DCI as a new parameter to measure the vigor of the peristalsis. A DCI ≥8000 mmHg/cm/sec is typically associated with symptoms, and a positive response to achalasia treatment. Multipeaked contractions were not associated with more symptoms or improved symptoms after treatment [16, 37]. The terms hypertensive peristalsis and nutcracker esophagus are not described anymore in the latest CC and have been replaced by the term Jackhammer esophagus [5].

Symptoms

The most common symptoms in patient with JHE are dysphagia (47%), noncardiac chest pain (29%) and cough, heartburn, and regurgitation (24%) [38]. Noncardiac chest pain is associated with higher DCI with average of 17,245 mmHg × s × cm [38].

Absent Contractility

Absent contractility is a motility disorder characterized by normal EGJ relaxation (IRP <15) with 100% absent peristalsis [5] (Fig. 9.5). Achalasia should be considered when IRP values are borderline and when there is evidence of esophageal

Fig. 9.5 Absent
contractility in scleroderma

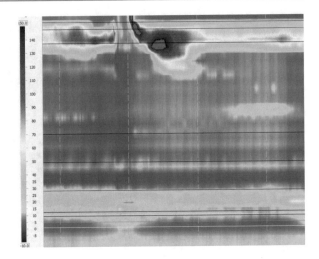

pressurization [5]. Although esophageal motor function is heterogeneous in patients with systemic scleroderma, absent contractility is the most common finding seen in 56% of patients [39]. This condition should be suspected when in addition to absent contractility they have associated hypotensive LES. Other systemic manifestations of the disease such as GERD, skin fibrosis, telangiectasias, sclerodactyly, Raynaud's disease, or pulmonary hypertension should prompt appropriate workup [40].

Clinical relevance of absent contractility is still not clear; however, it is important to rule it out when considering fundoplication procedures, due to the likelihood of this patients developing dysphagia afterwards [28].

Minor Disorders of Peristalsis

Minor disorders of peristalsis include ineffective esophageal motility (IEM) and fragmented peristalsis (FP) in the most updated version of the CC [5]. IEM is diagnosed when >50% of patients have a DCI measurement of <450 mmHg. This disorder can be seen in up to 50% of patients with GERD [41]. Although its clinical significance is unclear, this should be taken into consideration when evaluating a patient for antireflux surgical procedures. FP is diagnosed when at least 50% of contractions are fragmented which can be seen as area of lower pressure on HRM. Pressure breaks in HRM may be observed in symptomatic and asymptomatic patients [42]. Although the significance of small pressure breaks in the isobaric contour may be discounted, large breaks might be clinically relevant, and may be related to GERD [42]. The clinical significance of minor disorders of peristalsis is unclear.

Provocative Tests

The use of complementary provocative tests may be necessary for the diagnosis of esophageal motility disorders. The conventional use of ten 5 ml water swallows may not trigger abnormal findings of HRM [43]. Therefore, provocative tests using multiple rapid swallows and solid swallows may increase the sensitivity of the study [44–46]. The use of multiple rapid swallows consists in five swallows after the direct injection in the patient's mouth of 3 ml of water in 2–3-second intervals. The absence of smooth muscle contractions during the swallows followed by a strong contraction at the end of the swallow will typically be observed in the pressure plot [47–49]. Abnormal tests were found in 67% of patients with esophageal symptoms and normal findings on single swallows [28]. Solid swallows may be used as part of provocative testing. They are performed using 1 cm^3 bread swallows. Clinically, these tests are difficult to analyze because it generated complex pressure patterns and the food blouses are not transported in one single swallow. However, abnormalities detected during this test that trigger patient's complaint would provide direct pathophysiology for their symptoms [28].

Postsurgical Assessments

Patients with previous surgeries to the esophagus have an alteration of the normal anatomy, thereby changing the physiology and manometric findings in this population. For this reason, the presentation of new or recurrent symptoms in patients previously treated for esophageal disorders may be challenging.

In patients with fundoplications, there is an alteration of the distal high-pressure zone (DHPZ). The DHPZ corresponds to an area of 3–4 cm in the distal esophagus that acts as the antireflux barrier, and includes the LES and the crura of the diaphragm [50]. Identifying the strength of the DHPZ and its relation to the LES is useful information. LES complex HRM findings have been found to correlate well with anatomical status of the fundoplication [51]. An elevated DHPZ at the level of the LES are the normal expected findings after a wrap. An elevated single DHPZ at the LES with low pressure and normal relaxation suggests disrupted plication, while with high pressure and incomplete relaxation it suggests twisted fundoplication. The presence of dual DHPZ indicates inappropriate position of the wrap [50].

In achalasia, successful treatment can be observed by a loss of the DHPZ, and may show failure of treatment if there is a persistent high basal LES pressure [50].

References

1. Goyal RK, Chaudhury A. Physiology of normal esophageal motility. J Clin Gastroenterol. 2008;42:610–9.
2. Collman PI, Tremblay L, Diamant NE. The central vagal efferent supply to the esophagus and lower esophageal sphincter of the cat. Gastroenterology. 1993;104:1430–8.

3. Goyal RK, Rattan S, Said SI. VIP as a possible neurotransmitter of non-cholinergic non-adrenergic inhibitory neurones. Nature. 1980;288:378–80.
4. Yamato S, Spechler SJ, Goyal RK. Role of nitric oxide in esophageal peristalsis in the opossum. Gastroenterology. 1992;103:197–204.
5. Kahrilas PJ, Bredenoord AJ, Fox M, et al. The Chicago classification of esophageal motility disorders, v3.0. Neurogastroenterol Motil. 2015;27:160–74.
6. Moses PL, Ellis LM, Anees MR, et al. Antineuronal antibodies in idiopathic achalasia and gastro-oesophageal reflux disease. Gut. 2003;52:629–36.
7. Boeckxstaens GE. Achalasia: virus-induced euthanasia of neurons? Am J Gastroenterol. 2008;103:1610–2.
8. Dodds WJ, Dent J, Hogan WJ, Patel GK, Toouli J, Arndorfer RC. Paradoxical lower esophageal sphincter contraction induced by cholecystokinin-octapeptide in patients with achalasia. Gastroenterology. 1981;80:327–33.
9. O'Neill OM, Johnston BT, Coleman HG. Achalasia: a review of clinical diagnosis, epidemiology, treatment and outcomes. World J Gastroenterol. 2013;19:5806–12.
10. American Society for Gastrointestinal Endoscopy Standards of Practice Committee, Anderson MA, Appalaneni V, et al. The role of endoscopy in the evaluation and treatment of patients with biliary neoplasia. Gastrointest Endosc. 2013;77:167–74.
11. Spechler SJ, Souza RF, Rosenberg SJ, Ruben RA, Goyal RK. Heartburn in patients with achalasia. Gut. 1995;37:305–8.
12. Ponce J, Ortiz V, Maroto N, Ponce M, Bustamante M, Garrigues V. High prevalence of heartburn and low acid sensitivity in patients with idiopathic achalasia. Dig Dis Sci. 2011;56:773–6.
13. Crookes PF, Corkill S, DeMeester TR. Gastroesophageal reflux in achalasia. When is reflux really reflux? Dig Dis Sci. 1997;42:1354–61.
14. Eckardt VF, Stauf B, Bernhard G. Chest pain in achalasia: patient characteristics and clinical course. Gastroenterology. 1999;116:1300–4.
15. Fenster PE. Evaluation of chest pain: a cardiology perspective for gastroenterologists. Gastroenterol Clin N Am. 2004;33:35–40.
16. Kahrilas PJ, Shaheen NJ, Vaezi MF, et al. American Gastroenterological Association Medical Position Statement on the management of gastroesophageal reflux disease. Gastroenterology. 2008;135:1383–91, 91 e1-5.
17. Xiang H, Han J, Ridley WE, Ridley LJ. Bird's beak sign: achalasia. J Med Imaging Radiat Oncol. 2018;62 Suppl 1:58.
18. Ponds FA, van Raath MI, Mohamed SMM, Smout A, Bredenoord AJ. Diagnostic features of malignancy-associated pseudoachalasia. Aliment Pharmacol Ther. 2017;45:1449–58.
19. Roman S, Kahrilas PJ. Pseudoachalasia and laparoscopic gastric banding. J Clin Gastroenterol. 2011;45:745–7.
20. Lai CN, Krishnan K, Kim MP, Dunkin BJ, Gaur P. Pseudoachalasia presenting 20 years after Nissen fundoplication: a case report. J Cardiothorac Surg. 2016;11:96.
21. Neyaz Z, Gupta M, Ghoshal UC. How to perform and interpret timed barium esophagogram. J Neurogastroenterol Motil. 2013;19:251–6.
22. Vaezi MF, Baker ME, Richter JE. Assessment of esophageal emptying post-pneumatic dilation: use of the timed barium esophagram. Am J Gastroenterol. 1999;94:1802–7.
23. Lee JY, Kim N, Kim SE, et al. Clinical characteristics and treatment outcomes of 3 subtypes of achalasia according to the Chicago classification in a tertiary institute in Korea. J Neurogastroenterol Motil. 2013;19:485–94.
24. Andolfi C, Fisichella PM. Meta-analysis of clinical outcome after treatment for achalasia based on manometric subtypes. Br J Surg. 2019;106(4):332–41.
25. Carlson DA, Pandolfino JE. High-resolution manometry and esophageal pressure topography: filling the gaps of convention manometry. Gastroenterol Clin N Am. 2013;42:1–15.
26. Scherer JR, Kwiatek MA, Soper NJ, Pandolfino JE, Kahrilas PJ. Functional esophagogastric junction obstruction with intact peristalsis: a heterogeneous syndrome sometimes akin to achalasia. J Gastrointest Surg. 2009;13:2219–25.

27. van Hoeij FB, Smout AJ, Bredenoord AJ. Characterization of idiopathic esophagogastric junction outflow obstruction. Neurogastroenterol Motil. 2015;27:1310–6.
28. van Hoeij FB, Bredenoord AJ. Clinical application of esophageal high-resolution manometry in the diagnosis of esophageal motility disorders. J Neurogastroenterol Motil. 2016;22:6–13.
29. Ratuapli SK, Crowell MD, DiBaise JK, et al. Opioid-induced esophageal dysfunction (OIED) in patients on chronic opioids. Am J Gastroenterol. 2015;110:979–84.
30. Ortiz V, Garcia-Campos M, Saez-Gonzalez E, delPozo P, Garrigues V. A concise review of opioid-induced esophageal dysfunction: is this a new clinical entity? Dis Esophagus. 2018;31(5):doy003. https://doi.org/10.1093/dote/doy003.
31. Pandolfino JE, Roman S, Carlson D, et al. Distal esophageal spasm in high-resolution esophageal pressure topography: defining clinical phenotypes. Gastroenterology. 2011;141:469–75.
32. Behar J, Biancani P. Pathogenesis of simultaneous esophageal contractions in patients with motility disorders. Gastroenterology. 1993;105:111–8.
33. Rao SS. Diagnosis and management of esophageal chest pain. Gastroenterol Hepatol. 2011;7:50–2.
34. Fonseca EK, Yamauchi FI, Tridente CF, Baroni RH. Corkscrew esophagus. Abdom Radiol (NY). 2017;42:985–6.
35. Smout AJ, Breedijk M, van der Zouw C, Akkermans LM. Physiological gastroesophageal reflux and esophageal motor activity studied with a new system for 24-hour recording and automated analysis. Dig Dis Sci. 1989;34:372–8.
36. Roman S, Pandolfino JE, Chen J, Boris L, Luger D, Kahrilas PJ. Phenotypes and clinical context of hypercontractility in high-resolution esophageal pressure topography (EPT). Am J Gastroenterol. 2012;107:37–45.
37. Pandolfino JE, Ghosh SK, Rice J, Clarke JO, Kwiatek MA, Kahrilas PJ. Classifying esophageal motility by pressure topography characteristics: a study of 400 patients and 75 controls. Am J Gastroenterol. 2008;103:27–37.
38. Sloan JA, Mulki R, Sandhu N, Samuel S, Katz PO. Jackhammer esophagus: symptom presentation, associated distal contractile integral, and assessment of bolus transit. J Clin Gastroenterol. 2019;53(4):295–7.
39. Crowell MD, Umar SB, Griffing WL, DiBaise JK, Lacy BE, Vela MF. Esophageal motor abnormalities in patients with scleroderma: heterogeneity, risk factors, and effects on quality of life. Clin Gastroenterol Hepatol. 2017;15:207–13 e1.
40. Denton CP, Khanna D. Systemic sclerosis. Lancet. 2017;390:1685–99.
41. Abdel Jalil AA, Castell DO. Ineffective Esophageal Motility (IEM): the old-new frontier in esophagology. Curr Gastroenterol Rep. 2016;18:1.
42. Kumar N, Porter RF, Chanin JM, Gyawali CP. Analysis of intersegmental trough and proximal latency of smooth muscle contraction using high-resolution esophageal manometry. J Clin Gastroenterol. 2012;46:375–81.
43. Bogte A, Bredenoord AJ, Oors J, Siersema PD, Smout AJ. Reproducibility of esophageal high-resolution manometry. Neurogastroenterol Motil. 2011;23:e271–6.
44. Carlson DA, Ravi K, Kahrilas PJ, et al. Diagnosis of esophageal motility disorders: esophageal pressure topography vs. conventional line tracing. Am J Gastroenterol. 2015;110:967–77; quiz 78.
45. Pandolfino JE, Kwiatek MA, Nealis T, Bulsiewicz W, Post J, Kahrilas PJ. Achalasia: a new clinically relevant classification by high-resolution manometry. Gastroenterology. 2008;135:1526–33.
46. Pandolfino JE, Fox MR, Bredenoord AJ, Kahrilas PJ. High-resolution manometry in clinical practice: utilizing pressure topography to classify oesophageal motility abnormalities. Neurogastroenterol Motil. 2009;21:796–806.
47. Rohof WO, Salvador R, Annese V, et al. Outcomes of treatment for achalasia depend on manometric subtype. Gastroenterology. 2013;144:718–25; quiz e13-4.
48. Pratap N, Kalapala R, Darisetty S, et al. Achalasia cardia subtyping by high-resolution manometry predicts the therapeutic outcome of pneumatic balloon dilatation. J Neurogastroenterol Motil. 2011;17:48–53.

49. Salvador R, Costantini M, Zaninotto G, et al. The preoperative manometric pattern predicts the outcome of surgical treatment for esophageal achalasia. J Gastrointest Surg. 2010;14:1635–45.
50. Wang YT, Yazaki E, Sifrim D. High-resolution manometry: esophageal disorders not addressed by the "Chicago Classification". J Neurogastroenterol Motil. 2012;18:365–72.
51. Hoshino M, Srinivasan A, Mittal SK. High-resolution manometry patterns of lower esophageal sphincter complex in symptomatic post-fundoplication patients. J Gastrointest Surg. 2012;16:705–14.

Motility Disorders: Medical Modalities

10

Andrew M. Brown and Aurora D. Pryor

Motility Disorders and High-Resolution Manometry

Version 3.0 of the Chicago Classification (CC) of esophageal motility disorders, last updated in 2014, categorizes esophageal motility disorders using high-resolution manometry (HRM) with color pressure topography plots. The evaluation of HRM is based on the analysis of ten 5-ml swallows performed in the supine position, on patients without prior surgery affecting the esophagus or esophagogastric junction (EGJ) [1]. Using HRM, CC version 3.0 uses a tiered approach to define disorders of esophageal motility. It includes disorders of esophagogastric junction outflow, other major disorders of peristalsis, and minor disorders of peristalsis.

Disorders of the esophagogastric junction are further divided into achalasia (with subtypes I, II, and III), and EGJ outflow obstruction. Other major disorders of motility include absent contractility, distal esophageal spasm, and hypercontractile esophagus. Minor motility disorders, which are characterized by impaired esophageal bolus transit, are ineffective esophageal motility and fragmented peristalsis [1].

Evaluation of certain parameters of HRM correspond to esophageal physiology and enable the practitioner to make a diagnosis. Key parameters are described below.

1. Contractility is determined through the parameter distal contractile integral (DCI). This is a calculation that includes the amplitude, time, and length of the peristaltic wave. DCI classifies waves as failed (DCI <100 mmHg/s/cm), weak (DCI 100–450 mmHg/s/cm), ineffective (failed or weak), normal (DCI 450–8000 mmHg/s/cm), or hypercontractile (DCI >8000 mmHg/s/cm).
2. Distal latency (DL) is the timeframe of the peristaltic wave from the beginning of the swallow to an inflection point called the contractile deceleration point. Premature contractions have a DL <4.5 s.

A. M. Brown (✉) · A. D. Pryor
Department of Surgery, Stony Brook University Hospital, Stony Brook, NY, USA
e-mail: Andrew.brown@stonybrookmedicine.edu

© Springer Nature Switzerland AG 2021
N. Zundel et al. (eds.), *Benign Esophageal Disease*,
https://doi.org/10.1007/978-3-030-51489-1_10

Fig. 10.1 Normal esophageal motility on high-resolution manometry (HRM) [12]. (Image used with Permission from Dr. Alexandra Guillaume and Stony Brook University Hospital GI Motility Laboratory)

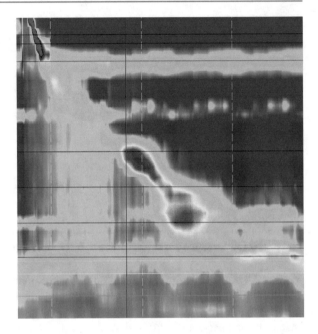

- Fragmented contractions have normal contraction vigor, but have a defect in the wave segment.
3. Lower esophageal sphincter (LES) relaxation is measured by the integrated relaxation pressure (IRP) that is measured by the mean pressure of 4 s of greatest post deglutitive relaxation in a 10-s gap, triggered at the beginning of a swallow. An IRP >15 mmHg [2].

Normal esophageal motility is represented in Fig. 10.1.

Major Disorders of Peristalsis

Achalasia

Achalasia is broadly defined by IRP, with an IRP >15 mmHg, and then is further divided into three subtypes by the patterns of nonperistaltic esophageal pressurization that accompanies the elevated IRP.

Type 1 achalasia (classic achalasia): Elevated IRP (>15 mmHg) with 100% failed peristalsis. A DCI <100 mmHg/s/cm or premature contractions with DCI <450 mmHg/s/cm satisfy criteria for failed peristalsis.

Type 2 achalasia (with esophageal decompression): Elevated IRP (>15 mmHg) with 100% failed peristalsis, and panesophageal pressurization with ≥20% of swallows. Contractions may be masked by esophageal pressurization and DCI should not be calculated.

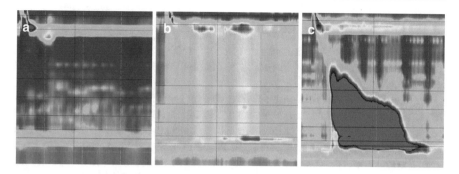

Fig. 10.2 Types 1–3 achalasia on HRM [1]. Panel (**a**) shows type 1 achalasia with impaired esophagogastric junction (EGJ) relaxation and aperistalsis. Panel (**b**) shows type 2 achalasia with impaired EGJ relaxation and pan pressurization of the esophagus. Panel (**c**) shows type 3 achalasia with impaired EGJ relaxation, and premature contractions with a DL <4.5 s. (Image used with Permission from Dr. Alexandra Guillaume and Stony Brook University Hospital GI Motility Laboratory)

Type 3 achalasia (spastic achalasia): Elevated IRP (>15 mmHg) with no normal peristalsis and premature (spastic) contractions with DCI >450 mmHg/s/cm with ≥20% of swallows. This may be mixed with panesophageal pressurization [1]. Achalasia is represented on HRM in Fig. 10.2.

Traditional management strategies for achalasia include pharmacologic, endoscopic, and surgical options. While numerous medications have been tried for the symptomatic relief of achalasia in adults, data suggests that there is limited long-term success. Current guidelines state that there is no convincing evidence for the use nitrates, calcium channel blockers, or phosphodiesterase inhibitors for symptom relief [3].

Nitrates act at the LES by making up for a long-term deficiency in the inhibitory neurotransmitter nitric oxide. This subsequently allows for a decrease in LES pressure [4]. Calcium channel blockers inhibit the uptake of intracellular calcium, which subsequently results in muscle relaxation. Use of both isosorbide dinitrate and nifedipine has led to the alleviation of symptoms in the short term, but long-term use of these medications promotes tolerance and diminishing effects over time [5]. Importantly, in a small subset of patients, (8.9%), with chronic nifedipine administration, there was sufficient clinical response, and esophageal manometry showed that the achalasia pattern had been replaced by a near-normal pattern [5]. This suggests there is a group of responders to this therapy. The use of Verapamil, while efficacious in lowering LES pressures, does not improve symptoms [6]. The use of both sublingual nitrates and calcium channel blockers is plagued by common side effects, including hypotension, headache, and peripheral edema, in as high as 30% of patients [7].

Phosphodiesterase inhibitors work through downstream actions to produce an inhibitory effect of on the smooth muscle and subsequent decrease in LES tone and residual pressure [8]. In a small study with 11 patients, Sildenafil leads to improved manometric findings in 9 patients, but symptomatic improvement in only 4 patients, of which 2 of the 4 had significant side effects requiring cessation of the medication [9]. Additional medications including aminophylline and terbutaline have been poorly studied [4].

Achalasia is best treated with surgical or endoscopic therapies. Pneumatic balloon dilation (PD), endoscopic botulinum toxin injection, Per Oral Endoscopic Myotomy (POEM), and heller myotomy (HM) have all been shown to be effective for relief of symptoms of achalasia [10]. While POEM and laparoscopic HM have been shown to be efficacious in treating symptoms of achalasia, there may be higher post-procedural acid exposure in the esophagus following POEM [11].

Esophagogastric Junction Outflow Obstruction

Esophagogastric junction outflow obstruction (EGJOO) is defined as an elevated IRP (>15 mmHg), with sufficient evidence of peristalsis such that criteria for types 1–3 achalasia are not met [1].

EGJOO can be further divided into two major categories, functional and mechanical EGJOO. Functional EGJOO is suspected in patients in which no mechanical cause is identified for the obstruction [12]. This is generally treated similarly to achalasia, with surgical and endoscopic interventions [13–15]. Botulinum toxin injection with pneumatic balloon dilation has had short-term successful outcomes [12].

Conversely, mechanical EGJOO has an underlying etiology that should be treated based on the cause. Common etiologies include eosinophilic esophagitis, which can effectively be treating with proton pump inhibitors (PPI) monotherapy as the first-line treatment, as well as corticosteroids [16]. Obesity caused EGJOO results from increased intra-abdominal pressures, and can be effectively treated with weight loss. Chronic daily opioid exposure has been shown to be present in almost a third of all EGJOO patients as defined by HRM [17]. Cessation of opioids may help mitigate the symptoms of esophageal dysfunction in these patients when there is not another cause identified. Figure 10.3 shows the topographic representation of EJGOO on HRM.

Hypercontractile Esophagus

Hypercontractile esophagus, also known as jackhammer esophagus, is defined by at least two swallows with DCI >8000 mmHg/s/cm. Hypercontractility may involve, or even be located to the lower esophageal sphincter [1].

Treatment for this condition is extremely varied, and given its low prevalence, few large studies have looked at treatment efficacy. A recent study by Kahn et al., in

Fig. 10.3 Esophagogastric outlet obstruction on HRM [12]. Impaired EGJ relaxation with normal peristalsis. (Image used with Permission from Dr. Alexandra Guillaume and Stony Brook University Hospital GI Motility Laboratory)

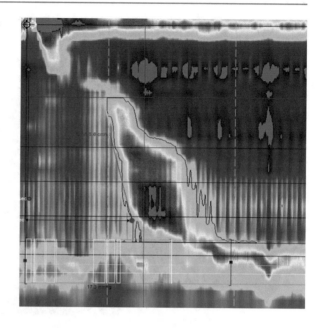

81 patients with jackhammer esophagus, found that treatment options included endoscopic dilation, Botox injection, PPI, surgical or endoscopic myotomy, calcium channel blockers, hyoscyamine, tadalafil, tricyclic antidepressants, peppermint oil, benzodiazepines, baclofen, and trazodone. These authors found that nonpharmacologic treatment (endoscopic treatment or myotomy) had significantly higher rates of symptomatic improvement, but this effect dissipated on long-term follow-up. No single pharmacologic agent proved to be superior [18]. Other research has found that pharmacological relaxation of the smooth muscle with phosphodiesterase-5 inhibitors or anticholinergic agents has shown symptomatic improvement [19]. Surgical and endoscopic options have also been tried with moderate results. Similar to esophageal spasm, POEM may be an effective tool for significant improvements in chest pain and dysphagia in this patient population [20]. Figure 10.4 shows HRM of hypercontractile esophagus.

Distal Esophageal Spasm

Distal esophageal spasm is defined by a normal IRP and with $\geq 20\%$ premature contractions (DL <4.5 s) with a DCI >450 mmHg/s/cm. Some normal peristalsis may be present [1, 2].

Pharmacologic treatment options have limited efficacy. Options include concentrated peppermint oil, nitrates or phosphodiesterase-5 inhibitors, calcium channel blockers, tricyclic antidepressants, endoscopic botulinum toxin injection, pneumatic dilation, and myotomy (surgical or endoscopic) [21]. In a small study with

Fig. 10.4 Hypercontractile esophagus on HRM
[2]. DCI >8000 mmHg/s/
cm in at least 20% of
swallows with a normal
DL. (Image used with
Permission from
Dr. Alexandra Guillaume
and Stony Brook
University Hospital GI
Motility Laboratory)

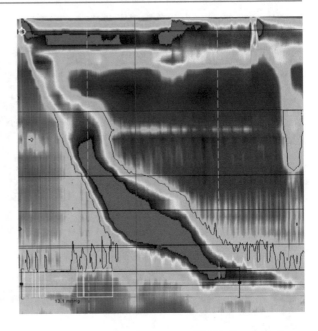

eight patients, peppermint reduced the number of simultaneous contractions found
on manometry [22]. Endoscopic and surgical options have traditionally had limited
impact, but there is some evidence that the POEM may be a viable option for the
treatment of chest pain and dysphagia in these patients, although the data is limited
[20]. Distal esophageal Spasm is represented on HRM in Fig. 10.5.

Absent Contractility

Absent contractility is characterized by 100% failed peristalsis with a normal
IRP. Achalasia should be considered when IRP values are borderline and when
there is evidence of esophageal pressurization [1].

Absent contractility has been shown to be associated with systemic sclerosis. A
recent study by Aggarwal et al. showed that in 122 patients with systemic sclerosis
who underwent HRM, 60% of patients had absent contractility [23]. There is no
available treatment to restore or improve peristalsis that has been well-proven.
Treatment of an underlying sclerotic condition and symptomatic management of
associated gastroesophageal reflux disease (GERD) remain the mainstay of management. This begins with PPI therapy, but symptom control has been attempted
with antireflux surgery, or gastric drainage procedures, although the data is limited
[2]. Absent contractility is seen in Fig. 10.6.

Fig. 10.5 Distal esophageal spasm on HRM [2]. Premature contractions (DL <4.5 s) in at least 20% of swallows. (Image used with Permission from Dr. Alexandra Guillaume and Stony Brook University Hospital GI Motility Laboratory)

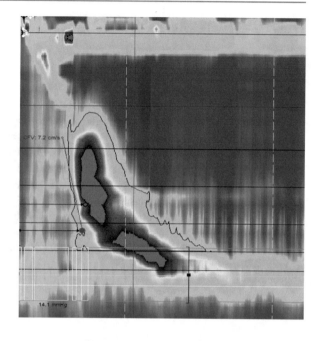

Fig. 10.6 Absent contractility on HRM [2]. Aperistalsis in the setting of a normal LES relaxation with an IRP <10 mmHg. (Image used with Permission from Dr. Alexandra Guillaume and Stony Brook University Hospital GI Motility Laboratory)

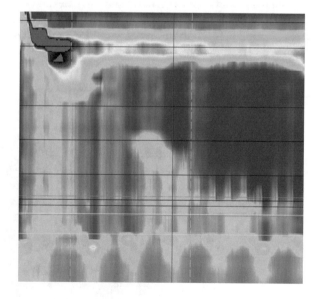

Minor Disorders of Peristalsis

Ineffective Esophageal Motility

Ineffective esophageal motility is defined by $\geq$50% ineffective swallows. Ineffective swallows can be either failed or weak with a DCI <450 mmHg/s/cm [1].

Treatment is aimed at the management of gastroesophageal reflux, with proton pump inhibitors with or without pro-kinetic agents. In a small study by Jeong et al., with 17 patients, only 41.2% of the patients had either a complete or satisfactory response to PPI treatment [24]. Mosapride, a prokinetic serotonin receptor agonist, significantly increases peristaltic contractions in healthy volunteers, and along with other prokinetic agents, are an area of future study [25]. Additional pharmacologic interventions have been studied without success. The anxiolytic buspirone did not lead to improvement, and treatment of GERD may be helpful when this disorder is secondary to reflux [2, 26]. HRM images of ineffective esophageal motility are seen in Fig. 10.7.

Fragmented Peristalsis

Fragmented peristalsis is defined by $\geq$50% fragmented contractions with a DCI >450 mmHg/s/cm [2].

Similar to ineffective esophageal motility, treatment is aimed at the management of GERD. Jeong et al., in only seven patients, found that 85.7% of patients symptomatically improved to treatment with PPIs [24]. Fragmented peristalsis is represented on HRM in Fig. 10.8.

Fig. 10.7 Ineffective esophageal motility on HRM [2]. Failed or weak peristalsis in at least 30% of swallows. (Image used with Permission from Dr. Alexandra Guillaume and Stony Brook University Hospital GI Motility Laboratory)

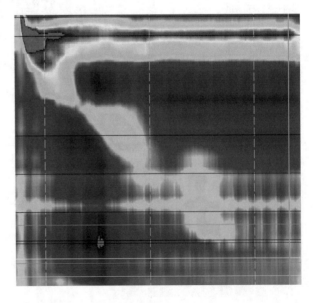

Fig. 10.8 Fragmented
peristalsis on HRM [2].
Fragmented peristalsis
with a 7 cm gap. (Image
used with Permission from
Dr. Alexandra Guillaume
and Stony Brook
University Hospital GI
Motility Laboratory)

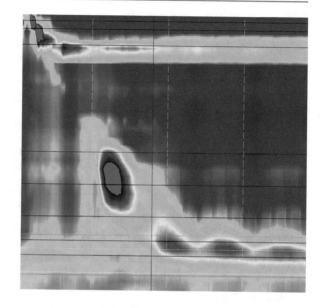

References

1. Kahrilas PJ, Bredenoord AJ, Fox M, et al. International High Resolution Manometry Working Group. The Chicago classification of esophageal motility disorders, v3.0. Neurogastroenterol Motil. 2015;27:160–74.
2. Schlottmann F, Patti MG. Primary esophageal motility disorders: beyond achalasia. Int J Mol Sci. 2017;18(7):1399.
3. Zaninotto G, Bennett C, Boeckxstaens G, et al. The 2018 ISDE achalasia guidelines. Dis Esophagus. 2018;31(9):1–29.
4. Lake JM, Wong RKH. Review article: the management of achalasia – a comparison of different treatment modalities. Aliment Pharmacol Ther. 2006;24(6):909–18.
5. Bortolotti M. Medical therapy of achalasia: a benefit reserved for few. Digestion. 1999;60(1):11–6.
6. Triadafilopoulos G, Aaronson M, Sackel S, et al. Medical treatment of esophageal achalasia. Dig Dis Sci. 1991;36:260–7.
7. Gelfond M, Rozen P, Gilat T. Isosorbide dinitrate and nifedipine treatment of achalasia: a clinical, manometric and radionuclide evaluation. Gastroenterology. 1982;83:963–9.
8. Bortolotti M, Mari C, Lopilato C, et al. Effects of sildenafil on esophageal motility of patients with idiopathic achalasia. Gastroenterology. 2000;111:253–7.
9. Eherer AJ, Schwetz I, Hammer HF, et al. Effect of sildenafil on oesophageal motor function in healthy subjects and patients with oesophageal motor disorders. Gut. 2002;50(6):758–64.
10. Kahrilas PJ, Bredenoord AJ, Carlson DA, et al. Advances in management of esophageal motility disorders. Clin Gastroenterol Hepatol. 2018;16(11):1692–700.
11. Sanaka MR, Thota PN, Parikh MP, et al. Peroral endoscopic myotomy leads to higher rates of abnormal esophageal acid exposure than laparoscopic Heller myotomy in achalasia. Surg Endosc. 2019;33(7):2284–92.
12. Samo S, Qayed E. Esophagogastric junction outflow obstruction: where are we now in diagnosis and management? World J Gastroenterol. 2019;25(4):411–7.

13. Van Hoeij FB, Smout AJ, Bredenoord AJ, et al. Characterization of idiopathic esophagogastric junction outflow obstruction. Neurogastroenterol Motil. 2015;27:1310–6.
14. Scherer JR, Kwiatek MA, Soper NJ, et al. Functional esophagogastric junction obstruction with intact peristalsis: a heterogenous syndrome sometimes akin to achalasia. J Gasgtrointest Surg. 2009;13:2219–25.
15. Perez-Fernandez MT, Santander C, Marinero A, et al. Characterization and follow-up of esophagogastric junction outflow obstruction detected by high resolution manometry. Neurogastroenterol Motil. 2016;28:116–26.
16. Molina-Infante J, Lucendo AJ. Proton pump inhibitor therapy for eosinophilic esophagitis: a paradigm shift. Am J Gastroenterol. 2017;112:1770–3.
17. Babaei A, Szabo A, Shad S, et al. Chronic daily opioid exposure is associated with dysphagia, esophageal outflow obstruction, and disordered peristalsis. Neurogastroenterol Motil. 2019;31(7):e13601.
18. Kahn A, Al-Qaisi MT, Obeid RA, et al. Clinical features and long-term outcome of lower esophageal sphincter-dependent and esophageal sphincter-independent jackhammer esophagus. Neurogastroenterol Motil. 2019;31(2):e13507.
19. Hong YS, Min YW, Rhee PL. Two distinct types of hypercontractile esophagus: classic and spastic jackhammer. Gut Liver. 2016;10:859–63.
20. Filicori F, Dunst CM, Sharata A, et al. Long-term outcomes following POEM for non-achalasia motility disorders of the esophagus. Surg Endosc. 2019;33(5):1632–9.
21. Khalaf M, Chowdhary S, Elias PS, et al. Distal esophageal spasm: a review. Am J Med. 2018;131(9):1034–40.
22. Pimentel M, Bonorris GG, Chow EJ, et al. Peppermint oil improves the manometric findings in diffuse esophageal spasm. J Clin Gastroenterol. 2001;33:27–31.
23. Aggarwal N, Lopez R, Gabbard S, et al. Spectrum of esophageal dysmotility in systemic sclerosis on high-resolution esophageal manometry as defined by Chicago classification. Dis Esophagus. 2017;30(12):1–6.
24. Jeong J, Kim SE, Park MI, et al. The effect of anti-reflux therapy on patients diagnosed with minor disorders of peristalsis in high-resolution manometry. Korean J Gastroenterol. 2017;69(4):212–9.
25. Fukazawa K, Furuta K, Adachi K, et al. Effects of mosapride on esophageal motor activity and esophagogastric junction compliance in healthy volunteers. J Gastroenterol. 2014;49:1307–13.
26. Scheerens C, Tack J, Rommel N. Buspirone, a new drug for the management of patients with ineffective esophageal motility? United European Gastroenterol J. 2015;3:261–5.

Esophageal Motility Disorders

Michael Jureller and Erin Moran-Atkin

Overview

Esophageal motility disorders are broad and present at various times in their natural course. This can make an exact diagnosis challenging. These various pathologies unfortunately have no definitive cure. All treatments, medical or surgical, are based on palliation and symptom relief [1].

The goal of this chapter is to provide an overview of the latest recommendations in the diagnosis, workup, and management in a spectrum of esophageal dysmotility syndromes.

History

The first account of surgical disease of the esophagus dates from 3600 BC to 2500 BC to the famed ancient Egyptian "Edwin Smith Papyrus," in which there is a description of "a gaping wound of the throat penetrating the gullet," and the repair of a cervical esophagus with assumingly a muscle flap, "Thou shouldst bind it with fresh meat the first day. Thou shouldst treat it afterwards with grease, honey, (and) lint every day, until he recovers" [2, 3].

Later, circa AD 0 Chinese scripts detail patients with esophageal cancer and associated dysphagia and dysmotility [4]. The first documented treatment of esophageal dysphagia, thought to be achalasia, was recorded in 1679 by Thomas Willis in which he described using a sponge-tipped whale bone to assist in passage of food

M. Jureller (✉) · E. Moran-Atkin
General Surgery, Montefiore Medical Center/Albert Einstein College of Medicine,
Bronx, NY, USA
e-mail: mjurelle@montefiore.org

© Springer Nature Switzerland AG 2021
N. Zundel et al. (eds.), *Benign Esophageal Disease*,
https://doi.org/10.1007/978-3-030-51489-1_11

bolus lodged in the esophagus [5, 6]. Later, in 1913, Heyrovsky published the first open surgical approach to "idiopathic dilation of the esophagus" in which he described a series of patients in which he performed an anastomosis of the distal esophagus to the gastric fundus [7]. Shortly afterward, Heller, De Bruine Groeneveldt, and Zaaijer described the esophagocardiomyotomy [8], which has since been modernized to what we refer to as the Heller myotomy. Since that time, minimally invasive techniques using endoscopy and robotics have emerged, which we will explore in this chapter. Presently, treatment for esophageal dysmotility syndromes ranges from behavioral, to pharmacologic, to endoscopic and surgical.

Initial Workup and Diagnosis

History and Physical Exam

As with all ailments, proper diagnosis begins with the careful history and physical examination of the patient. Most patients will complain of chest pain, and thus it is important to rule out acute coronary syndrome while proceeding with a workup. Particular attention should be paid to habits pertaining to diet and associated symptoms including chest pain and weight loss. Points to question in detail are any symptoms of dysphagia, retrosternal chest pain, immediate postprandial regurgitation, and halitosis [9, 10]. With achalasia, patients may complain of retrosternal pains when ingesting cold liquids and cold substances such as ice cream, which sit statically in the distal esophagus. If dysphagia is present, what is its quality? Has the dysphagia been progressive and does it favor solids or liquids? If gastric bloating, distension, and delayed postprandial emesis are endorsed, gastroparesis may be present. Upper respiratory tract complaints may be present as well, which are similar to those with gastrointestinal (GI) reflux disease such as cough, asthma, and even pulmonary fibrosis [11].

The Eckardt scoring system (Fig. 11.1) is traditionally used for patients with dysphagia and is a good and validated subjective marker for the need for treatment and can be followed postoperatively [12–15].

Physical examination, while important, is likely to be unremarkable. With the exception of signs of weight loss such as cachexia, temporal wasting, and thinning

Symptom	Score 0	1	2	3
Dysphagia	None	Occasional	Daily	Every meal
Regurgitation	None	Occasional	Daily	Every meal
Chest pain	None	Occasional	Daily	Several times per day
Weight loss (kg)	0	<5	5–10	>10

Fig. 11.1 Eckardt score graded 0–12 for subjective measurement of severity of dysphagia

of the thenar eminences, an examination is likely to be negative. It is of utmost importance to examine nodal basins, as esophageal and gastric cancers should be a part of the initial differential diagnosis. The findings of enlarged cervical, supraclavicular or periumbilical lymphadenopathy will drastically change the further workup and management.

Initial Testing

Upper GI Fluoroscopy

Fluoroscopic evaluation is the first test of choice and should be obtained on all patients being assessed for upper GI motility disorders. Contrast-enhanced video fluoroscopy should be performed prior to endoscopy to evaluate for diverticulum, since endoscopy in this setting can possibly result in perforation. Video fluoroscopy allows for visualization of esophageal dilation, length, the presence of diverticula or a hiatal hernia, as well as gastroesophageal reflux. Several pathognomonic signs can be present on an esophagram, most famously the "bird's beak" (Fig. 11.2) appearance of the esophagus at the lower esophageal sphincter [16].

The Rezende classification (Fig. 11.3), sorted between I and IV, has typically been used to communicate the extent of esophageal dilation and tortuosity [17].

EGD

Esophagogastroduodenoscopy (EGD) should be performed on all patients for all suspected esophageal motility disorders and most other pathologies of the foregut. There are multiple utilities for EGD including, importantly, its assessment for carcinoma. Additional pertinent findings on EGD are for the caliber and mucosal quality of the esophagus, if a hiatal hernia is present and the concomitant presence of *Helicobacter pylori* [11]. Biopsies should always be taken of any suspicious esophageal, gastric, or duodenal lesions.

Endoscopic findings particularly indicative of achalasia are numerous. In 2012, the Japan Esophageal Society established several typical findings including the dilation of the esophageal lumen, retained food bolus in the distal esophagus after their midnight fast, whitish thickening along the mucosa—a combination of adhesive debris from food and candida—functional stenosis of the gastroesophageal junction, and abnormal contractions of the esophageal body [18] (Fig. 11.4). An additional finding, a so-called "Pinstripe pattern" can also been seen in up to 60% of patients and is characterized by the longitudinal wrinkling of esophageal [19] (Fig. 11.5). On passage of the endoscope of the gastroesophageal junction, a typically popping sensation may be felt as the endoscope overcomes the pressure of the lower esophageal sphincter.

Fig. 11.2 Barium
swallow. Dilated
esophagus with retained
column of barium and a
"bird's beak sign"
suggestive of achalasia.
(Reproduced from Farrokhi
and Vaezi [106])

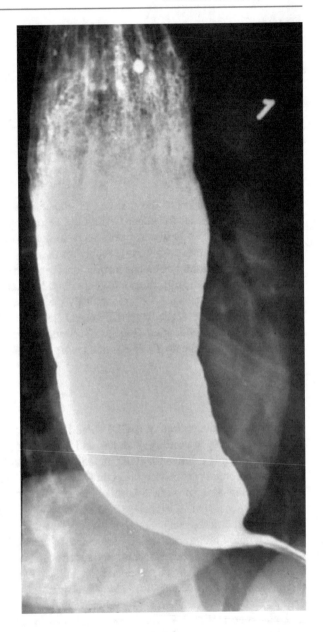

Manometry

Esophageal manometry for diagnosis of dysmotility syndromes is not only gold
standard but also helps classify dysmotility syndromes into several subclasses. The
advent and incorporation of high-resolution manometry (HRM) in the early 2000s
have been of invaluable help. Previous manometric studies limited recordings of

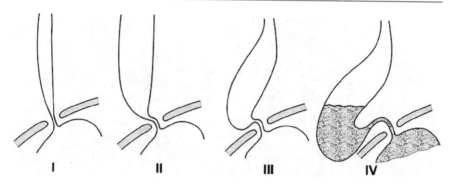

Fig. 11.3 Progression of esophageal dilation and contrast retention according to Rezende's classification of Chagastic megaesophagus. (Reproduced with permission from Griffiths et al. [102])

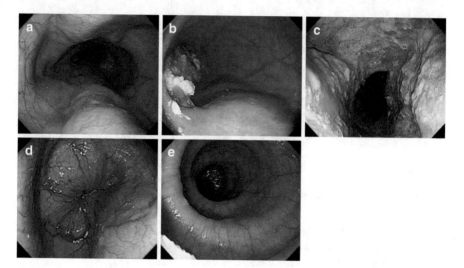

Fig. 11.4 Typical findings of achalasia on EGD (**a**) dilated esophagus, (**b**) retained food, (**c**) increased debris and bacterial overgrowth, (**d**) hypertrophic lower esophageal sphincter, (**e**) spastic paralysis. (Reproduced from Minami et al. [19])

esophageal pressure every 5–8 cm, whereas present HRM systems record pressures every 1 cm apart [20]. They are more accurate in providing a proper diagnosis and they generate colored output graphs that are easier to interpret and conceptualize in comparison to older linear plots [20].

The Chicago Classification v3.0 system [21], modified in 2015, gives the latest subdivisions of esophageal motility disorders based on HRM findings (Fig. 11.6). HRM has resulted in better diagnosis and differentiation of various esophageal motility disorders than traditional manometry [20].

Disorders can be simply subdivided into three main categories: (i) major disorders or peristalsis, (ii) minor disorders of peristalsis, and (iii) disorders with esophagogastric junction (EGJ) outflow obstruction [21].

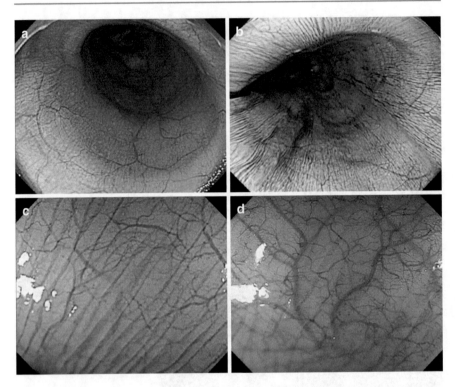

Fig. 11.5 Pinstripe pattern (**a**) minute superficial wrinkle on mucosal surface, (**b**) indigo carmine spray making the superficial structure clearer, (**c**) magnification after indigo carmine spraying, (**d**) narrow band imaging with magnification. (Reproduced from Minami et al. [19])

Some authors have started to use HRM intraoperatively to identify exact areas of esophageal hypertension to tailor the location of performed myotomy [22, 23]. However, multiple studies performed show varying results.

Several patient factors such as obesity, previous bariatric surgeries, diabetes, and possibly eosinophilic esophagitis can effect manometry studies and should be taken into account when evaluating a patient [24–28].

Differential of Dysmotility Syndromes

Achalasia

Achalasia has an incidence of approximately 1 in 100,000 per year. It does not discriminate against gender and has an increasing incidence later in life, but it can be present in the pediatric and young adult populations as well [29, 30].

Esophageal achalasia is defined by features from the Chicago Classification v3.0 system, and is a subdivision of EGJ outflow obstruction. Achalasia falls within a major disorder of peristalsis. It is defined by an elevation of the median integrated

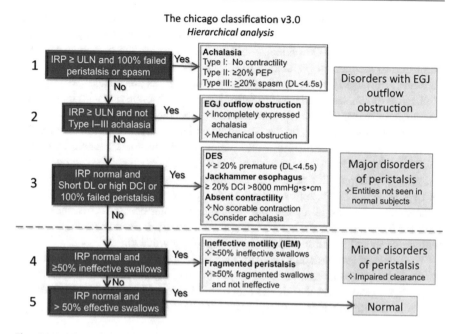

Fig. 11.6 Hierarchical algorithm for classification of motility disorders by the Chicago Classification. (Reproduced with permission from Kahrilas et al. [21])

relaxation pressure (IRP) with associated failed peristalsis or spasm. It can be broken down into three subtypes: type 1 achalasia is classical achalasia—100% failed peristalsis (distal contractile integral [DCI] <100 mmHg/s/cm) with failure of relaxation of the lower esophageal sphincter on swallowing (IRP >15 mmHg); type 2 has the added feature of increased panesophageal pressures on greater than 20% of swallows; and type 3 has the further added feature of esophageal spastic contractions (DCI >450 mmHg/s/cm) in greater than 20% of swallows. The differentiation of the subtypes is important as different surgical options are more efficacious than others depending on subtype [31].

The pathophysiology and mechanism of achalasia are still debated with several theories. There is some evidence that achalasia may be a consequence of infectious disease with an antecedent viral infection [31, 32] or due to the parasite *Trypanosoma cruzi*, the so-called Chagas disease, which will be highlighted later in this chapter. Otherwise, much of its mechanism is still idiopathic and under investigation. Histologically, there is proliferation of cytotoxic T-lymphocytes [33] and mast cell into the myenteric (Auerbach) plexus with neural loss and inflammation [34]. The aperistaltic segment of esophagus is likely due to failure of normal vagal motor function and dysfunctional cholinergic mechanisms. These alterations take time to develop, accounting for the various subtle symptoms of this disease and sometimes discrepancies in objective test results may explain for its delay in diagnosis [35, 36].

Long-term achalasia without treatment can progress to malnutrition, chronic aspiration, or eventual esophageal carcinoma. The malignant transformation, unlike in Barrett's esophagus with gastrointestinal reflux disease, has a higher prevalence of degeneration into squamous cell carcinoma. The prevalence for squamous cell carcinoma is 26 per 1000 patients—nearly 300-fold absolute risk increase when compared to the general population [37]. The risk for adenocarcinoma, while still elevated, is not nearly as outstanding as squamous cell. Its prevalence is nearly 4 per 1000 cases of achalasia and has an 18-fold increased absolute risk with its predilection potentially from nitrate concentration due to bacterial overgrowth [37]. Patients with at least 10-year history of disease should undergo endoscopic surveillance [37].

It is important to take history from a patient to rule out pseudoachalasia, usually hallmarked by extrinsic compression of the esophagus. Such causes can be a previous gastric fundoplication performed too tightly, a gastric band for weight loss [38], an overtightened LINX reflux management system [39], or dysphagia lusoria—extrinsic compression of an aberrant right subclavian artery [40]. It is not uncommon for those with achalasia to be diagnosed initially as having pseudoachalasia with reflux to and for those patients to undergo fundoplication.

Treatment of achalasia is vast—from pharmacologic management with calcium channel blockers to nitrates to relax the lower esophageal sphincter to endoscopic means to surgical. Treatment should best be individualized to the patient and degree of achalasia with consideration to potential comorbid conditions.

Chagas Disease

Chagas disease is caused by the parasite *Trypanosoma cruzi* and is mostly endemic to South America. The World Health Organization classifies it as a neglected tropic disease and in 2010, nearly six million people were thought to be infected [41]. The effects of Chagas disease is syndromic, causing dysfunction of the heart, viscera, brain, and other organs [41–43]. The exact mechanism of virulence is still under investigation, but is thought to involve over-excitatory effects of T lymphocytes, interferon gamma, tumor necrosis factor, and other cytokines [43]. Elevated levels of M2 acetylcholine muscarinic receptor autoantibodies have been identified at a higher rate compared to idiopathic achalasia—84% vs. 28%—which may play a role in the development of megaesophagus and the loss of Auerbach's and Meissner's plexuses [43].

Diagnosis involves a high index of suspicion when interviewing patients from endemic areas and confirmation using histology, polymerase chain reaction (PCR), and serology antigen assay [41, 42]. All patients with a confirmed diagnosis should have a cardiology consultation, with a minimum of a 12-lead echocardiogram (EKG). Workup of esophageal involvement is the same as other dysmotility disorders and is highlighted above but with the additional cavoite that manometry should be performed even in the setting of a normal esophagram [41]. Exact patterns on high-resolution manometry are currently being investigated and show mixed results. One study of symptomatic patients shows a decrease in esophageal body and lower esophageal sphincter pressure when compared to idiopathic achalasia, which may reflect more the degree of esophageal dilation, which is inversely related to transduced pressures on

HRM [44]. While, on the other hand, additional findings suggest that in the chronic phase of the disease (which can be relatively asymptomatic), there is a relatively hypotonic lower esophageal sphincter and hypertonic upper esophageal sphincter and may not correlate to a patient's degree of symptoms [45].

The risk for carcinoma of the esophagus is significantly higher in areas of the world where Chagas disease is endemic. Prevalence is as high has 56 per 1000 cases of achalasia patients. Mutations of the Fragile Histidine Triad Diadenosine Triphosphatase (FHIT) and tumor protein 53 (TP53) genes as well as abnormalities in chromosomes 7, 11, and 17 may be associated with degeneration to carcinoma [37].

The mainstay of treatment for Chagas disease remains medical with antiparasitic agents, namely benznidazole and nifurtimox [42]. It is paramount to work closely with infectious disease physicians who specialize in tropical diseases. Initial surgical treatment with Chagastic esophagus can be similar to that of idiopathic achalasia. One must be cautious however because some patients with Chagas disease can have an entity of gastroparesis, causing drastic worsening of reflux disease and gastric distension. In such cases, other surgical options such as the Serra-Dória procedure—cardioplasty with partial gastrectomy and Roux-en-Y reconstruction—should be entertained [46, 47]. In cases of megaesophagus an esophagocardioplasty (Fig. 11.7)—Grondhal's cardioplasty [46], or with a gastric patch—modified Thal procedure may be needed [48]. In other cases of end-stage disease, endoscopic mucosal resection [32] or a total esophagectomy may be necessary [47].

Systemic Sclerosis (Scleroderma)

Systemic sclerosis is an autoimmune syndrome with a predilection to females in the fourth through sixth decades of life. The esophagus is the most common gastrointestinal organ involved with the disease, and can occur in up to 90% of patients, 40–80% of whom are symptomatic [49]. At its root, there is fibroblastic and collagen proliferation in cellular tissue, leading to calcifications and sclerosis. A patient's

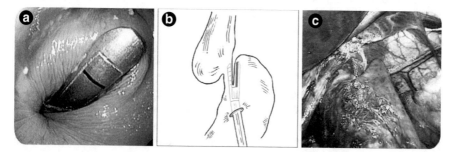

Fig. 11.7 Esophagocardioplasty. (**a**) endoscopic view of bottom jaw of the laparoscopic angled gun into the esophagus, (**b**) optimal positioning of the gastrotomy 4 cm below the gastroesophageal junction, (**c**) laparoscopic view of the stapler placement into the esophagus and fundus simultaneously. (Reproduced with permission from Griffiths et al. [102])

most typical complaint when there is esophageal involvement is gastrointestinal reflux disease and dysphagia [50].

Most diagnostic workup as detailed above reveals a hypotonic lower esophageal sphincter, aperistalsis, dilated esophagus, and acidic esophageal pH [51, 52].

Pharmacotherapy is first line of treatment, and should be managed primarily by a rheumatologist. The objective is to decrease symptoms of reflux and promote esophageal motility, done with a combination of proton pump inhibitors and prokinetic agents such as domperidone and buspirone [49].

Surgical management should be cautioned, especially in the treatment of reflux. Fundoplications alone should be contraindicated due to profound postoperative dysphagia. Other surgical choices such as the Roux-en-Y gastric bypass can be problematic as well if small bowel dysmotility is involved, but it may be the best option [49, 53]. As in Chagas disease, some patients with crippling quality of life may have indication for esophagectomy [54]. Regardless, surgical options should be reserved for patients who are refractory to medical management and for whom symptoms effect quality of life.

Other Spastic Disorders of the Esophagus

Distal esophageal spasm, hypercontractile esophagus, and aperistalsis are additional, but not a complete list of other esophageal motility disorders. High-resolution manometry is used to break down and subclassify this cohort and help to guide treatment [55] (Fig. 11.8).

Absent peristalsis characteristically has lack of esophageal motility with a normal lower esophageal sphincter. Patients with scleroderma will typically have this pattern of manometry and complain of regurgitation and reflux. Patients with long-standing severe gastroesophageal reflux disease (GERD) can also develop this pathology as a result of its ensuing fibrosis. Patients commonly have respiratory complaints such as cough, wheezing, and asthma; they can even progress to a state of pulmonary fibrosis [50]. The Chicago Classification subclassifies this cohort into four types of delayed peristalsis: absent, weak with large or small peristalsis defects, and frequent failed peristalsis. As one may imagine, fundoplication procedures may make this problem exceedingly worse and should be considered in a multidisciplinary fashion if chosen as part of therapy [56].

Hypertensive lower esophageal sphincter or esophagogastric junction outflow obstruction was most recently described by Code in 1960 [57]. Failure to previously identify this disease was probably due to failure to discriminate this pathology from achalasia [58]. Manometry shows an increased resting pressure of the lower esophageal sphincter greater than 15 mmHg but retains its ability to relax. Esophageal peristalsis is usually preserved, but can be diminished—but not to the extent as to meet criteria for achalasia.

Distal esophageal spasm is diagnosed in approximately 4–10% of patients on HRM and is more frequently seen in females and the elderly. This disorder was first proposed by Osgood in the 1880s in people who complained of chest and epigastric

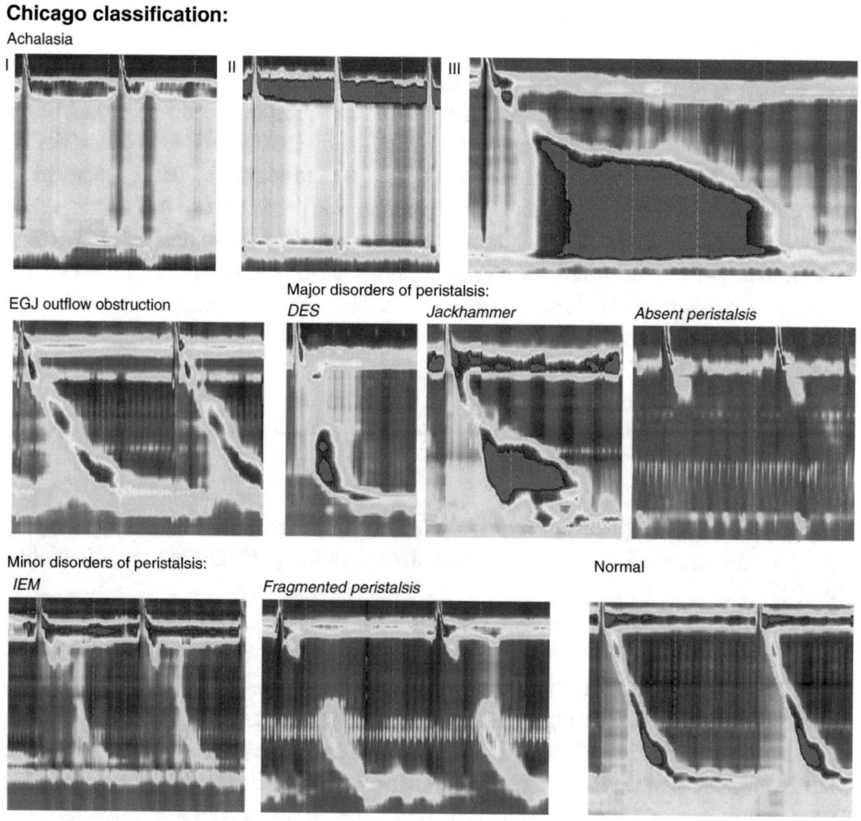

Chicago classification:

Achalasia

Fig. 11.8 Outputs of high-resolution manometry for various motility disorders, including sub-types of achalasia. Horizontal axis shows time, vertical axis shows length along the esophagus, colors from blue to red spectrum demonstrate increasing pressure. (Reproduced with permission from Rohof and Bredenoord [20])

pain with concomitant dysphagia [59]. Barium esophagram may show a "cork-screwing" pattern or pseudodiverticula. Manometry will show esophageal spasm in greater than 20% of swallows, usually in the distal esophagus, with a normal lower esophageal sphincter pressure [20, 60].

Hypercontractile esophagus, colloquially termed Jackhammer esophagus, is defined by greater than 20% of contractions being greater than 8000 mmHg/s/cm [21, 55]. The location of contraction along the esophagus is nonspecific, and can include the lower esophageal sphincter. It is present in 4.1% of patients who undergo manometry [61]. Most patients with this pathology will complain of chest pain and dysphagia.

Like achalasia, therapy is palliative and guided at treating dysphagia chest pain and reflux. Surgical therapy is explored after failure of initial medical and endo-scopic management. Because of the multifocal nature of this nonspecific esopha-geal disorders, balloon dilation and Botox injection have limited roles. Medical and endoscopic therapies are profoundly less efficacious than eventual surgical therapy [11].

There is limited prospective data on surgical options outside of achalasia, but similarly, authors agree on procedures involving myotomy and fundoplication. However, success rates in decreasing dysphagia and GERD are less successful than in achalasia. Furthermore, of considerable note is the length of esophageal myotomy needed in this patient cohort. The hypertrophic musculature and spasm occur along a greater length of the esophagus, and a transabdominal approach may result in a short myotomy. Thoracic approaches then are used to perform a long esophageal myotomy and gastric fundopexy [62–64]. This subset of patient may be benefit greatly from and endoscopic myotomy [65, 66], which will be discussed further later in this chapter.

Pharmacological Treatment

Esophageal motility disorders are not curative diseases. All treatments, whether medical, endoscopic, or surgical, are palliative with the goal of symptom alleviation [67, 68].

The mainstay of nonprocedural management is based on dietary habits and the use of calcium channel blockers and nitrates. The calcium channel blocker nifedipine is taken to relax the smooth muscle of the lower esophageal sphincter by inhibiting calcium reuptake. Resting pressure can be at times lowered by up to 60%. Side effects can occur in up to 30% of patients and could be cause for poor compliance. Mainly patients complain of dizziness, headache, and orthostatic hypotension [22]. These symptoms can be exacerbated if the patient is taking other antihypertensive agents. Nitrates behave similarly, resulting in increased relaxation of the lower esophageal sphincter and the increased passage of food bolus. The subjective patient improvement, however, was limited and full recommendations to clinic practice cannot be made.

Endoscopic Treatment for Achalasia

Endoscopic treatment for achalasia consists mainly of three procedures: Botox injection, pneumonic dilation, and per-oral endoscopic myotomy (POEM). Injection of botulinum toxin A into the lower esophageal sphincter is an attractive and logical treatment option. Unfortunately, its effects are short lived, lasting between 6 and 12 months [36]. Consequently, botulinum toxin causes scaring in the submucosal layers. This results in increased rate of perforation during later surgical myotomy [69, 70]. It is an increasingly controversial approach, and may only be appropriate to those who are unable to undergo general anesthesia and for whom life expectancy may be short [71].

Pneumatic dilation was introduced in the 1970s and 1980s and still is relevant in current treatment. Endoscopic treatment results in perforation with 1–3% of cases, half of which require surgery [72]. This risk increases both with each subsequent dilation and with the use of larger balloon dilators greater than 30 mm on initial dilation [36]. Treatment, however, can be quite robust, with maintained relief of dysphagia of 84% at one month, but may decline to 58% by 3 years [73]. Results may be best in those with type 2 achalasia. Balloon dilation is favored over bougie due to the ability to have direct visualization of the pathology, rather than blindly or with fluoroscopic guidance [74].

Surgical Treatment for Achalasia

Ernest Heller first described his operation in 1914 (on a patient he operated on in 1913) and was in fact different from his namesake procedure. In his original approach, he performed a myotomy both on the anterior and on the posterior esophageal surfaces [8]. The named procedure "Heller myotomy" is more similar to De Bruine Groeneveldt's description in which a single longitudinal anterior esophago-cardiomyotomy was performed, but without a gastric fundoplication. Presently, with the advent of laparoscopy and improvements in surgical technique, this has brought us to a single anterior myotomy with partial fundoplication, known today as a Heller's myotomy—today's gold standard in the United States [70, 75].

The application of a partial fundoplication has since reduced the rate of postoperative reflux from 32% to 8% [73]. Whether an anterior or posterior partial fundoplication is used has been a point of debate in the literature for some time. The majority of patients in literature-based searches has a Dor fundoplication, but this is likely favored based on surgeon preference rather than robust data [76].

Comparison meta-analysis of Heller myotomy and endoscopic balloon dilation favors surgical myotomy in reducing dysphagia, while having similar safety profiles and rates of reflux disease [72, 73]. The Heller myotomy has shown to decrease the rate of chest pain and dysphagia in up to 90% of patients, and depends somewhat on the stage of achalasia and subclassifications based on high-resolution manometry [73]. Perioperative complications and generally minimal and include perforation, wrap dysfunction, and dysphagia. Perforations are reported in approximately 1.6% of cases [70].

Since its advent, robotic surgery has been introduced to the foregut as well. While potentially having ergonomically advantages to the surgeon, outcomes data has not shown robotic-assisted Heller or transthoracic myotomy to be superior to laparoscopic [77, 78]. A recent publication, however, reported a decreased rate of complications with a robotic approached compared to traditional laparoscopic [79].

Peroral Endoscopic Myotomy

POEM is perhaps the champion of the nature orifice surgery movement and continues to gain traction. The procedure was first performed and described in 1980 by Ortega, Madureri, and Perez on a short series of treatments involving six dogs and

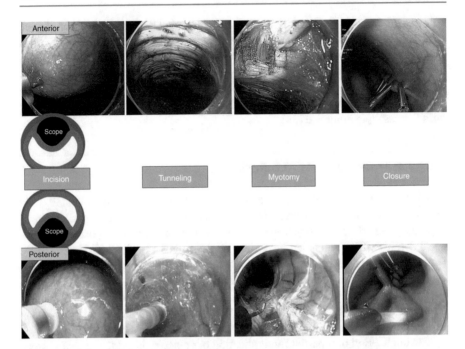

Fig. 11.9 Peroral endoscopic myotomy (POEM) procedure. Anterior POEM is performed in the 12 to 2 o'clock position, whereas posterior POEM is performed in the 5 to 6 o'clock position. Both approaches entail four stages: mucosotomy, submucosal tunneling, myotomy, and mucosal closure. (Reproduced with permission from Khashab et al. [107])

seventeen patients [80]. The technique, however, was abandoned for some time until it was reintroduced by Haruhiro Inoue in 2008 [81]. The procedure entails using a therapeutic gastroscope in which an esophageal submucosal tunnel is made approximately 4 cm proximal to the start of the myotomy and carried down 3–4 cm into the stomach distally. The circular fibers of the lower esophageal sphincter are identified and divided, and the mucosal defect is then closed endoscopically. Creation of the myotomy on the anterior or posterior surfaces of the esophagus seems to have equal efficacy [82] (Fig. 11.9).

Complications are minimal [83] in experienced hand and are limited to bleeding usually manageable with cautery and small perforations that can be controlled with endoclips. Rarely is conversion to laparoscopic/thoracoscopic or open procedures necessary. Obtaining an upper GI series on postoperative day 1 is not necessarily standard and may only be helpful if symptoms concerning for perforation are present such as tachycardia, shortness of breath, and chest or abdominal pain [84].

Inoue and his group's experience of 500 patients from 2008 to 2013 were successful in treating all variants of achalasia including sigmoid esophageal anatomy. They report significant improvement in Eckardt scores out to 3 years [81].

In comparing treatment-naive patients with achalasia, POEM had superior 2-year outcomes than endoscopic balloon dilation [60]. Specifically, 92% of patients who had POEM experienced improvement in dysphagia, compared to only 54% in the balloon dilation group. However, rates of reflux were higher in the POEM group—41% compared to 7%.

The use of POEM is gaining traction as for nonspecific esophageal motility disorders. The principle of an extended or long myotomy is well suited for POEM, since a submucosal tunnel can be easily initiated anywhere on the esophageal body and tailored towards manometric results. The use of a long myotomy, as advocated for in type III achalasia, can be accomplished nicely with POEM as shown in a recent series to have better success in this achalasia subtype when compared to Heller myotomy—98% vs. 80.8% success rate [13]. The success of POEM for type III achalasia, diffuse esophageal spasm, and jackhammer esophagus may be on the order of 92%, 88%, and 72%, respectively [65]. The decreased rate of success in jackhammer esophagus may be of a technical error if the lower esophageal sphincter is not included in the myotomy [85].

Recent reports demonstrate that POEM is more effective than Heller myotomy in relieving short-term dysphagia [86]. However, this does come at a price of increased levels of gastrointestinal reflux disease and asymptomatic esophagitis, which also increases in rate the further into the postoperative period the patient is [81, 86–88]. This result is not surprising as POEM is done without performing fundoplication [35]. These findings of increased GERD in patients who undergo POEM as compared to Heller myotomy are also seen on postoperative pH monitoring [86]. Interestingly, body mass index may not be a risk factor in the development of postoperative reflux in the POEM patient [89]. However, this may suggest that POEM can predispose a patient to the Barrett's metaplasia-dysplasia-carcinoma pathway. But until longer follow-up is established with POEM, this is still speculation. POEM has not been showed to be a carcinogenic procedure at this time.

Presently, POEM is still a highly specialized procedure and is not offered at all specialty centers. Most general surgery residents and many fellows who train in minimally invasive surgery are not exposed to this procedure. Thus, many who do POEM, learned the technique after their formal graduate medical education. It takes approximately 15–20 procedures, with appropriate faculty supervision to become facile and independent in POEM [35, 90].

Recurrent Dysphagia

Success of surgery is usually defined as postoperative Eckardt scores of less than 3 [12, 65, 91]. Surgical intervention for dysphagia is typically a robust intervention with lasting long-term results. There is, however, a small subset of patients who fail surgical intervention and have recurrent dysphagia. Preoperative predictors of failure may include higher Eckardt scores (≥9) and achalasia subset type III [91, 92]. POEM has a potential dysphagia recurrence rate of 10%, while laparoscopic myotomy is reported between 3.5% and 15%.

Reasons for recurrent dysphagia are multifactorial. Eventual failure of the Heller myotomy or recurrence of symptoms is due to incomplete myotomy (33%), myotomy fibrosis (27%), fundoplication disruption (13%), tight fundoplication (7%), or some combination of two (20%) [93]. Other lesser, but still possible, reasons for failure include overtightening of crural closure (if performed), peptic stricture, carcinoma, and even incorrect index diagnosis [94]. It can be easy to confuse gastroparesis, either undiagnosed or iatrogenic, from vagal nerve injury, as a possible cause of recurrence, as these patients will present with emesis and bloating with or without dysphagia.

Eckardt scores can be followed in patients to track their subjective complaints. As with following patients with reflux, it is important to correlate their subjective complaints with objective data [95]. Workup of recurrent dysphagia should be meticulous and mirror that of primary dysphagia [75, 94]. Again it starts with an upper GI contrast study. Evidence of the classic "bird's beak" appearance can be seen. HRM can often be misleading and unhelpful for a previously operated patient. Endoscopy can be both diagnostic and therapeutic. Pneumatic dilation, at times up to 40 mm, is typically the first intervention performed and its rate of success has been reported between 50% and 70% [96, 97]. Cross-sectional imaging, while not mandatory, can be helpful in defining anatomy and may provide insight to the etiology of what is provoking the recurrent dysphagia.

Unfortunately, some patients do not respond to repeat dilations, and their pathology can be lifestyle crippling. Many patients undergo repeat surgical intervention, such as redo Heller myotomy or POEM and therapy is usually successful [98–100]. Procedure selection is challenging and should be tailored to the patient. Redo myotomy is typically more difficult, as shown by increased rates of esophageal perforation, reported between 13% and 33% [98–100]. Presently, with more and more centers and surgeons becoming proficient in POEM, success rates on patients needing redo procedures approach that of primary POEM [99]. Importantly, when planning redo interventions, a previous primary Heller myotomy does not preclude a patient from having a secondary POEM, and vice versa [12].

Repeated recurrence despite persistent therapy usually leads to esophagectomy. Several salvage procedures, while are seldomly performed, do exist. Some surgeons and centers have experience with advanced techniques such as the modified Thal procedure, Serra-Dória operation [78, 95, 101, 102]. A newly published limited series describes resection of the dysfunctional gastroesophageal junction with esophagojejunostomy, using a Roux limb taken 30 cm from the ligament of Trietz and anastomosis of the in situ gastric remnant with biliopancreatic limb 60 cm down the Roux limb [103]. (insert pictures of operative anatomy).

Total Esophagectomy

Esophagectomy, while controversial, may be necessary for patients with end-stage disease of achalasia and dysmotility disorders [68]. Up to 5% of patients with disease, particularly achalasia, will undergo esophagectomy, most of them having previous endoscopic and myotomy procedures [1, 104]. Indications for total esophagectomy involve symptomatic features of end-stage disease, which are refractory to previous medical and surgical management. Such features include sigmoid esophagus >6 cm (the so-called dolicho-megaesophagus), disabling gastric reflux disease and dysphagia, malnutrition, recurrent aspiration pneumonia, airway compromise from extrinsic compression, recurrent bleeding, stricture, underlaying cancer, and if part of clinical trials [54, 67, 104].

Some authors report increased rates of bleeding, especially when a transhiatal approach is used, due to dense mediastinal adhesions from the chronic inflammatory state of the disease and previous procedures [105]. Laryngeal nerve anatomy and its displacement must be taken into account as well [68]. While most procedures are performed transthoracic as compared to transhiatal (73.9% vs. 26.1%) [1], both are acceptable and safe, especially since surgeons have become more experienced with minimally invasive and robotic approaches.

Esophagectomy has generally been tolerated well, especially at centers of excellence. Study of the Nationwide Inpatient Sample from 2000 to 2010 in comparing esophagectomy for achalasia compared to cancer showed decreased rates of mortality (3% vs. 8%) and postoperative complications were linked more to preoperative nutrition status rather than indication for surgery [67]. Pneumonia (15%) and anastomotic leak (7%) are the two most significant complications [1].

The choice of conduit for reconstruction is still of some debate. However, most surgeons and authors advocate for gastric interposition as first line conduit when available and is most used (95%), followed by colon and then small bowel [1, 54, 68, 104]. This is generally due to the robust vascular supply of the stomach and the need only for a single anastomosis when used.

Quality of life improves for the vast majority of discharged patients (75–100%) [1], with approximately 20–30% require further dilation due to anastomotic stricture and 20% complaining of dumping syndrome. Nearly all patients are able to normalize nutritional parameters and gain weight [104].

Conclusion

Esophageal motility disorders are a complicated pathology. Importantly, providers must be vigilant with a patient's preoperative workup. Obtaining all objective data possible and identifying the nuances are paramount, allowing a standardized, yet tailored approach to each patient. For achalasia, laparoscopic Heller myotomy remains the gold standard. However, for other pathologies such as nonspecific spastic disorder, achalasia type 3, and recurrent dysphagia after Heller myotomy, POEM continues to gain traction and more data on long-term outcomes are being published annually and is considered by some to be the procedure of choice.

Glossary
- Achalasia
- Adenocarcinoma
- Barrett's esophagus
- Chagas disease
- Chicago classification

- Distal esophageal spasm
- Dysphagia
- Dysphagia lusoria
- Eckardt score
- Edwin Smith Papyrus
- Ernst Heller
- Esophagectomy
- Esophagogastroduodenoscopy
- Gastroesophageal reflux disease
- Gastroparesis
- Haruhiro Inoue
- Heller myotomy
- High-resolution manometry
- Hypercontractile esophagus
- Jackhammer esophagus
- Modified Thal procedure
- Pinstripe pattern
- Pneumatic dilation
- Por oral endoscopy myotomy
- Pseudoachalasia
- Roux en Y gastric bypass
- Rezende classification
- Scleroderma
- Serra-Dória procedure
- Squamous cell carcinoma
- Thomas Willis
- Trypanosoma Cruzii
- Upper GI fluoroscopy

References

1. Aiolfi A, Asti E, Bonitta G, Siboni S, Bonavina L. Esophageal resection for end-stage achalasia. Am Surg. 2018;84(4):506–11.
2. Eslick GD. Esophageal cancer: a historical perspective. Gastroenterol Clin N Am. 2009;38(1):1–15. https://doi.org/10.1016/j.gtc.2009.01.003.
3. Breasted JH. The Edwin Smith Surgical Papyrus, no. Vol. 1, xxiv+596 pages, 8 plates. Chicago: The University of Chicago Press; 1930.
4. Karamanou M, Markatos K, Papaioannou TG, Zografos G, Androutsos G. Hallmarks in history of esophageal carcinoma. J BUON. 2017;22(4):1088–91.
5. Brewer LA. History of surgery of the esophagus. Am J Surg. 1980;139(6):730–43. https://doi.org/10.1016/0002-9610(80)90375-X.
6. Willis ST. Pharmaceutice Rationalis sive Diatriba do Medicamentorum Oerationibus in Humano Corpore. London: Hagae Comitis; 1674.
7. Heyrovsky H. Idiopathic dilation of the esophagus. In: Hare HA, Martin E, editors. The Therapeutic gazette. vol. 37, no. 3. Detroit: E.G. Swift; 1913. p. 746–7.
8. Andreollo NA, Lopes LR, Malafaia O. Heller's myotomy: a hundred years of success! Arq Bras Cir Dig. 2014;27(1):1–2.
9. Mittal S. Achalasia – A SAGES Wiki Article. 2008:1–6.
10. Hamer PW, Lamb PJ. The management of achalasia and other motility disorders of the oesophagus. In: Griffin SM, Lamb PJ, editors. Oesophagogastric surgery: a companion to specialist surgical practice. 6th ed. Philadelphia: Elsevier; 2019. p. 251–60.

11. Vaezi MF, Ph D, Richter JE. Diagnosis and management of achalasia. Am J Gastroenterol. 1999;94(12):3406–12. https://doi.org/10.1111/j.1572-0241.1999.01639.x.
12. van Hoeij FB, et al. Management of recurrent symptoms after per-oral endoscopic myotomy in achalasia. Gastrointest Endosc. 2018;87(1):95–101. https://doi.org/10.1016/j.gie.2017.04.036.
13. Kumbhari V, et al. Peroral endoscopic myotomy (POEM) vs laparoscopic Heller myotomy (LHM) for the treatment of Type III achalasia in 75 patients: a multicenter comparative study. Endosc Int Open. 2015;3(03):E195–201. https://doi.org/10.1055/s-0034-1391668.
14. Shemmeri E, Aye RW, Farivar AS, Bograd AJ, Louie BE. Use of a report card to evaluate outcomes of achalasia surgery: beyond the Eckardt score. Surg Endosc. 2019;34(4):1856–62. https://doi.org/10.1007/s00464-019-06952-2.
15. Gockel I, Junginger T. The value of scoring achalasia: a comparison of current systems and and the impact on treatment--the Surgeon's viewpoint. Am Surg. 2007;73(4):327–31.
16. Amiraian DE, DiSantis DJ. The esophageal bird's beak sign. Abdom Radiol. 2017;42(5):1608–9. https://doi.org/10.1007/s00261-016-1028-9.
17. Teles Filho RV, De Azevêdo LHS, De Matos Abe G. 35 years of the classification of rezende: the importance of esophagogram in the context of Chagas disease in Brazil. Arq Gastroenterol. 2019;56(1):106–7. https://doi.org/10.1590/s0004-2803.201900000-05.
18. Matsubara H, et al. Descriptive rules for achalasia of the esophagus, June 2012: 4th edition. Esophagus. 2017;14(4):275–89. https://doi.org/10.1007/s10388-017-0589-1.
19. Minami H, et al. New endoscopic indicator of esophageal achalasia: 'pinstripe pattern. PLoS One. 2015;10(2):1–10. https://doi.org/10.1371/journal.pone.0101833.
20. Rohof WOA, Bredenoord AJ. Chicago classification of esophageal motility disorders: lessons learned. Curr Gastroenterol Rep. 2017;19(8):37. https://doi.org/10.1007/s11894-017-0576-7.
21. Kahrilas PJ, et al. The Chicago classification of esophageal motility disorders, v3.0. Neurogastroenterol Motil. 2015;27(2):160–74. https://doi.org/10.1111/nmo.12477.
22. Chuah SK, et al. Bridging the gap between advancements in the evolution of diagnosis and treatment towards better outcomes in achalasia. Biomed Res Int. 2019;2019:8549187. https://doi.org/10.1155/2019/8549187.
23. Triantafyllou T, et al. Long-term outcome of myotomy and fundoplication based on intra-operative real-time high-resolution manometry in achalasia patients. Ann Gastroenterol. 2019;32(1):46–51. https://doi.org/10.20524/aog.2018.0326.
24. George NS, et al. Distribution of esophageal motor disorders in diabetic patients with dysphagia. J Clin Gastroenterol. 2017;51(10):890–5. https://doi.org/10.1097/MCG.0000000000000894.
25. Shiroky J, Jimenez Cantisano BG, Schneider A. Esophageal motility disorders after bariatric surgery. Dysphagia. 2013;28(3):455–6. https://doi.org/10.1007/s00455-013-9475-8.
26. Weiss AH, Iorio N, Schey R. Esophageal motility in eosinophilic esophagitis. Rev Gastroenterol Mex (Engl Ed). 2015;80(3):205–13. https://doi.org/10.1016/j.rgmxen.2015.05.002.
27. Côté-Daigneault J, Poitras P, Rabasa-Lhoret R, Bouin M. Plasma leptin concentrations and esophageal hypomotility in obese patients. Can J Gastroenterol Hepatol. 2015;29(1):49–51. https://doi.org/10.1155/2015/490818.
28. Tolone S, Savarino E, Yates RB. The impact of bariatric surgery on esophageal function. Ann N Y Acad Sci. 2016;1381(1):98–103. https://doi.org/10.1111/nyas.13107.
29. Mayberry J. Epidemiology and demographics of achalasia. Gastrointest Endosc Clin N Am. 2001;11(2):235–48.
30. Sonnenberg A. Hospitalization for achalasia in the United States 1997 – 2006. Dig Dis Sci. 2009;54(8):1680–5. https://doi.org/10.1007/s10620-009-0863-8.
31. Rohof WO, et al. Outcomes of treatment for achalasia depend on manometric subtype. Gastroenterology. 2013;144(4):718–25. https://doi.org/10.1053/j.gastro.2012.12.027.
32. de Aquino JLB, Said MM, Pereira DR, do Amaral PC, Lima JCA, Leandro-Merhi VA. Surgical treatment analysis of idiopathic esophageal achalasia. Arq Bras Cir Dig. 2015;28(2):98–101. https://doi.org/10.1590/S0102-67202015000200003.

33. Villanacci V, et al. An immunohistochemical study of the myenteric plexus in idiopathic achalasia. J Clin Gastroenterol. 2010;44(6):407–10. https://doi.org/10.1097/MCG.0b013e3181bc9ebf.

34. Goldblum JR, Whyte RI, Orringer MB, Appelman HD. Achalasia: a morphologic study of 42 resected specimens. Am J Surg Pathol. 1994;18(4):327–37.

35. Kahrilas PJ, Katzka D, Richter JE. Clinical practice update: the use of per-oral endoscopic myotomy in achalasia: expert review and best practice advice from the AGA Institute. Gastroenterology. 2017;153(5):1205–11. https://doi.org/10.1053/j.gastro.2017.10.001.

36. Esposito D, Maione F, D'Alessandro A, Sarnelli G, De Palma GD. Endoscopic treatment of esophageal achalasia. World J Gastrointest Endosc. 2016;8(2):30–9. https://doi.org/10.4253/wjge.v8.i2.30.

37. Tustumi F, et al. Esophageal achalasia: a risk factor for carcinoma. A systematic review and meta-analysis. Dis Esophagus. 2017;30(10):1–8. https://doi.org/10.1093/dote/dox072.

38. Le Page PA, Kwon S, Lord SJ, Lord RV. Esophageal dysmotility after laparoscopic gastric band surgery. Obes Surg. 2014;24(4):625–30. https://doi.org/10.1007/s11695-013-1134-5.

39. Skubleny D, et al. LINX® magnetic esophageal sphincter augmentation versus Nissen fundoplication for gastroesophageal reflux disease: a systematic review and meta-analysis. Surg Endosc. 2017;31(8):3078–84. https://doi.org/10.1007/s00464-016-5370-3.

40. Levitt B, Richter JE. Dysphagia lusoria: a comprehensive review. Dis Esophagus. 2007;20(6):455–60. https://doi.org/10.1111/j.1442-2050.2007.00787.x.

41. Pérez-Molina JA, Molina I. Chagas disease. Lancet. 2018;391(10115):82–94. https://doi.org/10.1016/S0140-6736(17)31612-4.

42. Bern C. Chagas' disease. N Engl J Med. 2015;373(5):456–66. https://doi.org/10.1056/NEJMra1410150.

43. Bilder CR, Goin JC. Gastrointestinal involvement in Chagas disease. NeuroGastroLATAM Rev. 2018;1(4):168–79. https://doi.org/10.24875/ngl.17000002.

44. Vicentine FPP, Herbella FAM, Allaix ME, Silva LC, Patti MG. Comparison of idiopathic achalasia and Chagas' disease esophagopathy at the light of high-resolution manometry. Dis Esophagus. 2014;27(2):128–33. https://doi.org/10.1111/dote.12098.

45. Sánchez-Montalvá A, et al. High resolution esophageal manometry in patients with Chagas disease: a cross-sectional evaluation. PLoS Negl Trop Dis. 2016;10(2):1–11. https://doi.org/10.1371/journal.pntd.0004416.

46. Ponciano H, Cecconello I, Alves L, Ferreira BD, Gama-Rodrigues J. Cardioplasty and Roux-en-Y partial gastrectomy (Serra-Dória procedure) for reoperation of achalasia. Arq Gastroenterol. 2004;41(3):155–61. https://doi.org/10.1590/s0004-28032004000300004.

47. de Oliveira GC, da Rocha RLB, Coelho-Neto J d S, Terciotti-Junior V, Lopes LR, Andreollo NA. Esophageal mucosal resection versus esophagectomy: a comparative study of surgical results in patients with advanced megaesophagus. Arq Bras Cir Dig. 2015;28(1):28–31. https://doi.org/10.1590/S0102-67202015000100008.

48. Alves APR, De Oliveira PG, De Oliveira JM, De Mesquita DM, Dos Santos JHZ. Long-term results of the modified thal procedure in patients with chagasic megaesophagus. World J Surg. 2014;38(6):1425–30. https://doi.org/10.1007/s00268-013-2445-3.

49. Denaxas K, Ladas SD, Karamanolis GP. Evaluation and management of esophageal manifestations in systemic sclerosis. Ann Gastroenterol. 2018;31(2):165–70. https://doi.org/10.20524/aog.2018.0228.

50. Denton CP, Khanna D. Systemic sclerosis. Lancet. 2017;390(10103):1685–99. https://doi.org/10.1016/S0140-6736(17)30933-9.

51. Weston S, Thumshirn M, Wiste J, Camilleri M. Clinical and upper gastrointestinal motility features in systemic sclerosis and related disorders. Am J Gastroenterol. 1998;93(7):1085–9. https://doi.org/10.1111/j.1572-0241.1998.00334.x.

52. Aggarwal N, Lopez R, Gabbard S, Wadhwa N, Devaki P, Thota PN. Spectrum of esophageal dysmotility in systemic sclerosis on high-resolution esophageal manometry as defined by Chicago classification. Dis Esophagus. 2017;30(12):1–6. https://doi.org/10.1093/dote/dox067.

53. Kent MS, et al. Comparison of surgical approaches to recalcitrant gastroesophageal reflux disease in the patient with scleroderma. Ann Thorac Surg. 2007;84(5):1710–6. https://doi.org/10.1016/j.athoracsur.2007.06.025.
54. Mormando J, Barbetta A, Molena D. Esophagectomy for benign disease. J Thorac Dis. 2018;10(3):2026–33. https://doi.org/10.21037/jtd.2018.01.165.
55. Schlottmann F, Patti MG. Primary esophageal motility disorders: beyond achalasia. Int J Mol Sci. 2017;18(7):1399. https://doi.org/10.3390/ijms18071399.
56. Bakhos CT, Petrov RV, Parkman HP, Malik Z, Abbas AE. Role and safety of fundoplication in esophageal disease and dysmotility syndromes. J Thorac Dis. 2019;11(4):S1610–7. https://doi.org/10.21037/jtd.2019.06.62.
57. Code CF, Schlegel JF, Kelley ML, Olsen AM, Ellis FH. Hypertensive gastroesophageal sphincter. Mayo Clin Proc. 1960;35:391–9, PMID 13810841.
58. Howell M, Moran-Atkin E. Motility disorders of esophagus and surgical interventions. In: Carrau RL, Murry T, Howell RJ, editors. Comprehensive management of swallowing disorders. 2nd ed. San Diego: Plural Publishing; 2016.
59. Osgood H. œsophagismus, oesophagus. Bost Med Surg J. 1889;120:401–5. https://doi.org/10.1056/NEJM188904251201701.
60. Ponds FA, et al. Effect of peroral endoscopic myotomy vs pneumatic dilation on symptom severity and treatment outcomes among treatment-naive patients with achalasia: a randomized clinical trial. JAMA. 2019;322(2):134–44. https://doi.org/10.1001/jama.2019.8859.
61. Roman S, Tutuian R. Esophageal hypertensive peristaltic disorders. Neurogastroenterol Motil. 2012;24(Suppl 1):32–9. https://doi.org/10.1111/j.1365-2982.2011.01837.x.
62. Inose T, et al. Surgical treatment for nonspecific esophageal motility disorders. Surg Today. 2013;43(8):877–82. https://doi.org/10.1007/s00595-012-0356-9.
63. Nomura T, et al. Thoracoscopic long myotomy in the prone position to treat rapid esophageal contractions with normal latency. J Clin Gastroenterol. 2015;49(4):320–2. https://doi.org/10.1097/MCG.0000000000000123.
64. Nomura T, Iwakiri K, Uchida E. Thoracoscopic treatment of a patient with jackhammer esophagus. Dig Endosc. 2014;26(6):753–4. https://doi.org/10.1111/den.12339.
65. Khan MA, et al. Is POEM the answer for management of spastic esophageal disorders? A systematic review and meta-analysis. Dig Dis Sci. 2017;62(1):35–44. https://doi.org/10.1007/s10620-016-4373-1.
66. Dawod E, Saumoy M, Xu MM, Kahaleh M. Peroral endoscopic myotomy (POEM) in jackhammer esophagus: a trick of the trade. Endoscopy. 2017;49(10):E254–5. https://doi.org/10.1055/s-0043-115887.
67. Molena D, Mungo B, Stem M, Feinberg RL, Lidor AO. Outcomes of esophagectomy for esophageal achalasia in the United States. J Gastrointest Surg. 2014;18(2):310–7. https://doi.org/10.1007/s11605-013-2318-y.
68. Molena D, Yang SC. Surgical management of end-stage achalasia. Semin Thorac Cardiovasc Surg. 2012;24(1):19–26. https://doi.org/10.1053/j.semtcvs.2012.01.015.
69. Patti MG, et al. Effects of previous treatment on results of laparoscopic Heller myotomy for achalasia. Dig Dis Sci. 1999;44(11):2270–6. https://doi.org/10.1023/A:1026660921776.
70. Stefanidis D, Richardson W, Farrell T, Kohn G, Augenstein V, Fanelli R. Guidelines for the surgical treatment of esophageal corresponding author: Dimitrios Stefanidis. Surg Endosc. 2012;26(2):296–311. https://doi.org/10.1007/s00464-011-2017-2.
71. Simchuk EJ, Alderson D. Oesophageal surgery. World J Gastroenterol. 2001;7(6):760–5. https://doi.org/10.3748/wjg.v7.i6.760.
72. Illés A, et al. Is heller myotomy better than balloon dilation? A meta-analysis. J Gastrointestin Liver Dis. 2017;26(2):121–7. https://doi.org/10.15403/jgld.2014.1121.262.myo.
73. Campos GM, et al. Endoscopic and surgical treatments for achalasia: a systematic review and meta-analysis. Ann Surg. 2009;249(1):45–57. https://doi.org/10.1097/SLA.0b013e31818e43ab.

74. Josino IR, et al. Endoscopic dilation with bougies versus balloon dilation in esophageal benign strictures: systematic review and meta-analysis. Gastroenterol Res Pract. 2018;2018:5874870. https://doi.org/10.1155/2018/5874870.
75. DeMeester SR. Per-oral endoscopic myotomy for achalasia. J Thorac Dis. 2017;9(Suppl 2):S130–4. https://doi.org/10.21037/jtd.2016.09.39.
76. Rebecchi F, Allaix ME, Schlottmann F, Patti MG, Morino M. Laparoscopic Heller myotomy and fundoplication: what is the evidence? Am Surg. 2018;84(4):481–8.
77. Kim SS, Guillen-Rodriguez J, Little AG. Optimal surgical intervention for achalasia: laparoscopic or robotic approach. J Robot Surg. 2019;13(3):397–400. https://doi.org/10.1007/s11701-018-0865-7.
78. Zilberstein B, Franciss MY, Genovesi A, Volpe P, Domene CE, Barchi LC. Pioneer robotic Serra-Doria operation for recurrent achalasia after Heller's Cardiomyotomy: a 'new quondam' procedure. J Laparoendosc Adv Surg Tech A. 2017;27(5):524–8. https://doi.org/10.1089/lap.2017.0076.
79. Ali AB, et al. Robotic and per-oral endoscopic myotomy have fewer technical complications compared to laparoscopic Heller myotomy. Surg Endosc. 2020;34(7):3191–6. https://doi.org/10.1007/s00464-019-07093-2.
80. Ortega JA, Madureri V, Perez L. Endoscopic myotomy in the treatment of achalasia. Gastrointest Endosc. 1980;26(1):8–10. https://doi.org/10.1016/S0016-5107(80)73249-2.
81. Inoue H, et al. Per-oral endoscopic myotomy: a series of 500 patients. J Am Coll Surg. 2015;221(2):256–64. https://doi.org/10.1016/j.jamcollsurg.2015.03.057.
82. Khashab MA, et al. Peroral endoscopic myotomy: anterior versus posterior approach: a randomized single-blinded clinical trial. Gastrointest Endosc. 2020;91(2):288–97.e7. https://doi.org/10.1016/j.gie.2019.07.034.
83. Haito-Chavez Y, et al. Comprehensive analysis of adverse events associated with per oral endoscopic myotomy in 1826 patients: an international multicenter study. Am J Gastroenterol. 2017;112(8):1267–76. https://doi.org/10.1038/ajg.2017.139.
84. El Khoury R, et al. Evaluation of the need for routine esophagram after peroral endoscopic myotomy (POEM). Surg Endosc. 2016;30(7):2969–74. https://doi.org/10.1007/s00464-015-4585-z.
85. Bechara R, Ikeda H, Inoue H. Peroral endoscopic myotomy for Jackhammer esophagus: to cut or not to cut the lower esophageal sphincter. Endosc Int Open. 2016;04(05):E585–8. https://doi.org/10.1055/s-0042-105204.
86. Schlottmann F, Luckett DJ, Fine J, Shaheen NJ, Patti MG. Laparoscopic Heller myotomy versus peroral endoscopic myotomy (POEM) for achalasia: a systematic review and meta-analysis. Ann Surg. 2018;267(3):451–60. https://doi.org/10.1097/SLA.0000000000002311.
87. Repici A, et al. GERD after per-oral endoscopic myotomy as compared with Heller's myotomy with fundoplication: a systematic review with meta-analysis. Gastrointest Endosc. 2018;87(4):934–43.e18. https://doi.org/10.1016/j.gie.2017.10.022.
88. Swanstrom LL, Kurian A, Dunst CM, Sharata A, Bhayani N, Rieder E. Long-term outcomes of an endoscopic myotomy for achalasia: the POEM procedure. Ann Surg. 2012;256(4):659–67. https://doi.org/10.1097/SLA.0b013e31826b5212.
89. Sanaka MR, et al. Obesity does not impact outcomes or rates of gastroesophageal reflux after peroral endoscopic myotomy in achalasia. J Clin Gastroenterol. 2019;00(00):1–6. https://doi.org/10.1097/MCG.0000000000001235.
90. Hungness ES, Sternbach JM, Teitelbaum EN, Kahrilas PJ, Pandolfino JE, Soper NJ. Peroral endoscopic myotomy (POEM) after the learning curve: durable long-term results with a low complication rate. Ann Surg. 2016;264(3):508–15. https://doi.org/10.1097/SLA.0000000000001870.
91. Shea GE, et al. Long-term dysphagia resolution following POEM versus Heller myotomy for achalasia patients. Surg Endosc. 2020;34(4):1704–11. https://doi.org/10.1007/s00464-019-06948-y.

92. Ren Y, et al. Pre-treatment Eckardt score is a simple factor for predicting one-year peroral endoscopic myotomy failure in patients with achalasia. Surg Endosc. 2017;31(8):3234–41. https://doi.org/10.1007/s00464-016-5352-5.
93. Iqbal A, et al. Laparoscopic re-operation for failed Heller myotomy. Dis Esophagus. 2006;19(3):193–9. https://doi.org/10.1111/j.1442-2050.2006.00564.x.
94. Weche M, Saad AR, Richter JE, Jacobs JJ, Velanovich V. Revisional procedures for recurrent symptoms after Heller myotomy and per-oral endoscopic myotomy. J Laparoendosc Adv Surg Tech A. 2020;30(2):1–7. https://doi.org/10.1089/lap.2019.0277.
95. Galvani C, et al. Symptoms are a poor indicator of reflux status after fundoplication for gastroesophageal reflux disease: role of esophageal functions tests. Arch Surg. 2003;138(5):514–9. https://doi.org/10.1001/archsurg.138.5.514.
96. Amani M, Fazlollahi N, Shirani S, Malekzadeh R, Mikaeli J. Assessment of pneumatic balloon dilation in patients with symptomatic relapse after failed Heller myotomy: a single center experience. Middle East J Dig Dis. 2015;8(1):57–62. https://doi.org/10.15171/mejdd.2016.08.
97. Saleh CMG, Ponds FAM, Schijven MP, Smout AJPM, Bredenoord AJ. Efficacy of pneumodilation in achalasia after failed Heller myotomy. Neurogastroenterol Motil. 2016;28(11):1741–6. https://doi.org/10.1111/nmo.12875.
98. Fumagalli U, et al. Repeated surgical or endoscopic myotomy for recurrent dysphagia in patients after previous myotomy for achalasia. J Gastrointest Surg. 2016;20(3):494–9. https://doi.org/10.1007/s11605-015-3031-9.
99. Orenstein SB, et al. Peroral endoscopic myotomy (POEM) leads to similar results in patients with and without prior endoscopic or surgical therapy. Surg Endosc. 2015;29(5):1064–70. https://doi.org/10.1007/s00464-014-3782-5.
100. James DRC, et al. The feasibility, safety and outcomes of laparoscopic re-operation for achalasia. Minim Invasive Ther Allied Technol. 2012;21(3):161–7. https://doi.org/10.3109/13645706.2011.588798.
101. de Aquino JLB, Said MM, Leandro-Merhi VA, Ramos JPZ, Ichinoche L, Guimarães DM. Esophagocardioplasty as surgical treatment in relapsed non advanced megaesophagus. Arq Bras Cir Dig. 2012;25(1):20–4. https://doi.org/10.1590/S0102-67202012000100005.
102. Griffiths EA, Devitt PG, Jamieson GG, Myers JC, Thompson SK. Laparoscopic stapled cardioplasty for end-stage achalasia. J Gastrointest Surg. 2013;17(5):997–1001. https://doi.org/10.1007/s11605-012-2111-3.
103. Ithurralde-Argerich J, Cuenca-Abente F, Faerberg A, Rosner L, Duque-Seguro C, Ferro D. Resection of the gastroesophageal junction and Roux-en-Y reconstruction as a new alternative for the treatment of recurrent achalasia: outcomes in a short series of patients. J Laparoendosc Adv Surg Tech A. 2020;30(2):1–6. https://doi.org/10.1089/lap.2019.0300.
104. Aiolfi A, Asti E, Bonitta G, Bonavina L. Esophagectomy for end-stage achalasia: systematic review and meta-analysis. World J Surg. 2018;42(5):1469–76. https://doi.org/10.1007/s00268-017-4298-7.
105. Miller DL, Allen MS, Trastek VF, Deschamps C, Pairolero PC. Esophageal resection for recurrent achalasia. Ann Thorac Surg. 1995;60(4):922–6. https://doi.org/10.1016/0003-4975(95)00522-M.
106. Farrokhi F, Vaezi MF. Idiopathic (primary) achalasia. Orphanet J Rare Dis. 2007;2:38.
107. Khashab MA, et al. Peroral endoscopic myotomy anterior versus posterior approach: a randomized single-blinded clinical trial. Gastrointest Endosc. 2020;91(2):288–97.e7. https://doi.org/10.1016/j.gie.2019.07.034.

The Endoscopic Treatment of Esophageal Motility Disorders

12

Vitor Ottoboni Brunaldi and Manoel Galvao Neto

Introduction

Esophageal dysmotility disorders include several benign diseases of the esophagus that impair adequate conduction of the food bolus to the stomach. Esophageal food transport may be didactically divided into four phases. The first phase is the accommodation—when the esophagus receives and accepts the bolus from the oropharynx. The second phase is the compartmentalization—when medullary programmed peristalsis of the proximal esophagus leads the bolus into the distal esophagus. The third phase is the esophageal emptying—when the bolus is expelled from the esophagus and into the stomach that is mainly mediated by post-transition zone myenteric plexus programmed peristalsis. The final phase is the ampullary emptying—when the lower esophageal sphincter (LES) returns to its preperistaltic state, that is closed, shortened, and intrahiatal [1]. Abnormalities in any of the aforementioned phases may elicit symptoms.

High-resolution manometry (HRM) findings were recently standardized by the Chicago Classification that restructured the classification of the esophageal motility disorders. It has gained broad acceptance worldwide while it divides disorders into major (achalasia, esophagogastric junction [EGJ] obstruction, distal esophageal spasm, jackhammer esophagus, absent contractility, end-stage achalasia) and minor ones (ineffective esophageal motility and fragmented peristalsis). The HRM is based on three key metrics: the integrated relaxation pressure (IRP), the distal contractile integral (DCI), and the distal latency (DL) [2]. The combination of different

V. O. Brunaldi (✉)
Gastrointestinal Endoscopy Unit, Gastroenterology Department,
University of São Paulo Medical School, Sao Paulo, Brazil
e-mail: vitor.brunaldi@usp.br

M. Galvao Neto
Surgery Department, ABC University, Sao Paolo, Brazil

abnormalities in those three topographic metrics is indicative of specific motility disorders [3].

Achalasia is the main esophageal dysmotility disorder characterized by degeneration of the inhibitory myenteric ganglion cells of the esophagus [4]. Its central condition is impaired LES relaxation. The HRM helps to identify three types of achalasia based on the other pressure parameters: type I, no esophageal peristalsis; type II, pan-esophageal pressurization; and type III, premature spastic distal contractions. Furthermore, preservation of the peristalsis in the context of an impaired LES relaxation suggests a fourth phenotypic diagnosis: outlet obstruction such as postoperative pseudoachalasia [5]. That is particularly important since the best therapeutic approach and response to treatment may differ according to the subtype of achalasia [6].

It is a rare disease with an incidence of around 1.6 per 100,000 and prevalence around 10.8 per 100,000 [7]. More than 90% of patients suffer from dysphagia but other frequent symptoms are regurgitation, heartburn, and chest pain [8]. The HRM is the main diagnostic tool but upper endoscopy and upper contrast studies may also corroborate and help classify the severity of the disease, especially in an altered anatomy context [3, 9, 10].

The exact physiopathology of the achalasia is not well understood but viral infection, genetic inheritance, and autoimmune diseases have been proposed as triggers for esophageal achalasia [4]. In Southern countries, such as Brazil, a parasite called *Trypanosoma cruzi* transmitted by an insect—the barbeiro—may infect the esophagus, destroy esophageal ganglia, ultimately leading to the chagasic achalasia [9, 11]. Since no other obvious etiologic causes for achalasia have been unequivocally identified to date, all but chagasic achalasia are still referred to as idiopathic.

In spite of the etiology, the classic gold-standard treatment for achalasia is the surgical Heller's myotomy, typically associated with a fundoplication to avoid long-term gastroesophageal reflux disease (GERD) [9]. However, several endoscopic techniques have been reported to address achalasia, each with different efficacy and safety profiles. Botulinum toxin (BTx) injection at the esophagogastric junction (EGJ), pneumatic dilation (PD) with large balloons, and most recently the peroral endoscopic myotomy (POEM) are the main endoscopic treatment modalities [12–14]. The aim of this chapter is to review and summarize the current role of these endoluminal approaches to treat achalasia and other dysmotility disorders.

Botulinum Toxin (BTx) Injection

The BTx is a neurotoxin that acts through a strong binding to the presynaptic cholinergic-nerve terminals, ultimately inhibiting the acetylcholine release from nerve endings [15]. It impairs muscular contractility and may also lower smooth muscle tone in the gastrointestinal (GI) tract [16]. In 1994, Pasricha et al described the first human use of the BTx injections in the EGJ to treat achalasia. Ten patients with achalasia underwent one to three sessions of BTx injections. Six patients presented clinical improvement sustained up to 1 year, three had an initial improvement but relapsed within 2 months, and one did not improve (treatment failure) [16].

A posterior study from the same working group was published 2 years later. Among the 31 patients who underwent BTx injections, 28 improved initially but only 20 had a sustained improvement beyond 3 months (so-called responders). Ultimately, 19 out of the 20 responders relapsed at a median follow-up of 468 days (153–840 days) [12].

However, in time, robust data from controlled randomized trials succeeded in proving the superiority of either the surgical approach (Heller's myotomy) or the pneumatic dilation (PD) over the BTx injection. Vaezi et al enrolled 42 patients that were randomly allocated to either BTx injection or PD. The pneumatic dilation carried the same initial failure rate but higher remission rates at 12 months (70% × 32%, $p < 0.05$). Moreover, PD significantly reduced symptom scores, lowered LES pressure and the esophageal barium column height, while BTx resulted only in a reduction in symptom scores [17]. Accordingly, a recent systematic review published in the Cochrane Database included seven randomized studies comparing those two endoscopic modalities. The authors firmly concluded that PD was more effective than BTx in the long term (greater than 6 months) [18].

As to comparisons with the Heller's procedure, Zaninotto et al randomly allocated 40 patients to BTx injections in the EGJ and 40 to surgical myotomy in 2004. Except for slightly lower symptom scores favoring surgery, most results were comparable at 6 months. Nonetheless, 65% of BTx patients recurred at 2 years; thus, the probability of being symptom-free at 2 years was 87.5% after myotomy and 34% after BTx ($p < 0.05$) [19].

Consequently, the transient effect of the BTx diminished significantly its role in the endoscopic armamentarium against achalasia. Currently, most authors consider BTx only for patients not amenable to more invasive procedures such as PD, POEM, or surgery [13, 20].

Pneumatic Dilation

The pneumatic dilation of the LES is usually performed under both endoscopic and fluoroscopic guidance. A prior upper GI endoscopy with esophageal chromoscopy is strongly recommended due to the high risk of squamous cell cancer in achalasia patients [21]. Initially, the distance from the EGJ to the superior dental arch is endoscopically measured and later used to help to position the mid portion of the balloon exactly over the LES. Then, the endoscopist places a large diameter, catheter-based, noncompliant, over-the-scope balloon (Fig. 12.1) across the EGJ using fluoroscopy and the previous measurement. The balloon is gradually inflated using a handheld manometer up to 1.4 psi to reach 30 mm in diameter (Fig. 12.2). Further sessions dilation up to 40 mm may be needed in cases of relapse or poor initial response. This specific technique has been described to have less serious adverse events and mortality than the surgical myotomy [22].

Fig. 12.1 Picture of the handheld manometer and the achalasia balloon

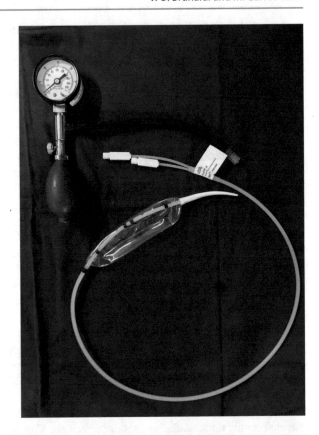

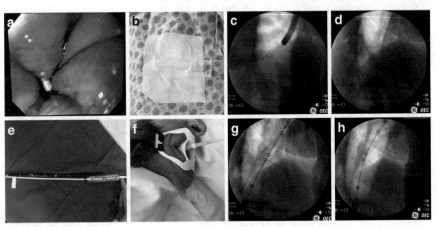

Fig. 12.2 Pneumatic dilation procedure: (**a**) endoscopic identification of the esophagogastric junction; (**b** and **c**) placement of external radiopaque marks at the esophagogastric junction (EGJ); (**d**) placement of the metallic guidewire in the antrum towards the esophagogastric junction; (**e**) marking the balloon with tape according to the distance from the superior dental arch to the EGJ; (**f** and **g**) introduction of the balloon over the wire until both marks match; (**h**) fluoroscopic appearance of the inflated pneumatic balloon

Browne and McHardy published the first description of PD to treat achalasia in 1939 [23] and Benedict EB reported the first comparison of dilation and surgical myotomy in 1964 [24]. Decades later, the good outcomes of the PD rendered this modality a plausible alternative to the surgical myotomy [25, 26].

The most robust article to date is a European multicenter controlled trial comparing the endoscopic dilation and the laparoscopic Heller's myotomy (LHM). Published in 2011, this study enrolled 201 newly diagnosed patients allocated either to PD ($n = 95$) or to LHM ($n = 106$) who were followed for a mean of 43 months. The therapeutic success rates (Eckardt score ≤ 3 [27]) for the PD group were 90% and 86% at 1 and 2 years, respectively, while 93% and 90% for the LHM group in the intention-to-treat analysis ($p = 0.46$). Accordingly, there was no difference between groups regarding LES pressure, the height of the barium-contrast column, and quality of life at 2 years. The perforation rate during PD was 4% and the rate of mucosal tears during LHM was 12% ($p = 0.28$). This study concluded that there were no relevant differences in terms of efficacy and safety of the PD compared to the LHM [28]. The following study with a 5-year evaluation confirmed those finding at a longer term except for a need for redilation of 25% in the PD group [29]. A recent meta-analysis also reported similar results [26].

As a consequence of the aforementioned data, the endoscopic pneumatic balloon dilation of the LES remains as a relevant alternative to surgical myotomy [20].

Peroral Endoscopic Myotomy (POEM)

The first description of an endoscopic esophageal myotomy was reported in an animal study by Pasricha et al in 2007 [30]. In 2010, Inoue et al published the first human feasibility study describing the POEM in 17 patients [31]. Despite being a recently developed procedure, it has gained worldwide acceptance. Despite the lack of controlled studies, series as large as 1000 patients are currently available, which hardly classify POEM as an experimental procedure [14].

This procedure is usually performed under general anesthesia with the patient in left lateral decubitus or supine position. The first step of the procedure is to measure the distance between the superior dental arch and the EGJ. Around 6 to 10 cm cranially to the EGJ, the operator injects saline with indigo carmine to create a submucosal cushion and then incise the mucosa. Using a cone-shaped cap attached to the end of the scope, the endoscopist manages to enter the submucosal space and dissects this layer caudally up to 2–4 cm below the EGJ. Then, under complete endoscopic visualization and control, the muscularis propria layer of the stomach just below the LES, the LES itself, and the muscularis propria layer of the esophagus are cut in a distal-to-proximal fashion. Finally, the mucosal incision is closed using a sequence of endoclips [32] (Fig. 12.3). Several technical particularities exist among different centers and experts, namely, anterior or posterior wall tunneling [33], full-thickness (circular and longitudinal) or circular-only myotomy [34], and length of the myotomy [35]. However, there is still no consensus among studies on the impact of those technical dissimilarities in short- or long-term outcomes.

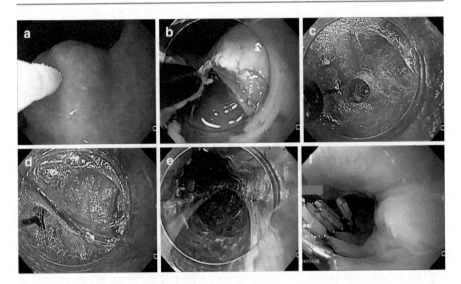

Fig. 12.3 The peroral endoscopic myotomy (POEM) procedure: (**a**) injection at the mid esophagus to create a submucosal cushion; (**b**) mucosal incision; (**c** and **d**) submucosal tunneling; (**e**) full-thickness endoscopic myotomy showing the longitudinal muscular layer completely cut; (**f**) final mucosal clipping. (Gentle courtesy from Dr. José Eduardo Brunaldi)

In spite of the lack of randomized controlled trials (RCTs) comparing POEM to LHM, robust data certify the effectiveness of POEM in most clinical scenarios. In 2015, Inoue et al. reported a series of 500 POEM cases. Approximately 82% of patients had nonsigmoid esophagus but almost 40% had previously undergone treatment for achalasia (PD, BTx injection or LHM). At 2 months, the authors reported significant reductions in Eckardt score (6.0 ± 3.0 vs. 1.0 ± 2.0, $p < 0.0001$) and in LES pressure (25.4 ± 17.1 vs. 13.4 ± 5.9 mmHg, $p < 0.0001$), both sustained at 3 years post-POEM. As a long-term adverse effect, 16.8% and 21.3% of patients presented GERD at 2 months and 3 years, respectively [32].

Although full text is not available yet, a randomized trial including 133 therapy-naïve patients comparing POEM to PD was published in 2017. At 1 year, 92.2% of POEM patients had clinical remission (Eckardt score ≤ 3) versus 70% of PD patients ($p < 0.01$). There were two serious adverse events in the PD group (1 perforation, 1 chest pain requiring admission) and none in the POEM group. However, 48% of POEM patients had esophagitis versus 13% of PD patients ($p < 0.01$) after proton pump inhibitor (PPI) cessation at 1-year follow-up.

Patel et al recently published a systematic review and meta-analysis assessing the efficacy and safety of POEM to treat achalasia. In a noncomparative analysis, the article included 22 studies with a total of 1122 patients. The pooled average pre- and post-POEM Eckardt score were 6.8 ± 1.0 and 1.2 ± 0.6 ($p < 0.01$), respectively. Accordingly, the authors demonstrated reductions by 66% and 80% in the LES pressure and timed barium esophagogram column height, respectively. Three comparative noncontrolled studies were also included in this meta-analysis. Comparisons with LHM showed similar total adverse events rate and incidence of perforation but shorter length of stay and operative time for POEM [36]. Another systematic review exclusively investigated comparisons with LHM. Fifty-three studies enrolling 5834 patients undergoing LHM and 21 articles with 1958 patients undergoing POEM were included. The predicted probabilities for improvement in dysphagia at 12 and 24 months were 93.5% and 92.7% for POEM versus 91.0% and 90.0% for LHM (both $p = 0.01$). However, patients who underwent POEM were more likely to develop GERD symptoms, erosive esophagitis, and altered pH monitoring compared to LHM. In contrast to the previous systematic review, the authors found the length of hospital stay to be 1.03 days longer after POEM than LHM ($p = 0.04$) [37]. Nonetheless, there are still no controlled data comparing those two therapeutic modalities but a few ongoing trials shall fill this gap in the near future and might confirm the aforementioned results.

Reliable international experiences have also demonstrated good efficacy and safety profile of POEM to address achalasia in the pediatric population [38], in patients who relapsed or failed primary POEM [39], and to treat cases of failed LHM [40, 41].

The main shortcoming of the POEM is the development of GERD. The destruction of the most important antireflux mechanism without associating a fundoplication ultimately favors gastric content reflux into the distal esophagus. Studies report GERD in up to 46% of patients after POEM [20]. A recent systematic review including 45 studies and more than 4000 individuals compared POEM to LHM in terms of GERD. The pooled rate of esophagitis assessed by upper endoscopy was 29.4% and 7.6% after POEM and LHM, respectively. The pooled rate estimate of abnormal acid exposure at pH monitoring was 39% and 16.8% after POEM and LHM, respectively [42]. Therefore, strict follow-up focused on preventing long-term complications of GERD is strongly recommended for POEM patients.

In an attempt to address this drawback, Inoue et al reported a series of 21 cases associating a NOTES fundoplication with the standard POEM. After performing the full-thickness myotomy, the endoscopist managed to enter the abdominal cavity incising the peritoneum at the anterior wall of the stomach. Using a combination of an endoloop and endoclips, the fundus was retracted at the EGJ thus creating a fundoplication. The authors reported no immediate or delayed complications of the procedure. Accordingly, length of stay and use of analgesia were similar to the conventional POEM. The fundoplication added a mean of 51 minutes to the procedure. At 2 months, 20/21 patients (95%) had a wrap across the EGJ consistent with an intact plication [43]. Despite being the only available study to date describing this technique, the rationale is exciting. Further studies are needed to assess its effectiveness at preventing long-term GERD.

Treatment Options According to the HRM

The introduction of the HRM in the management of esophageal motility disorders allowed the identification of new predictive factors for good response to treatment. The subdivision of types of achalasia is one of the most important among them. In spite of the treatment modality, the type II achalasia has good response rates over 90% in most studies. On the contrary, type III carries the worst outcome: good outcome rates as low as 30% for endoscopic treatments other than POEM and as low as 69% for LHM. Finally, the type I achalasia has intermediate outcomes [6, 44–46].

In fact, since the Chicago Classification was released [2], it was possible to create phenotypes instead of purely labeled diseases, thus allowing guidance according to the topographic finding. In this sense, that is the major advantage of the POEM procedure: the possibility to increase the length of the myotomy as needed and eventually even guide by the HRM findings. Khan et al recently published a meta-analysis pooling data from uncontrolled POEM series and analyzed response rates according to the manometric diagnoses. Contrary to previous data, the authors showed a pooled response rate of 92% for type III achalasia with a mean myotomy length of 17 cm. Moreover, this same treatment provided good responses in 72% of patients with Jackhammer esophagus and in 88% of patients with distal esophageal spasm. Such long myotomy rendering POEM effective in these contexts corroborates the rationale of treating according to HRM topographic findings on a case-by-case basis [47].

In this sense, a very experienced group from Japan created a therapeutic algorithm grouping motility disorders according to specific topographic findings that ultimately define treatment particularities. Tuason and Inoue proposed the categorization of disorders in three groups: group 1 (achalasia type I, type II, and EGJ outflow obstruction), group 2 (type III achalasia), and group 3 (Diffuse esophageal spasm and Jackhammer esophagus). The best approach differs according to the group: group 1 should undergo standard POEM, group 2 should undergo extended myotomy, and group 3 should undergo LES-preserving myotomy of the esophageal body [20] (Fig. 12.4). This algorithm is novel and currently, no controlled data derives from it. Nevertheless, it seems extremely accurate at customizing treatment according to the origin of the disorder.

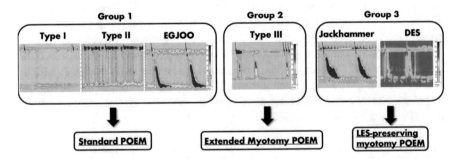

Fig. 12.4 Therapeutic algorithm for peroral endoscopic myotomy according to high-resolution manometry findings. (Gentle courtesy from Dr. Ricardo Brandt and Dr. Leticia Roque). EGJOO esophagogastric junction outflow obstruction, DES diffuse esophageal spasm, POEM peroral endoscopic myotomy, LES lower esophageal sphincter

Once again, controlled data are needed to prove the effectiveness and safety of POEM compared to LHM. In the meantime, robust non-controlled data may support the routine employment of POEM to treat achalasia. Finally, future randomized controlled trials must assess the impact of the aforementioned customization of the endoscopic approach on long-term efficacy. As to other endoscopic treatments, botulinum toxin injection at the EGJ has currently very limited indications but PD is still firmly established as a plausible alternative to surgery especially for type II achalasia.

References

1. Lin Z, Yim B, Gawron A, Imam H, Kahrilas PJ, Pandolfino JE. The four phases of esophageal bolus transit defined by high-resolution impedance manometry and fluoroscopy. Am J Physiol Gastrointest Liver Physiol. 2014;307:G437–44.
2. Kahrilas PJ, Bredenoord AJ, Fox M, Gyawali CP, Roman S, Smout AJPM, Pandolfino JE. The Chicago classification of esophageal motility disorders, v3.0. Neurogastroenterol Motil. 2015;27:160–74.
3. Kahrilas PJ, Bredenoord AJ, Carlson DA, Pandolfino JE. Advances in Management of Esophageal Motility Disorders. Clin Gastroenterol Hepatol. 2018;16:1692–700.
4. Park W, Vaezi MF. Etiology and pathogenesis of achalasia: the current understanding. Am J Gastroenterol. 2005;100:1404–14.
5. Kahrilas PJ, Bredenoord AJ, Fox M, Gyawali CP, Roman S, Smout AJPM, Pandolfino JE. Expert consensus document: advances in the management of oesophageal motility disorders in the era of high-resolution manometry: a focus on achalasia syndromes. Nat Rev Gastroenterol Hepatol. 2017;14:677–88.
6. Pandolfino JE, Kwiatek MA, Nealis T, Bulsiewicz W, Post J, Kahrilas PJ. Achalasia: a new clinically relevant classification by high-resolution manometry. Gastroenterology. 2008;135:1526–33.
7. Sadowski DC, Ackah F, Jiang B, Svenson LW. Achalasia: incidence, prevalence and survival. A population-based study. Neurogastroenterol Motil. 2010;22:e256–61.
8. Fisichella PM, Raz D, Palazzo F, Niponmick I, Patti MG. Clinical, radiological, and manometric profile in 145 patients with untreated achalasia. World J Surg. 2008;32:1974–9.
9. Herbella FAM, Aquino JLB, Stefani-Nakano S, et al. Treatment of achalasia: lessons learned with Chagas' disease. Dis Esophagus. 2008;21:461–7.
10. Ramos AC, Murakami A, Lanzarini EG, Neto MG, Galvao M. Achalasia and laparoscopic gastric bypass. Surg Obes Relat Dis. 2009;5:132–4.
11. de Lima MA, Cabrine-Santos M, Tavares MG, Gerolin GP, Lages-Silva E, Ramirez LE. Interstitial cells of Cajal in chagasic megaesophagus. Ann Diagn Pathol. 2008;12:271–4.
12. Pasricha PJ, Rai R, Ravich WJ, Hendrix TR, Kalloo AN. Botulinum toxin for achalasia: long-term outcome and predictors of response. Gastroenterology. 1996;110:1410–5.
13. Vaezi MF, Pandolfino JE, Vela MF. ACG clinical guideline: diagnosis and management of achalasia. Am J Gastroenterol. 2013;108:1238–49; quiz 1250.
14. Bechara R, Onimaru M, Ikeda H, Inoue H. Per-oral endoscopic myotomy, 1000 cases later: pearls, pitfalls, and practical considerations. Gastrointest Endosc. 2016;84:330–8.
15. Jankovic J, Brin MF. Therapeutic uses of botulinum toxin. N Engl J Med. 1991;324:1186–94.
16. Pasricha PJ, Ravich WJ, Hendrix TR, Sostre S, Jones B, Kalloo AN. Treatment of achalasia with intrasphincteric injection of botulinum toxin. A pilot trial. Ann Intern Med. 1994;121:590–1.
17. Vaezi MF, Richter JE, Wilcox CM, Schroeder PL, Birgisson S, Slaughter RL, Koehler RE, Baker ME. Botulinum toxin versus pneumatic dilatation in the treatment of achalasia: a randomised trial. Gut. 1999;44:231–9.

18. Leyden JE, Moss AC, MacMathuna P. Endoscopic pneumatic dilation versus botulinum toxin injection in the management of primary achalasia. Cochrane Database Syst Rev. 2014;(12):CD005046.
19. Zaninotto G, Annese V, Costantini M, et al. Randomized controlled trial of botulinum toxin versus laparoscopic heller myotomy for esophageal achalasia. Ann Surg. 2004;239:364–70.
20. Tuason J, Inoue H. Current status of achalasia management: a review on diagnosis and treatment. J Gastroenterol. 2017;52:401–6.
21. Tustumi F, Bernardo WM, da Rocha JRM, Szachnowicz S, Seguro FC, Bianchi ET, Sallum RAA, Cecconello I. Esophageal achalasia: a risk factor for carcinoma. A systematic review and meta-analysis. Dis Esophagus. 2017;30:1–8.
22. Lynch KL, Pandolfino JE, Howden CW, Kahrilas PJ. Major complications of pneumatic dilation and Heller myotomy for achalasia: single-center experience and systematic review of the literature. Am J Gastroenterol. 2012;107:1817–25.
23. Browne DC, McHardy G. A new instrument for use in esophagospasm. J Am Med Assoc. 1939;113:1963–4.
24. Benedict EB. Bougienage, forceful dilatation, and surgery in treatment of achalasia. A comparison of results. JAMA. 1964;188:355–7.
25. Pandolfino JE, Gawron AJ. Achalasia: a systematic review. JAMA. 2015;313:1841–52.
26. Bonifacio P, de Moura DTH, Bernardo WM, de Moura ETH, Farias GFA, Neto ACM, Lordello M, Korkischko N, Sallum R, de Moura EGH. Pneumatic dilation versus laparoscopic Heller's myotomy in the treatment of achalasia: systematic review and meta-analysis based on randomized controlled trials. Dis Esophagus. 2019;32(2) https://doi.org/10.1093/dote/doy105.
27. Eckardt VF. Clinical presentations and complications of achalasia. Gastrointest Endosc Clin N Am. 2001;11:281–92, vi.
28. Boeckxstaens GE, Annese V, des Varannes SB, et al. Pneumatic dilation versus laparoscopic Heller's myotomy for idiopathic achalasia. N Engl J Med. 2011;364:1807–16.
29. Moonen A, Annese V, Belmans A, et al. Long-term results of the European achalasia trial: a multicentre randomised controlled trial comparing pneumatic dilation versus laparoscopic Heller myotomy. Gut. 2016;65:732–9.
30. Pasricha PJ, Hawari R, Ahmed I, Chen J, Cotton PB, Hawes RH, Kalloo AN, Kantsevoy SV, Gostout CJ. Submucosal endoscopic esophageal myotomy: a novel experimental approach for the treatment of achalasia. Endoscopy. 2007;39:761–4.
31. Inoue H, Minami H, Kobayashi Y, Sato Y, Kaga M, Suzuki M, Satodate H, Odaka N, Itoh H, Kudo S. Peroral endoscopic myotomy (POEM) for esophageal achalasia. Endoscopy. 2010;42:265–71.
32. Inoue H, Sato H, Ikeda H, Onimaru M, Sato C, Minami H, Yokomichi H, Kobayashi Y, Grimes KL, Kudo S. Per-Oral endoscopic myotomy: a series of 500 patients. J Am Coll Surg. 2015;221:256–64.
33. Tan Y, Lv L, Wang X, Zhu H, Chu Y, Luo M, Li C, Zhou H, Huo J, Liu D. Efficacy of anterior versus posterior per-oral endoscopic myotomy for treating achalasia: a randomized, prospective study. Gastrointest Endosc. 2018;88:46–54.
34. Wang X-H, Tan Y-Y, Zhu H-Y, Li C-J, Liu D-L. Full-thickness myotomy is associated with higher rate of postoperative gastroesophageal reflux disease. World J Gastroenterol. 2016;22:9419–26.
35. Familiari P, Calì A, Landi R, Gigante G, Boskoski I, Barbaro F, Tringali A, Zurita SA, Perri V, Costamagna G. Tu2041 long vs short POEM for the treatment of achalasia. Interim analysis of a randomized controlled trial. Gastrointest Endosc. 2016;83:AB624.
36. Patel K, Abbassi-Ghadi N, Markar S, Kumar S, Jethwa P, Zaninotto G. Peroral endoscopic myotomy for the treatment of esophageal achalasia: systematic review and pooled analysis. Dis Esophagus. 2016;29:807–19.
37. Schlottmann F, Luckett DJ, Fine J, Shaheen NJ, Patti MG. Laparoscopic Heller Myotomy versus Peroral Endoscopic Myotomy (POEM) for achalasia: a systematic review and meta-analysis. Ann Surg. 2018;267:451–60.

38. Lee Y, Brar K, Doumouras AG, Hong D. Peroral endoscopic myotomy (POEM) for the treatment of pediatric achalasia: a systematic review and meta-analysis. Surg Endosc. 2019;33(6):1710–20. https://doi.org/10.1007/s00464-019-06701-5.
39. Tyberg A, Seewald S, Sharaiha RZ, et al. A multicenter international registry of redo per-oral endoscopic myotomy (POEM) after failed POEM. Gastrointest Endosc. 2017;85:1208–11.
40. Tyberg A, Sharaiha RZ, Familiari P, et al. Peroral endoscopic myotomy as salvation technique post-Heller: international experience. Dig Endosc. 2018;30:52–6.
41. Fernandez-Ananin S, Fernandez AF, Balague C, Sacoto D, Targarona EM. What to do when Heller's myotomy fails? Pneumatic dilatation, laparoscopic remyotomy or peroral endoscopic myotomy: a systematic review. J Minim Access Surg. 2018;14:177–84.
42. Repici A, Fuccio L, Maselli R, et al. GERD after per-oral endoscopic myotomy as compared with Heller's myotomy with fundoplication: a systematic review with meta-analysis. Gastrointest Endosc. 2018;87:934–943.e18.
43. Inoue H, Ueno A, Shimamura Y, et al. Peroral endoscopic myotomy and fundoplication: a novel NOTES procedure. Endoscopy. 2019;51:161–4.
44. Rohof WO, Salvador R, Annese V, et al. Outcomes of treatment for achalasia depend on manometric subtype. Gastroenterology. 2013;144:714–8.
45. Salvador R, Costantini M, Zaninotto G, et al. The preoperative manometric pattern predicts the outcome of surgical treatment for esophageal achalasia. J Gastrointest Surg. 2010;14:1635–45.
46. Pratap N, Kalapala R, Darisetty S, et al. Achalasia cardia subtyping by high-resolution manometry predicts the therapeutic outcome of pneumatic balloon dilatation. J Neurogastroenterol Motil. 2011;17:48–53.
47. Khan MA, Kumbhari V, Ngamruengphong S, et al. Is POEM the answer for management of spastic esophageal disorders? A systematic review and meta-analysis. Dig Dis Sci. 2017;62:35–44.

Redo Interventions in Failed Procedures

Kelly R. Haisley and Lee L. Swanström

Introduction

Esophageal motility disorders can present with a wide array of clinical symptoms and dynamic differences in esophageal function, which makes recognition of treatment failures complicated. While achalasia is the best defined disorder of esophageal motility, there are other diagnoses that fall outside the achalasia definition, including esophageal outflow obstruction, major disorders of peristalsis (diffuse esophageal spasm (DES), hypercontractile esophagus, absent contractility), and minor disorders of peristalsis (ineffective esophageal motility, fragmented peristalsis) [1]. While esophageal relaxing medications such as calcium channel blockers or endoscopic approaches such as Botox or dilation are often applied for short-term symptom relief, surgical myotomy is the most commonly applied technique (thoracoscopic, laparoscopic, or endoscopic) for definitive management of esophageal motility disorders. Esophageal myotomy is effective for both hyper-contractile disorders (in which cutting the muscle decreases its ability to spasm) and hypocontractile disorders (in which cutting the LES allows for easier bolus clearance either by weak peristalsis or gravity). With appropriate initial workup and a fastidious surgical technique, myotomy can have an 80–90% initial clinical response rate when applied to appropriately selected patients [2].

Nevertheless, some patients will develop recurrent symptoms after myotomy. The recommended treatment course after a failed motility procedure is not well defined and no randomized trials have been conducted to date [3]. Management choices depend primarily on the patient's clinical symptoms, severity of disease, and the cause of the treatment failure. Depending on individual factors, treatment options may include medical management, pneumatic dilation, surgical revision, or conversion to an alternate surgical procedure [3].

K. R. Haisley (✉) · L. L. Swanström
Gastrointestinal and Minimally Invasive Surgery, The Oregon Clinic, Portland, OR, USA

© Springer Nature Switzerland AG 2021
N. Zundel et al. (eds.), *Benign Esophageal Disease*,
https://doi.org/10.1007/978-3-030-51489-1_13

Rates of Motility Treatment Failure

Despite high rates of early treatment success, recurrent dysphagia or other symptoms will return in approximately 10–20% of patients in the years following their index operation. Despite these relatively high rates of recurrent symptoms, the need for operative re-intervention remains low. In a retrospective analysis of more than 12,000 patients undergoing Heller myotomy over a 38-year period, Gouda and colleagues showed a rate of reoperation of only 6.2% [4]. Of note, these re-interventions generally did not take place until 8–9 years after the initial operation, indicating either a late recurrence or that many patients live with these symptoms for an extended period before getting treatment [3].

POEM (per-oral endoscopic myotomy) is a newer treatment for motility disorders, with less than 10 years of outcomes data, and therefore less knowledge of the causes of treatment failures and rates of re-intervention in POEM patients. A recent 5-year follow-up by Teitelbaum et al. suggests that there is a small but significant worsening of symptoms between 2 and 5 years, though the clinical relevance of this remains to be seen. However, only three patients of 36 (0.8%) in this study required re-intervention in this period, two for recurrent dysphagia and one for the new onset of GERD (gastroesophageal reflux disease) [5]. Longer term outcomes and rates of re-intervention remain to be defined.

In total, these data suggest a moderate rate of recurrent symptoms (20–30%) following operative treatment for motility disorders, but a low rate of need for intervention following surgical myotomy (0.8–6.2%).

Symptoms of Motility Treatment Failure

The clinical course after surgical myotomy can be challenging to follow as symptoms and recovery are highly subjective. A well myotomized esophagus, in the setting of either primary aperistalsis due to achalasia or induced aperistalsis due to a long myotomy, will never truly function normally, and as such, some degree of swallowing abnormality is likely to persist for many patients who have had these procedures. However, failure to have any improvement after myotomy, or worsening dysphagia after a period of improvement, should raise clinical concern for treatment failure. By far the most common presenting symptom of a failed motility procedure is dysphagia, with a mean time to recurrence of approximately 1.5 years after the index operation [6]. Other less specific symptoms can also certainly develop, including persistent chest pain or gastroesophageal reflux disease (GERD) symptoms such as heartburn or regurgitation. The presenting symptom will depend somewhat on the reason for treatment failure and should help guide the clinical workup.

Table 13.1 Indications for re-intervention after motility procedures

Incomplete myotomy	50%
Gastroesophageal reflux disease	30%
Megaesophagus	16%
Others	4%

Reasons for Motility Treatment Failure

There can be a number of reasons for treatment failure after surgical myotomy (Table 13.1), and the optimal treatment approach will ultimately depend on the etiology of the failure, the impact on quality of life, and the patient's surgical risk profile. The specific reason for recurrence may also predict the likelihood of successful intervention. Veenstra and colleagues showed that while re-intervention for dysphagia related to an incomplete myotomy or a failed fundoplication will have long-term success rates of approximately 75%, those rates drop dramatically to 0–40% if the cause of the recurrent dysphagia is related to a mucosal stricture or significant fibrosis [7]. For these reasons, a thorough investigation and understanding of the cause of treatment failure is essential in designing an appropriate treatment plan.

Incorrect Indication for Initial Surgery

Given the challenges in diagnosing motility disorders, it sometimes occurs that a treatment failure is related to a simple misunderstanding of the primary motility disorder prior to the index operation. Esophagogastric junction outflow obstruction (EJGOO) can be a particularly challenging clinical entity. While an elevated IRP is characteristic of both EGJOO and achalasia, EGJOO is a distinctly different clinical entity than achalasia, as peristalsis is typically preserved and the LES failure may be intermittent. EGJOO can be caused by a number of different clinical entities, such as GERD, PEH, or even cancer. Recent reports suggest that in the setting of EGJOO, in spite of traditional approaches focusing on relieving the obstruction with endoscopic dilation, Botox, POEM, or laparoscopic myotomy, relatively few patients respond well in terms of symptom resolution and surgical treatment should be considered with caution [1]. In fact, a myotomy in EGJOO can even cause worsening symptoms if, for example, their true underlying disease process was GERD. For this reason, review of the initial workup and motility is an important key in treating these patients.

Primary Surgical Failure

If the patient fails to have the expected response from their procedure in the immediate postoperative period, a primary surgical issue should be considered. This may include incomplete myotomy or a problem with the fundoplication. Certainly a grace period to allow for resolution of postoperative swelling and general recovery should be allowed, though some authors prefer revisional surgery as the first step in the treatment algorithm if dysphagia is early onset (<3 months) rather than any attempts at endoscopic dilation [3]. Later presentations of dysphagia are less likely to be due to a primary surgical failure and treatment will depend more on the determined specific cause of the symptoms.

Incomplete Myotomy

Incomplete myotomy is the most common indication for re-intervention after a surgical myotomy, responsible for around 50% of all revisional operations [4]. This should certainly be the first suspicion when evaluating a patient with recurrent dysphagia after myotomy and can be related to either inadequate proximal or distal extent of the myotomy. Studies have shown that an extended myotomy at the initial procedure reduces relapse rates from 17% to 5% and the need for re-intervention from 7% to basically 0% [3]. When incomplete myotomy is suspected as the cause of symptoms, surgical extension of the myotomy, either laparoscopically or endoscopically, is likely to be effective. While this can certainly occur in achalasia if the myotomy is not extended all the way through the high pressure zone, it is particularly likely in cases of non-achalasia motility disorders, such as diffuse esophageal spasm (DES) and Jackhammer esophagus that involve the entire esophagus. As the problematic portion of the esophagus may extend well above a traditional LES myotomy, a classic laparoscopic Heller myotomy (LHM) may result in an incomplete myotomy being performed, simply due to the technical limitations of extending a long myotomy from an abdominal approach. While VATS can be performed to lengthen this dissection, it does add some morbidity. POEM can be more effective in this regard, but incomplete myotomy is still possible if there is missed division of circular fibers or incomplete proximal or distal extension due to misidentification of landmarks or measurements.

Gastroesophageal Reflux Disease (GERD)

New or recurrent GERD is always a concern after myotomy and is the second most common indication for late reoperation in this population, making up 30% of redo cases [3]. This is a particular concern in pneumatic dilation and POEM, which typically do not include any fundoplication. Even in the case of a myotomy with fundoplication, wraps do have a progressive rate of failure, which can lead to the development of post-myotomy GERD. Furthermore, although current approaches for LHM generally include a fundoplication, this was not always the case in previous eras and its presence cannot necessarily be assumed [4].

The rates of increased acid exposure in the distal esophagus after POEM are consistently around 30% on objective testing, nearly twice that of the early rates reported for LHM patients with fundoplication [8]. It should be noted, however, that quality of life scores seem to be fairly similar between the two groups and that most patients with post-myotomy GERD (POEM or LHM) are easily managed with medications alone [9]. Reflux can also be the cause of dysphagia (due to esophagitis or peptic strictures), in which case aggressive PPI therapy is indicated as first-line treatment before surgical re-intervention [3]. However, in rare cases, revisional surgery may be required if symptoms are severe or if patients have a contraindication to long-term acid suppression medication.

Failed Fundoplication

In patients undergoing LHM with fundoplication, wrap failures can cause significant symptoms. A loose or dehisced fundoplication can lead to GERD, as mentioned above, while a slipped, overly tight, or herniated fundoplication may be associated with dysphagia or pain. Wrap failure is the reason for reoperation in approximately 25% of failed Heller myotomies [7]. In these cases, treatment may need to be focused on the wrap rather than the myotomy.

Ineffective Esophageal Motility/Pan-Aperistalsis

Many severe dysmotility disorders, aside from achalasia, are part of a progressive disease process that can lead to the subsequent deterioration of the motor function of other parts of the GI tract, including proximal esophagus, stomach, and small and large intestines. Therefore, recurrent dysphagia or regurgitation may develop even in the face of a successful LES myotomy [4]. Treatment options for generalized ineffective motility or pan-aperistalsis are less robust as there is no available method to restore esophageal motility once lost. Treatment goals in these cases should focus on esophageal emptying, chest pain mitigation, and controlling reflux. In these cases, expectation management is extremely important. Despite aggressive and appropriate treatment, these complex cases can lead to progressive dilation with megaesophagus and end-stage failure, which eventually becomes the indication for surgery in 16.2% of patients who require revision after LHM [4]. When the esophagus progresses to this point, esophagectomy may be the best option for the patient.

Esophageal Cancer Development

Patients with achalasia have an elevated risk of squamous cell carcinoma due to chronic stasis, inflammation, and increased exposure to carcinogens in the diet. This risk persists even in treated patients and may be as high as 3%—considerably higher than the general population. This stresses the importance of continued lifelong surveillance of all patients who have undergone myotomy for achalasia [3, 4]. In addition, increased acid exposure in the distal esophagus from GERD after myotomy can also theoretically put the patient at risk of intestinal metaplasia (IM) and the development of adenocarcinoma. When identified, these patients should be treated along standard esophageal metaplasia/dysplasia/cancer protocols regardless of their concomitant motility disorder [10].

Other Causes of Treatment Failure

Other possible causes of recurrent symptoms after surgical myotomy include but are not limited to diverticulum, healing/closure of the myotomy, and acute surgical complications such as bleeding and seroma/abscess.

Patient Workup

When a patient returns with persistent or recurrent symptoms after surgical myotomy, the first priority is to complete a thorough workup to identify the cause of the failure and to tailor a specific treatment plan for the patient moving forward [11].

Upper Gastrointestinal Series (UGI) +/− Barium Tablet

An UGI is an important starting point in understanding treatment failure after motility surgery. Contrast evaluation provides valuable information about the anatomy of the esophagus, particularly if the preoperative films are available for comparison. UGI can identify many fundoplication issues, hiatal hernias and will document anatomic evolution of the esophagus such as sigmoidization or end-stage dilation that could add to the difficulty of any redo interventions, particularly POEM (Fig. 13.1). It will further allow for the identification of any diverticulization that may have

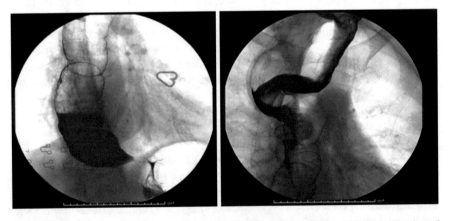

Fig. 13.1 UGI series showing recurrent achalasia with significant dilation and sigmoidization of the esophagus 15 years after laparoscopic Heller myotomy

developed from an intrathoracic myotomy site and could be contributing to symptoms. UGI may show also the presence of esophageal spasm, which can be a valuable diagnostic tool, particularly if the patient is symptomatic at the time of the test.

A formal timed barium swallow in addition to the standard UGI is extremely helpful in the setting of motility disorders, as this will quantify the degree of delayed emptying and can be an objective follow-up tool for success or failure. A barium tablet may be particularly useful to assess the location of any transit delay if solid dysphagia is the main presenting symptom.

UGI may be particularly helpful in identifying which patients are likely to benefit from redo myotomy, with those patients who have limited dilation and tortuosity being more likely to respond to redo myotomy, while those with massive esophageal dilation or significant tortuosity being more likely to benefit from esophageal resection [12].

Esophagogastroduodenoscopy (EGD)

Upper endoscopy (EGD) should be performed in all patients with recurrent symptoms after motility surgery to evaluate for structural abnormalities or other unexpected pathology (especially cancer) that could be causing symptoms. As discussed above, GERD may lead to esophagitis, ulcers, or strictures that may be better managed with medical therapy once diagnosed. Retained food or liquid in the esophagus or stomach on EGD is also helpful in understanding the degree of delayed esophageal or gastric emptying. If a fundoplication is present, its position and structure can be evaluated with visual inspection to determine if a wrap failure is present. Sometimes, an incomplete myotomy can be appreciated by feeling resistance to passage of the scope, hinting at the location of the failure. In cases where there is question, functional luminal imaging (Endoflip, Medtronic, Ireland) measurements can be taken to help better define any areas of narrowing and identify if an incomplete myotomy is present based on a persistent waist of high resistance [13].

High-Resolution Manometry (HRM)

High-quality manometry is essential to the understanding of the relationship of motility disorders of the esophagus and symptoms. While motility studies are certainly important before undertaking an initial operation, they are extremely valuable in understanding treatment failure, as they may detect a misdiagnosis in the initial surgery or a clinical change over time. Repeating manometry can allow for a comparison of the LES pattern and pressure before and after surgery to assess for incomplete myotomy and the degree of remaining peristalsis. In cases of Jackhammer esophagus or DES, motility will show whether hyper-contractile or spastic segments remain proximal to the area of the previous myotomy, or if new proximal spasm has developed. High-resolution manometry with impedance in combination

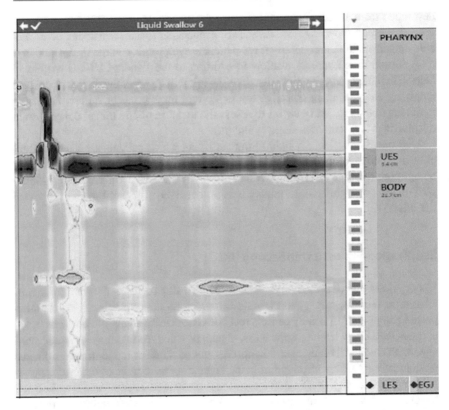

Fig. 13.2 High-resolution manometry performed 15 years after a laparoscopic Heller myotomy in a patient with recurrent dysphagia to solids with the catheter unable to be threaded past the LES with pan-esophageal pressurization from fluid stasis

with the revised Chicago classification provides the most comprehensive evaluation of esophageal function and should be a part of a standard foregut workup (Fig. 13.2) [14].

pH/Impedance

If post-myotomy GERD is suspected, it is important to confirm its presence through objective pH testing as many of the symptoms and even some manometric findings of motility disorders can be caused by reflux [1]. Contrarily, it is also well described that GERD symptoms, and even lack of symptoms, are extremely unreliable indicators of true gastroesophageal reflux [15]. A 48-h Bravo pH can be placed at the time of EGD, or standard 24-h pH testing can provide similar information. Impedance testing can be included with a standard pH to evaluate for non-acid fluid reflux, though this data can be somewhat difficult to interpret in the setting of the esophageal stasis that is common in esophageal dysmotility disorders and the data should be interpreted with caution and by an expert.

Gastric Emptying Study (GES)

Patients with esophageal motility disorders may have dysmotility in other parts of the GI tract as well. In the case of gastroparesis or delayed gastric emptying (DGE), backup in the stomach can cause overflow reflux into the esophagus. Patients with this problem typically complain of bloating, nausea, and early satiety in addition to their more classic reflux symptoms. If this is suspected or confirmed, treatment may be best focused on improving gastric emptying rather than simply esophageal interventions [16].

Medical Treatments

Medical options for failed motility procedures are somewhat limited, though in the setting of mild symptoms or high-risk patients, conservative treatment may be best in some scenarios. If spasm, as evidenced by noncardiac chest pain, is a primary issue, either new or persistent, esophageal relaxants such as calcium channel blockers (Nifedipine) may be effective in a partially myotomized esophagus, even if the patient had incomplete relief with these medications prior to their myotomy. Narcotics should be avoided whenever possible in the case of esophageal pain as they are unlikely to be effective and carry significant side effects and risks and can actually worsen esophageal contraction strength or induce spastic peristalsis [17]. Botox is generally not recommended after a myotomy due to high failure rates and development of fibrosis [3].

Pneumatic Dilation (PD)

Pneumatic dilation is a good initial treatment choice in patients with recurrent dysphagia after myotomy, with 64–80% of recurrent patients (whether LHM or POEM) having good results with PD [3]. PD is reported to have a high short-term success rate of approximately 85% after failed Heller but requires a mean of 2.5 treatments (range 1–3) [3]. Presumably, some of this effect would deteriorate over time, as is the case in treatment naive achalasia patients who undergo pneumatic dilation, in whom long-term effectiveness is only around 60% [3]. If pneumatic dilation is to be undertaken after a myotomy, timing is important. The risk of perforation is highest in the first 4 months after surgery, and it should be avoided in this time frame if possible. If early dilation is needed, it can be still acceptable to dilate to 35–40 mm, but it should be recognized that there is significant scar tissue, which will increase the risk of esophageal perforation with more aggressive dilations [3]. After two dilations, if the patient is not improved, it should be considered a treatment failure and surgical revision should be considered. Savary or wire guided dilations are also acceptable but are less effective and should be used with caution in cases of sigmoid esophagus.

Many patients who undergo PD will continue to progress to needing formal surgical re-intervention, whether by LHM or POEM. While there is no data to suggest that a previous PD complicates success rates of a redo LHM, there is some conflicting data on whether PD may lead to decreased success rates of POEM, but this data is somewhat limited, particularly in the redo population [18, 19].

Revision of the Index Operation

Redo Heller Myotomy

Redo Heller myotomy has been considered the mainstay of treatment for recurrent dysphagia following LHM [3]. In the past, the majority of both primary and revisional operations were performed open, though this has been largely replaced by laparoscopic intervention since the 1990s [4]. Since 1995, more than 50% of Heller myotomies being performed are done laparoscopically; however, only 2.3% of reoperations are performed with minimally invasive approaches [4]. Nonetheless, laparoscopic revisional Heller myotomy has been effectively applied in multiple institutions with good outcomes [3, 6, 7]. These studies report between 73% and 89% clinical success rate of redo laparoscopic Heller myotomy [3, 18]. Case reports of even second and third time re-myotomy have been published in an effort to preserve the esophagus, but such operations should certainly only be undertaken by very experienced surgeons [7].

When performing a redo LHM, the myotomy is best performed in a new orientation compared to the initial myotomy, preferably to the right side in case of eventual need for an esophagectomy, in order to preserve the future gastric conduit. As the most common reason for revision is an incomplete myotomy, one should ensure that the myotomy is extended adequately both proximally and distally.

The rate of complications in redo LHM is higher than that in primary operations, with a conversion to open rate as high as 6% [3]. Intraoperative mucosal perforation is perhaps the greatest risk of redo LHM and occurs in as many as 20% of these cases, fortunately such perforations when recognized intraoperatively seem to have no clinical impact. There is no clear indication that previous pneumatic dilation increases the risk of perforation [3]. In addition, the surgeon should be aware of the type of fundoplication that was performed at the index operation as the risk of mucosal injury is higher in patients who had a Toupet or no fundoplication compared to those who had a Dor, probably because the exposed mucosa has adhered to the undersurface of the left lobe of the liver [12]. However, with careful technique, any mucosal perforations can generally be identified and repaired primarily without a major negative impact on the patient's course [7].

Redo POEM

Redo POEM has been shown to be technically possible, though compared to the first-time POEM, clinical success rates are somewhat lower (around 85%) and complication rates are slightly higher (around 17%) [20]. If this is to be undertaken, the submucosal tunnel and myotomy should be performed in a new location relative to the initial myotomy. While this approach is feasible, it should be noted that these operations are often more complex, particularly in the case of sigmoid esophagus, and can require more than double the operative time of a first-time operation [19].

Redo Fundoplication

Whether to perform a fundoplication at the time of a revision is a matter of some debate. In the setting of a failed wrap, particularly due to herniation, slippage, or dehiscence, a revision of the fundoplication is reasonable and may be what is necessary to relieve symptoms, particularly if the wrap failure is felt to be the main problem. In this situation, as long as the original myotomy is adequate, there may be no need to extend this at the time of take-back, and the focus of surgery can be on correcting the wrap alone. The results of repeat motility should be taken into consideration when deciding on the type of fundoplication to perform, though in general a partial wrap is always recommended, either posterior (Toupet) or anterior (Dor) [21]. In rare cases in which the patient has completely preserved peristalsis and severe reflux (e.g., a patient misdiagnosed as achalasia who had an inappropriate myotomy), a full fundoplication may be possible, but this should be considered very carefully.

There are patients, however, who may actually be harmed by a fundoplication at the time of a re-operative motility procedure, specifically those with megaesophagus, significant tortuosity, or following multiple previous interventions. If esophageal preservation is being attempted, a fundoplication may produce too much resistance at the GE junction and lead to worsening esophageal deterioration. In this rare clinical setting, a fundoplication may not necessarily be recommended [3].

Conversion to Alternate Surgical Procedure

Conversion from LHM to POEM

In cases where the patient's indication for revision is related to incomplete myotomy, correction to a POEM is an attractive alternative to a redo LHM as it allows for the creation of an extended myotomy more easily and less invasively than a laparoscopic revision. POEM is particularly interesting following LHM as most of these patients have already had an anti-reflux procedure as part of their initial operation, thus minimizing the risk of GERD following the POEM, which has been a theoretical criticism of the procedure [3].

Multiple centers have shown POEM to be safe and effective after a Heller myotomy with a 98–100% technical success and 81–100% clinical response rate [18, 22–24]. While this is slightly lower than that of first-time POEM in patients without a previous Heller myotomy, it also appears to be slightly higher than the success rates of redo LHM (73–89%), though no head-to-head randomized trials have been performed [18, 24]. There do not appear to be increased complications in performing POEM in a patient with a previous LHR compared to a patient with no previous myotomy [18]. Use of POEM is reported to have shorter OR time, less blood loss, less post-procedural pain, shorter length of stay, and faster return to activities compared to redo LHM [3, 18].

When performing POEM in a patient with previous surgical myotomy, the anterior wall of the esophagus should be avoided so as to stay away from the previous scar tissue and dissection plane. While some authors recommend a posterior approach, a lateral or 3 o'clock position will also allow for avoidance of both the anterior dissection plane and the posterior major mediastinal structures and aorta [22].

Conversion from POEM to Heller Myotomy

Heller myotomy is a reasonable approach for patients with persistent dysphagia after POEM, as long as it is determined that the reason for dysphagia can be addressed by a more targeted intervention on the LES, such as an incomplete myotomy near the GE junction. It is also a valid approach if the patient is suffering from uncontrollable reflux in addition to dysphagia and the workup suggests that a fundoplication is needed.

As POEM is typically performed in the lateral esophagus, this leaves the anterior myotomy plane undisturbed and a traditional Heller myotomy can usually be performed in the standard fashion. Limited reports regarding the feasibility of LHM after POEM have shown it to be safe and effective [25].

Creation of a New Fundoplication

Most POEM patients and even some Heller myotomy patients will not have a fundoplication created as part of their index operation. While POEM patients who do have GERD are usually well controlled with medications, those with severe symptoms or contraindications to long-term acid suppression medications may benefit from a surgical fundoplication. If this is the case, and the myotomy appears to be functioning well, it is reasonable to consider a primary surgical fundoplication if they are meeting other clinical indications for intervention (objectively confirmed reflux, symptoms, appropriate risk profile). Again, a partial fundoplication is favored in the setting of a previously myotomized esophagus.

Other novel techniques have been proposed, particularly endoscopic fundoplications, either a transoral incisionless fundoplication (TIF) [26] or POEM-fundoplication [27], but their safety and efficacy in the setting of previous myotomy have not yet been fully evaluated.

Esophagectomy

In previous eras, primary myotomy failure was considered an indication for esophagectomy [12]. However, more recent studies have shown that esophageal preservation is possible even in second and third time redo procedures in experienced hands [7]. Nevertheless, progression to end-stage esophageal dilation, persistent chest pain, very late onset dysphagia, or even severe refractory GERD may sometimes require a "last resort" esophagectomy. While this treatment is very effective in eliminating the symptoms of dysphagia, particularly in patients with megaesophagus, it carries a relatively high complication and mortality rate and should not be generally considered as a primary treatment approach. It should, however, remain in the treatment algorithm for patients who have failed multiple less invasive procedures, and it can provide favorable long-term outcomes [28].

Robotics

The role of robotics in foregut surgery continues to evolve and data remains somewhat limited. However, small studies have suggested that the 3D visualization with the robot and fine motor abilities may be of particular benefit in myotomy and revisional operations. Small series have suggested a decreased rate of mucosal perforation in the first-time Heller myotomy and decreased conversion to open in redo surgeries when comparing the robotic approach to the laparoscopic approach, though additional data is needed to confirm these findings [29].

Conclusion

Revisional motility surgery can be a difficult endeavor in regard to both diagnostic subtleties and technical challenges. However, with appropriate workup and a clear understanding of various motility disorders and the reason that treatments can and do fail, revisional motility surgery can provide good clinical outcomes. The best results in revisional motility operations are obtained at centers that can provide an expert multidisciplinary approach familiar with the subtleties and challenges of revisional motility surgery [11]. Successfully managing these patients requires a thoughtful workup and careful treatment algorithm (Fig. 13.3).

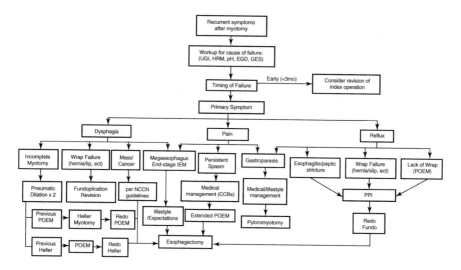

Fig. 13.3 Treatment algorithm for recurrent symptoms after motility surgery

References

 1. Schlottmann F, Patti MG. Primary Esophageal motility disorders: beyond achalasia. Int J Mol Sci. 2017;18(7):1399.
 2. Awaiz A, Yunus RM, Khan S, Memon B, Memon MA. Systematic review and meta-analysis of perioperative outcomes of peroral endoscopic myotomy (POEM) and laparoscopic Heller myotomy (LHM) for achalasia. Surg Laparosc Endosc Percutan Tech. 2017;27(3):123–31.
 3. Fernandez-Ananin S, Fernández AF, Balagué C, Sacoto D, Targarona EM. What to do when Heller's myotomy fails? Pneumatic dilatation, laparoscopic remyotomy or peroral endoscopic myotomy: a systematic review. J Minim Access Surg. 2018;14(3):177–84.
 4. Gouda BP, Nelson T, Bhoyrul S. Revisional surgery after heller myotomy for treatment of achalasia: a comparative analysis focusing on operative approach. Indian J Surg. 2012;74(4):309–13.
 5. Teitelbaum EN, Dunst CM, Reavis KM, Sharata AM, Ward MA, DeMeester SR, Swanström LL. Clinical outcomes five years after POEM for treatment of primary esophageal motility disorders. Surg Endosc. 2018;32(1):421–7.
 6. Mandovra P, Kalikar V, Patel A, Patankar RV. Redo laparoscopic Heller's cardiomyotomy for recurrent achalasia: is laparoscopic surgery feasible? J Laparoendosc Adv Surg Tech A. 2018;28(3):298–301.
 7. Veenstra BR, Goldberg RF, Bowers SP, Thomas M, Hinder RA, Smith CD. Revisional surgery after failed esophagogastric myotomy for achalasia: successful esophageal preservation. Surg Endosc. 2016;30(5):1754–61.
 8. Repici A, Fuccio L, Maselli R, et al. GERD after per-oral endoscopic myotomy as compared with Heller's myotomy with fundoplication: a systematic review with meta-analysis. Gastrointest Endosc. 2018;87(4):934–943.e18.
 9. Chan SM, Wu JC, Teoh AY, Yip HC, Ng EK, Lau JY, Chiu PW. Comparison of early outcomes and quality of life after laparoscopic Heller's cardiomyotomy to peroral endoscopic myotomy for treatment of achalasia. Dig Endosc. 2016;28(1):27–32.
10. National Comprehensive Cancer Network. Esophageal and Esophagogastric Junction Cancers (Version 2.2018). https://www.nccn.org/professionals/physician_gls/pdf/esophageal.pdf.
11. Patti MG, Allaix ME. Recurrent symptoms after Heller myotomy for achalasia: evaluation and treatment. World J Surg. 2015;39(7):1625–30.
12. Loviscek MF, Wright AS, Hinojosa MW, Petersen R, Pajitnov D, Oelschlager BK, Pellegrini CA. Recurrent dysphagia after Heller myotomy: is esophagectomy always the answer? J Am Coll Surg. 2013;216(4):736–43; discussion 743-4.
13. Yoo IK, Choi SA, Kim WH, Hong SP, Cakir OO, Cho JY. Assessment of clinical outcomes after peroral endoscopic myotomy via esophageal distensibility measurements with the endoluminal functional lumen imaging probe. Gut Liver. 2019;13(1):32–9.
14. Bredenoord AJ, Fox M, Kahrilas PJ, Pandolfino JE, Schwizer W, Smout AJ, International High Resolution Manometry Working Group. Chicago classification criteria of esophageal motility disorders defined in high resolution esophageal pressure topography. Neurogastroenterol Motil. 2012;24 Suppl 1:57–65.
15. Khajanchee YS, O'Rourke RW, Lockhart B, Patterson EJ, Hansen PD, Swanstrom LL. Postoperative symptoms and failure after antireflux surgery. Arch Surg. 2002;137(9):1008–13.
16. Zihni AM, Dunst CM, Swanström LL. Surgical Management for Gastroparesis. Gastrointest Endosc Clin N Am. 2019;29(1):85–95.
17. Ratuapli SK, Crowell MD, DiBaise JK, et al. Opioid-induced esophageal dysfunction (OIED) in patients on chronic opioids. Am J Gastroenterol. 2015;110(7):979–84.
18. Ngamruengphong S, Inoue H, Ujiki MB, et al. Efficacy and safety of peroral endoscopic myotomy for treatment of achalasia after failed Heller myotomy. Clin Gastroenterol Hepatol. 2017;15(10):1531–7.

19. Louie BE, Schneider AM, Schembre DB, Aye RW. Impact of prior interventions on outcomes during per oral endoscopic myotomy. Surg Endosc. 2017;31(4):1841–8.
20. Tyberg A, Seewald S, Sharaiha RZ, et al. A multicenter international registry of redo per-oral endoscopic myotomy (POEM) after failed POEM. Gastrointest Endosc. 2017;85(6):1208–11.
21. Siddaiah-Subramanya M, Yunus RM, Khan S, Memon B, Memon MA. Anterior dor or posterior toupet with Heller myotomy for achalasia cardia: a systematic review and meta-analysis. World J Surg. 2019;43(6):1563–70.
22. Vigneswaran Y, Yetasook AK, Zhao JC, Denham W, Linn JG, Ujiki MB. Peroral endoscopic myotomy (POEM): feasible as reoperation following Heller myotomy. J Gastrointest Surg. 2014;18(6):1071–6.
23. Onimaru M, Inoue H, Ikeda H, et al. Peroral endoscopic myotomy is a viable option for failed surgical esophagocardiomyotomy instead of redo surgical Heller myotomy: a single center prospective study. J Am Coll Surg. 2013;217(4):598–605.
24. Kristensen HØ, Kirkegård J, Kjær DW, Mortensen FV, Kunda R, Bjerregaard NC. Long-term outcome of peroral endoscopic myotomy for esophageal achalasia in patients with previous Heller myotomy. Surg Endosc. 2017;31(6):2596–601.
25. Giulini L, Dubecz A, Stein HJ. Laparoscopic Heller myotomy after failed POEM and multiple balloon dilatations: better late than never. Chirurg. 2017;88(4):303–6.
26. Chimukangara M, Jalilvand AD, Melvin WS, Perry KA. Long-term reported outcomes of transoral incisionless fundoplication: an 8-year cohort study. Surg Endosc. 2018;33(4):1304–9.
27. Inoue H, Ueno A, Shimamura Y, et al. Peroral endoscopic myotomy and fundoplication: a novel NOTES procedure. Endoscopy. 2019;51(2):161–4.
28. Gockel I, Kneist W, Eckardt VF, Oberholzer K, Junginger T. Subtotal esophageal resection in motility disorders of the esophagus. Dig Dis. 2004;22(4):396–401.
29. Rebecchi F, Allaix ME, Morino M. Robotic technological aids in esophageal surgery. J Vis Surg. 2017;3:7.

Diverticulum: Workup and Evaluation

14

Juan S. Barajas-Gamboa and Matthew Kroh

Introduction

The esophagus is a muscular tube with the primary function of delivering swallowed material (food and fluid) from the mouth to the stomach. It has an average length of 25 cm measured from its origin at the neck level below the cricoid cartilage [1].

Anatomically, three different regions can be identified: the cervical esophagus, the thoracic esophagus, and the abdominal esophagus. Functionally, the esophagus can be divided into three areas: the upper esophageal sphincter (UES), the esophageal body, and the lower esophageal sphincter (LES). The coordination of these areas is crucial to ensure propulsion of the alimentary bolus from the pharynx into the stomach [2].

The esophagus is composed of two groups of muscles, the outer layer of longitudinal muscles and the inner layer of circular muscles. The outer longitudinal muscles are responsible for contraction and allow the esophagus to shorten and elongate. The inner circular layer is responsible for the squeezing motion that affects peristalsis and closure of the esophageal sphincters. Benign esophageal diseases include a spectrum of nonmalignant diseases including gastroesophageal reflux disease (GERD), motility disorders, hiatal hernia, Barrett's esophagus, and diverticula of different anatomic locations [3].

J. S. Barajas-Gamboa
Department of General Surgery, Digestive Disease Institute, Cleveland Clinic Abu Dhabi, Abu Dhabi, United Arab Emirates

M. Kroh (✉)
Department of General Surgery, Digestive Disease Institute, Cleveland Clinic Abu Dhabi, Abu Dhabi, United Arab Emirates

Cleveland Clinic Lerner College of Medicine, Cleveland Clinic, Cleveland, OH, USA
e-mail: KrohM@ClevelandClinicAbuDhabi.ae; krohm@ccf.org

© Springer Nature Switzerland AG 2021
N. Zundel et al. (eds.), *Benign Esophageal Disease*,
https://doi.org/10.1007/978-3-030-51489-1_14

Esophageal diverticulum (ED) is a mucosal pouch that protrudes from the esophageal lumen. ED is classified according to its location (pharyngoesophageal, midesophageal, or epiphrenic), the layers of the esophagus that are involved (true or false), and the mechanism of formation (pulsion or traction) [1].

ED is a rare clinical finding with a low prevalence of 0.06–3.6% based on previous population studies published. Most patients with ED are asymptomatic. However, patients may present with dysphagia, heartburn, chest pain, belching, pharyngeal bolus, halitosis, and cough. Treatment includes both nonsurgical and surgical approaches based on a patient's symptoms and overall fitness, anatomic location, and associated diseases. The objective of this chapter is to describe the general approach to workup and evaluation of ED [2, 3].

Clinical Presentation

Zenker Diverticulum

Zenker diverticulum (ZD), also known as pharyngoesophageal diverticula, was described first by Dr. Abraham Ludlow in 1764. However, the common namesake is from German pathologist, Frederick Albert von Zenker, who published in 1878 a series of 27 patients with pharyngoesophageal diverticulum. ZD is the most common esophageal diverticulum. The prevalence is reported between 0.01% and 0.11% of the population, with approximately 50% of cases presenting in the seventh and eighth decades; women are predominantly affected [4].

Clinical manifestations include, in order of frequency, esophageal dysphagia, regurgitation of undigested food, aspiration, halitosis, and changes in voice. The most common complications of this anatomical abnormality are the risk of aspiration and the development of pulmonary conditions such as pneumonia as well as potential perforation of the diverticulum. ZD is unlikely related to malignancy development, however is associated with hiatal hernia, gastroduodenal ulcers, and achalasia [5].

ZD arises within the inferior pharyngeal constrictor, between the oblique fibers of the thyropharyngeus muscle and through or above the more horizontal fibers of the cricopharyngeus muscle (the upper esophageal sphincter). Killian's triangle is the named area of weakness through which most pharyngoesophageal diverticula protrude. Some authorities report that ZD is an acquired abnormality. The physiologic mechanism of this includes some degree of incoordination in the swallowing mechanism, with an abnormally high intrapharyngeal pressure leading to protrusion of esophageal mucosa and submucosa through the esophageal wall. Over time, and with repeated mechanism, this results in subsequent diverticulum formation [6, 7].

As a structural abnormality, treatment is most commonly procedural based. Most of the described interventions have in common techniques to relieve the relative obstruction distal to the pouch through cricopharyngeal myotomy. The different procedures involve the division of the cricopharyngeus muscle, followed by resection, imbrication, and obliteration of the diverticulum. Success rate is achieved in more than 90% of the cases overall, with low morbidity. Twenty percent of patients may require reintervention to achieve acceptable clinical outcomes, depending on technique used and experience of the proceduralist [8].

Midthoracic Diverticulum

Midthoracic diverticulum (MD) also known as midesophageal diverticulum is commonly associated with mediastinal granulomatosis disease (histoplasmosis or tuberculosis). MD is considered a true diverticulum due to the involvement of layers of the esophageal wall [1, 3].

This rare and uncommon condition is found in less than 4% of fluoroscopic esophagograms in adults. Described first by Rokitansky in 1840, MD is typically located within 4–5 cm of the carina. These diverticula are usually asymptomatic and most do not require interventions [9].

MD is thought to arise from adhesions between inflamed mediastinal lymph nodes and the esophagus. By contraction, the adhesions create pull on the esophageal wall with eventual diverticulum development. Patients with this clinical condition are typically asymptomatic and may present as an unsuspected finding. However, a subset will develop dysphagia, belching, retrosternal pain, regurgitation, heartburn, and/or weight loss. Complications are rare and include aspiration and esophagobronchial fistula. Carcinoma has also been reported [10].

Only symptomatic diverticula require treatment. Larger and symptomatic diverticula usually require surgery resection or diverticulopexy. After a complete preoperative workup including esophageal manometry in the absence of motor abnormality, diverticulectomy alone is recommended. Without definitive evidence, some authorities perform a simultaneous Heller myotomy with resection. The physiological purpose of distal myotomy is to relieve any potential obstruction and minimize the risk of staple line leak secondary to early postoperative esophageal lumen pressurization [11].

Repeat intervention may be necessary for first failures of therapy. For elective cases, reported mortality rate varies widely from 0% to 9%. Mortalities were found to be related to mediastinitis due to leakage from the esophageal closure, and pulmonary complications such as aspiration pneumonia [11].

Epiphrenic Diverticulum

Epiphrenic diverticulum (ED) was first described by Mondiere in 1833, who initially proposed that ED was secondary to increased intraluminal pressure. ED is typically single; however, up to 10% of patients may have two or more esophageal diverticula. Rarely, ED may be congenital (Ehlers-Danlos syndrome) or due to trauma [12].

ED appears in the distal third of the esophagus, within 10 cm of the gastroesophageal junction, and is associated with motor disorders including achalasia, hypertensive lower esophageal sphincter, diffuse esophageal spasm, and nonspecific motor disorders [13].

Patient symptoms may emanate from combination of abnormal peristalsis with a poorly relaxing lower esophageal sphincter. Clinical manifestations include vomiting, chest pain, epigastric pain, anorexia, weight loss, cough, halitosis, and noisy swallowing. The relationship between symptoms and the diverticulum size is unclear. Treatment of ED requires esophageal myotomy extending from the neck of the diverticulum onto the gastric cardia for a distance of 1.5–3.0 cm. Diverticulectomy, fundoplication, or repair of the hiatal hernia may also be necessary depending on the associated conditions and defect size [14].

ED is often asymptomatic and do not always require surgical treatment. The success rate with surgical approaches including minimally invasive techniques is about 85%. Not infrequently, patients may require more than one procedure to achieve acceptable clinical improvements. Morbidity is related to potential leakage from the suture line [15].

Intramural Pseudodiverticulosis

Intramural pseudodiverticulosis (IP) is a rare benign abnormality of the esophageal wall, characterized by dilatation of the submucosal glands. IP is not considered a true diverticulum. There is an increased risk of esophageal carcinoma in these patients. IP was first reported in 1960 by Mendl et al., and close to 200 cases have been published worldwide. Over three-fourths of cases of IP occur in the proximal or midesophagus [3, 5].

The pathogenesis remains unclear; however, histologically submucosal glands and excretory ducts have been identified in pathology specimens. IP impacts teens and individuals in their fifties and sixties. Men are slightly more affected than women. Patients with previous medical history of diabetes mellitus, esophageal candidiasis, reflux esophagitis, chronic alcohol abuse, and corrosive acid injury have a higher risk of IP. Several reports suggest a direct correlation between benign esophageal diseases; however, other authors refer to an association with esophageal cancer. Furthermore, over 90% of patients with this condition have an accompanying stricture [5].

Considering the condition involves changes in the wall of the esophagus and reduction of the lumen, the symptoms are primarily related to swallowing. Some patients present with esophageal bleeding, vomiting with blood, and melena [16]. Difficulty swallowing solids is a typical symptom. Weight loss and anorexia is also commonly found.

Treatment of IP is directed toward accompanying conditions and relieving symptoms. Interventions are often limited to endoscopic dilatations and care of underlying esophageal conditions, including acid suppression therapy or treatment of fungal infections. Surgical approaches are exclusively considered in rare cases and advanced stage disease. Cho et al. reported that IP symptoms were markedly improved by dilating the esophageal stricture accompanied with pseudodiverticulosis [17].

Evaluation

Zenker Diverticulum

Contrast upper tract fluoroscopy is the preferred clinical imaging (dynamic study) for diagnosis of ZD, typically with anteroposterior and lateral films. At the level of the sternoclavicular joint, a typical outpunching on the dorsal surface of the esophagus is visualized; size and position can be assessed [5, 7]. Esophagogastroduodenoscopy (EGD) may also diagnose ZD and to exclude other pathology. Computed tomography (CT) scan is also considered a valuable alternative in the evaluation process. Manometry is not useful in routine diagnosis [9] (Fig. 14.1).

Midthoracic Diverticulum

Barium swallow is an appropriate study to identify the MD. Manometry is useful to identify the cause of the diverticulum and directing therapy. However, this may be difficult to perform if there is obstruction of passage of the motility catheter by the diverticulum [3, 4]. CT scan is also useful to identify other associated esophageal or extra-esophageal abnormalities [11] (Fig. 14.2).

Epiphrenic Diverticulum

Diagnostic evaluation includes a barium swallow, upper endoscopy, CT scan, and esophageal manometry [7]. Barium swallow determines the size and demonstrates where the diverticulum is located, which has implications in the accessibility of the

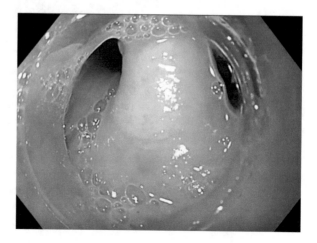

Fig. 14.1 Zenker diverticulum view in the esophagogastroduo-denoscopy

Fig. 14.2 Midthoracic
diverticulum view in
barium swallow

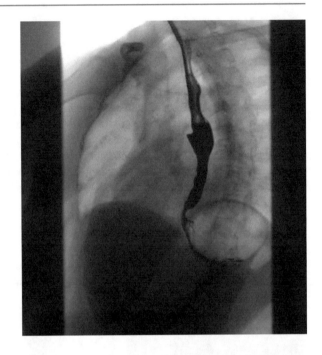

Fig. 14.3 Epiphrenic
diverticulum view in the
esophagogastroduo-
denoscopy

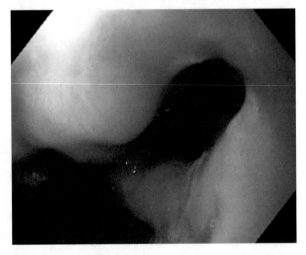

diverticulum based on surgical approach. Esophageal manometry is used to classify
the underlying motility disorder [12]. It is important to note that manometry results
may not always be abnormal. Considering the correlation between ED and esophageal dysmotility, normal manometry results should not be used to define the surgical
management of the diverticulum alone (Fig. 14.3).

Intramural Pseudodiverticulosis

IP is commonly diagnosed at the time of EGD. Endoscopic findings show evidence of pseudodiverticulae, which are numerous resembling pits in the wall, generally located in the upper esophagus [4]. Barium swallow is also used to evaluate IP [2]. The appearance is commonly flask shaped, located along the entire esophagus, and sometimes seen in longitudinal rows, parallel to the long axis of the esophagus. Due to the nature of this condition, esophageal biopsies are required. Manometry may provide information to assist in the diagnosis as IP is associated with motility disturbances [7].

Conclusions

Esophageal diverticula are rare entities in the spectrum of benign foregut diseases. Assessment includes history and radiographic imaging, endoscopy, and often complementary tests such as manometry and pH monitoring. In most cases, presence of a lesion is not, per se, an indication for intervention, and this should be weighed with patient symptoms, qualify of life, potential complications, operative risks, and availability of a local surgical expert, considering the rarity of the disease.

References

1. Sonbare DJ. Pulsion diverticulum of the oesophagus: more than just an out pouch. Indian J Surg. 2015;77(1):44–8. https://doi.org/10.1007/s12262-013-0955-8. Epub 2013 Aug 2.
2. Meyer GW, Castell DO. Evaluation and management of diseases of the esophagus. Am J Otolaryngol. 1981;2(4):336–44.
3. Lallemant Y. Esophageal diverticula. Cah Coll Med Hop Paris. 1969;10(14):1109–24.
4. Baker ME, Zuccaro G Jr, Achkar E, et al. Esophageal diverticula: patient assessment. Semin Thorac Cardiovasc Surg. 1999;11(4):326–36.
5. Costantini M, Zaninotto G, Rizzetto C, et al. Oesophageal diverticula. Best Pract Res Clin Gastroenterol. 2004;18(1):3–17.
6. do Nascimento FA, Lemme EM, Costa MM. Esophageal diverticula: pathogenesis, clinical aspects, and natural history. Dysphagia. 2006;21(3):198–205.
7. Jang KM, Lee KS, Lee SJ, et al. The spectrum of benign esophageal lesions: imaging findings. Korean J Radiol. 2002;3(3):199–210.
8. Valenza V, Perotti G, Di Giuda D, et al. Scintigraphic evaluation of Zenker's diverticulum. Eur J Nucl Med Mol Imaging. 2003;30(12):1657–64. Epub 2003 Sep 9.
9. Kumar VV, Amin MR. Evaluation of middle and distal esophageal diverticuli with transnasal esophagoscopy. Ann Otol Rhinol Laryngol. 2005;114(4):276–8.
10. Herbella FA, Dubecz A, Patti MG. Esophageal diverticula and cancer. Dis Esophagus. 2012;25(2):153–8. https://doi.org/10.1111/j.1442-2050.2011.01226.x. Epub 2011 July 21.
11. Rice TW, Baker ME. Midthoracic esophageal diverticula. Semin Thorac Cardiovasc Surg. 1999;11(4):352–7.
12. Cohen JT, Postma GN, Koufman JA. Epiphrenic diverticulum. Ear Nose Throat J. 2003;82(5):354–5.

13. Smith CD. Esophageal strictures and diverticula. Surg Clin North Am. 2015;95(3):669–81. https://doi.org/10.1016/j.suc.2015.02.017. Epub 2015 Apr 15.
14. Bagheri R, Maddah G, Mashhadi MR, et al. Esophageal diverticula: analysis of 25 cases. Asian Cardiovasc Thorac Ann. 2014;22(5):583–7. https://doi.org/10.1177/0218492313515251. Epub 2013 Dec 9.
15. Tobin RW. Esophageal rings, webs, and diverticula. J Clin Gastroenterol. 1998;27(4):285–95.
16. Thomas ML, Anthony AA, Fosh BG, et al. Oesophageal diverticula. Br J Surg. 2001;88(5):629–42.
17. Khan N, Ismail F, Van de Werke IE. Oesophageal pouches and diverticula: a pictorial review. S Afr J Surg. 2012;50(3):71–5.

Esophageal Diverticula

15

Andrew T. Strong and Jeffrey L. Ponsky

Introduction

Esophageal diverticula are outpouchings of esophageal mucosa and submucosa classified based on both anatomic location and presumed mechanism leading to their formation and enlargement. Possible locations include hypoesophageal (pharyngoesophageal), mid-esophageal, or epiphrenic. Mechanisms of formation are traction and pulsion. Traction diverticula result from pulling forces that originate external to the esophagus. Classic examples are inflammatory reactions and scar tissue formation from anterior spinal fixation and stabilization hardware or mediastinal lymphadenopathy. Pulsion diverticula result from a pushing forces created from pressurization of the esophageal lumen, with mucosa herniating through weaknesses in esophageal musculature. The most common esophageal diverticulum is widely known by its eponymous designation, a Zenker's diverticulum. A Zenker's diverticulum is a pulsion diverticulum that occurs in the posterolateral esophagus in a natural weakness located superior to the cricopharyngeus muscle and inferior to the thyropharyngeus (both are portions of the inferior constrictor muscle), known as Killian's triangle. Presentations and symptoms of esophageal diverticula vary somewhat by location within the esophagus. Diagnosis of esophageal diverticula typically follows a similar algorithm and is primarily made using barium contrast esophagrams. Hypopharyngeal diverticula will be discussed in detail, as there has been a wide array of advances in surgical approach over the past two decades and these are the most common. Other esophageal diverticula, including mid-esophageal and epiphrenic diverticula, will be discussed briefly as well. We use the term diverticulum throughout this chapter; however, most diverticula discussed are in fact

A. T. Strong · J. L. Ponsky (✉)
Digestive Disease and Surgery Institute, Cleveland Clinic, Cleveland, OH, USA

Cleveland Clinic Lerner College of Medicine of Case Western Reserve University, Cleveland, OH, USA
e-mail: ponskyj@ccf.org

pseudodiverticula, wherein the mucosa and submucosa are herniated. True diverticula of the esophagus do exist that involve all layers of the esophageal wall. However, these are quite rare and are primarily traction-type diverticula of the proximal and middle esophagus.

Incidence of Esophageal Diverticula

Hypopharyngeal diverticula are the most common diverticula of the esophagus, they and make up more than 70% of all esophageal diverticula. A prototypical patient presenting with a symptomatic hypopharyngeal diverticulum will be a male sexagenarian or septuagenarian. While presentation at a younger age is possible, hypopharyngeal diverticula noted under the age of 40 is virtually unheard of [1, 2]. Most published series report incidence of symptomatic hypopharyngeal diverticula, and as such the true prevalence including asymptomatic individuals is likely unknown. The best estimates of incidence that are published originate from England, with an estimated incidence of roughly 2 hypopharyngeal diverticula per 100,000 persons per year [1, 3]. Prior studies have noted geographic variation in terms of incidence of hypopharyngeal diverticula, which appear to occur with greater frequency in Europe, the United States, and Canada when compared to Japan and Indonesia, which may be related to variations in neck length [1, 4]. Mid-esophageal diverticula comprise 10–15% of esophageal diverticula [5]. As opposed to hypopharyngeal diverticula, mid-esophageal diverticula may arise from both pulsion and traction mechanisms, and as such may also be either pseudodiverticula or true diverticula involving all layers of the esophagus. Mid-esophageal diverticula are often related to other disorders such as mediastinal lymphadenopathy, which may be either extrinsic or intrinsic to the esophagus. Epiphrenic diverticula make up the remainder of esophageal diverticula and are quite rare. Only hundreds of epiphrenic diverticula are reported in the literature [6]. Increased use of upper endoscopy and cross-sectional imaging over the past three decades have led increased detection of smaller, asymptomatic diverticula at all levels of the esophagus.

Pathophysiology of Hypopharyngeal Diverticula

The classically described Zenker's diverticulum occurs superior to the cricopharyngeus in the previously described Killian's triangle above the cricopharyngeal muscle and inferior to the thyropharyngeus [7]. This occurs at the level of the sixth cervical vertebrae. Two other rarer types of hypopharyngeal diverticula exist. One is a herniation within the cricopharyngeus muscle where the upper oblique fibers of the cricopharyngeus diverge from the lower transverse fibers (Killian-Jamieson triangle), known as Killian's diverticulum. The second occurs at the inferior border of the cricopharyngeus and above the confluence of the longitudinal muscle fibers of the esophagus (Larimer's triangle), known as Larimer's diverticulum. All produce similar symptoms and are treated similarly. They are collectively referred to as hypopharyngeal diverticula (see Fig. 15.1).

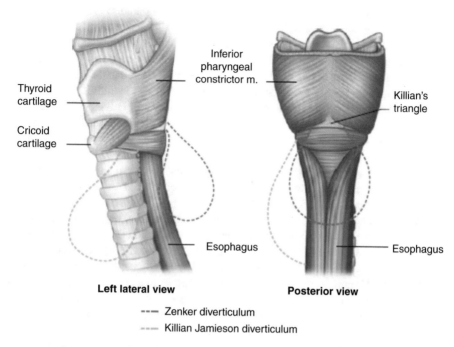

Fig. 15.1 Potential anatomic locations of hypopharyngeal diverticula in relation to musculature of the pharynx and proximal esophagus. (Reproduced from Kroh and Reavis [134]; Fig. 18.1)

The etiologic origin of hypopharyngeal diverticula has been a matter of debate since it was first described by Zenker as a pulsion diverticulum. Specifically, it was unclear if there was an antecedent disorder of coordination, muscle tone, or compliance that initiated the process of diverticulization through over pressurization of the hypopharyngeal region. Contemporary understanding is derived from both video-fluorometric and manometric studies and focus on two abnormalities: anatomic weakness of the muscles of the posterior pharynx adjacent to the upper esophageal sphincter, and/or muscular dysfunction of the upper esophageal sphincter. The best evidence comes from studies published in the early 1990s where a 6 cm sleeve catheter for manometry with concurrent videofluorometric recording was performed in patients with symptomatic hypopharyngeal diverticula [8, 9]. The experiments showed that there was full manometric relaxation realized by the upper esophageal sphincter, as defined by the hypopharyngeal wall losing contact with the recording catheter. However, videofluorimetry revealed that relaxation was incomplete, and specifically was reduced in comparison to controls. This resulted in increased pressure through the segment as a food bolus passed, which was termed intrabolus pressure [8, 9]. Thus, incomplete relaxation of the upper esophageal sphincter led to increased hypopharyngeal pressurization, in particular in response to food bolus. Histologic studies and muscle contractility studies of the cricopharyngeus offer additional supporting evidence for this theory [10]. Compared to normal controls, patients with hypopharyngeal diverticula have slower and weaker muscular contraction with delayed relaxation of the cricopharyngeus. This is partially related to more predominate type 1 muscle fibers [10]. Enzymatic function studies of histologic sections have demonstrated decreased acetylcholinesterase and fewer neurofilaments, suggesting denervation may play a role as well [10]. In addition, histologic samples of the cervical mucosa show an increase in overall collagen fibers and a decrease in elastin content in the muscularis mucosa of the cervical esophagus, which may indicate that the mucosa is also less compliant [11]. Worth noting for these studies, however, is that the majority have been performed in patients that have already developed symptomatic hypopharyngeal diverticula, thus it is difficult to determine if noted changes were present and contributed to the formation of diverticula, or occured secondarily after development of the diverticulum. While it is most likely that a constellation of neuromuscular and histological changes must exist to initiate the pathologic process leading to formation of a hypopharyngeal diverticulum, a unifying theory does not yet exist. The ideal study to discover that condition once would have to obtain functional studies, dynamic anatomic studies, and histological samples from the hypopharynx and its associated musculature and regular time points from a population with normal baseline structure and function of their inferior pharynx and proximal esophagus, following by *post hoc* analysis to compare those that eventually developed diverticula to those that did not. It is unlikely, however, that a study of that nature could be feasibly accomplished.

Theories of impaired musculature relaxation and discoordination do not stand opposed to complementary theories that anatomic variations may also contribute. The hypopharynx has an inherent defect that behaves as a natural point of weakness occurring between the oblique fibers of the thyropharyngeus and the horizontal fibers of the cricopharyngeus, also known as Killian's triangle. Jos van Overbeek proposed individuals with longer necks may have a larger Killian's triangle. This may also explain regional variations in incidence, as individuals from Western countries, where hypopharyngeal diverticula are more common, tend to have both longer necks and a longer pharynx [4]. However, this has not been supported by anatomic studies [12].

More recent technological advances shine new light on this subjection. The advent of high-resolution video manometry has led to new classification schema for motility disorders of the esophagus. High-resolution manometry studies detailing the pharyngeal phase of swallowing are currently limited; however, comparison between patients with hypopharyngeal diverticula and normal controls may better elucidate and/or classify the nature of motility disorders associated with hypopharyngeal diverticula. Impedance planimetry may also offer new insight. Impedance planimetry uses an electrode area on a catheter surrounded by a balloon containing a conductive fluid. Signal processing is able to use the change the minor alteration in the electric field produced by the changes in the balloon diameter to reconstruct a profile of the upper esophageal sphincter. Measures of esophageal distensibility, diameter, relaxation time, and pressure may be determined within the upper esophageal sphincter [8, 13, 14].

Symptoms of Hypopharyngeal Diverticula

The predominant symptom of hypopharyngeal diverticula is progressive dysphagia, which is present the vast majority of patients. There are two mechanisms that may underlie dysphagia. The first is the aforementioned impaired relaxation of the upper esophageal sphincter. The second is an effect of content of a food bolus preferentially filling the diverticulum, impeding distension of the esophageal lumen by mass effect. Filling of the diverticulum may also distort the esophagus, as the weight of the contents of diverticulum causes traction and angulation of the esophagus. In addition to dysphagia, regurgitation of undigested food even hours after ingestion may occur. There are numerous reports of pills being found within hypopharyngeal diverticula at the time of operative intervention, which would reduce the efficacy of medications, since they are undigested. Other symptoms include halitosis, belching, cervical borborygmi, globus pharyngeus, and recurrent respiratory infections from unprovoked aspiration events. Boyce's sign is a physical exam finding of a gurgling mass present in the lateral neck, which, while rare, is pathognomonic for hypopharyngeal diverticula.

Diagnosis of Hypopharyngeal Diverticula

When symptoms are present, diagnosis of hypopharyngeal diverticulum is typically made by barium esophagography (see Fig. 15.2). In most cases flexible endoscopic evaluation is also pursued to rule out other causes for dysphagia, in particular neoplasm (see Fig. 15.3). Given the increased use of both endoscopic investigations and cross-sectional imaging, there is a proportion of hypopharyngeal diverticula that are discovered incidentally in asymptomatic individuals. Diverticula vary in size, and presumably grow slowly over time. Measures of diverticular size from the operating room correlated well with radiographic studies, but do not correlated well with dimensions determined endoscopically [15]. A number of authors have attempted to classify hypopharyngeal diverticula in terms of size and presumed disease severity [7]. These are summarized in Table 15.1, though their utility in a clinical setting is relatively limited.

Fig. 15.2 Lateral view of the neck obtained from a barium esophagram demonstrating a typical appearance of a hypopharyngeal diverticulum. The inset depicts where size of the diverticulum is measured radiographically

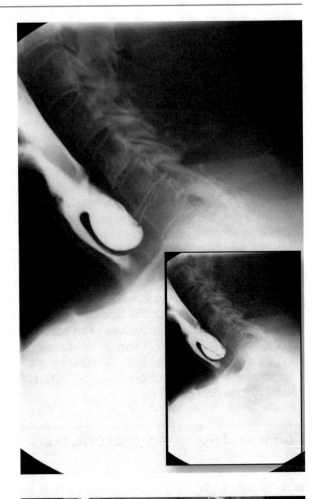

Fig. 15.3 Endoscopic view of a hypopharyngeal diverticulum. In this image, an endoscopic cap has been attached to the end of the endoscope. The esophageal lumen (E) appears on the left of the image, and the diverticulum (D) on the right, separated by the common wall or septum, which contains the cricopharyngeus muscle

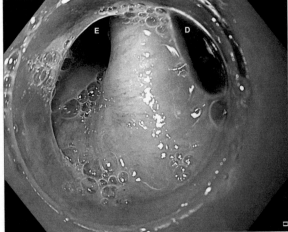

Table 15.1 Classification systems for Zenker's diverticulum

Author/year	Basis	Stage 1	Stage 2	Stage 3	Stage 4
Lahey/1930	Appearance only	Small mucosal propulsion with *spherical shape*	*Pear* shape	*Glove-fingered shape*	(No stage 4)
Brombart and Monges/1964	Appearance/ size and phase of deglutition	*Thorn-like* diverticulum (2–3 mm) visible only during contraction phase of upper esophageal sphincter	*Club-like* diverticulum (7–8 mm) visible only during contraction phase of the upper esophageal sphincter	*Bar-shaped* diverticulum (>1 cm in length) without esophageal compression	Compression of the esophagus with ventral displacement
Morton and Bartley/1993	Size	<2 cm	2–4 cm	>4 cm	(No stage 4)
Van Overbeck and Groote/1994	Size	One vertebral body	One to three vertebral bodies	More than three vertebral bodies	(No stage 4)

Notes: Adapted from Scher and Puscas [7]

Treatment of Hypopharyngeal Diverticula and Defining Treatment Success

Surgical treatment of hypopharyngeal diverticula is generally reserved for individuals with symptoms. Both open transcervical and transoral options exist to treat hypopharyngeal diverticula, with the best outcomes for smaller diverticula. Increases in the use of cross-sectional imaging and endoscopy have increased the diagnosis of small diverticula that are asymptomatic. While these do not warrant surgical repair when asymptomatic, patients should be followed to expedite repair early, when diverticula are smaller and result in less severe complications. In most studies, the primary outcome has been resolution of symptoms, as this is the most clinically meaningful outcome. However, metrics to track this quantitatively or semiquantitatively are varied by study. There are a number of scoring systems that have been validated that assess severity of dysphagia and degrees of dysfunction. A full review of these scoring systems is outside the scope of this chapter, and they are of greatest utility in the research setting. In general, with current surgical techniques, greater than 95% of patients should expect to garner symptomatic relief after surgical intervention, though durability of symptom resolution will vary.

Recurrence may be defined based on symptoms or radiography. However, similar to paraesophageal hernia, radiographic evidence of recurrence may not correlate with symptomatic recurrence. The authors advise caution when interpreting studies that quote recurrence rates, as they are a function of both follow-up time and the definition used to define recurrence in that particular manuscript. This is particularly important in the literature that has emerged using flexible endoscopic techniques in the past decade, as some patients undergo "multiple sessions" of endoscopic intervention in a short time frame, with the recurrence quoted as the recurrence from the time of full symptom resolution to relapse, as opposed to the first intervention. Also, given that there may be underlying an esophageal motility disorder in conjunction with hypopharyngeal diverticula, some recurrence of symptoms may be attributable to dysmotility and not the presence of a new or recurrent diverticulum.

Historical Perspectives on Surgical Management of Hypopharyngeal Diverticula

An investigation into the management of hypopharyngeal diverticulum includes a history of surgical innovation and ingenuity spanning more than a century. Both open and transoral techniques have been developed and will be detailed. Given the rarity of this condition, the bulk of the accumulated evidence is comprised of case series and retrospective comparison studies. The evidence that is summarized below demonstrates that there is a tremendous heterogeneity in techniques and devices employed both historically and contemporarily. While the past two decades have seen new application of a flexible endoscope, surgical treatment of hypopharyngeal must simultaneously address two separate issues: division of cricopharyngeus muscle to decrease pharyngeal pressurization and eliminating the ability of the pouch to fill. The latter may be accomplished either by resection, inversion, suspension, or elimination of the common wall shared by the diverticulum and esophagus.

Open Surgical Approaches for Hypopharyngeal Diverticula

Open Hypopharyngeal Diverticulectomy

Some of the earliest descriptions of surgical therapy for hypopharyngeal diverticula came in 1830, with a description by Bell (of Bell's palsy fame). The described technique was the surgical creation of a diverticulocutaneous fistula [12]. The first recorded attempt at this surgical technique came in 1877, and resulted in the patient's death [12]. The following decade saw the first attempts at surgical resection through a left lateral neck incision, which again resulted in the patient's death from mediastinal sepsis [12]. Early series of single stage diverticulectomy and esophageal closure were beset by frequent, and often fatal mediastinal sepsis [16]. One of the earliest publications on the surgical treatment of hypopharyngeal diverticula that was published in 1910 included 60 patients from multiple centers and prior publication. The pooled mortality rate reported in that manuscript was 16.6%, with numerous additional complications including bleeding, pneumonia, recurrent laryngeal nerve paralysis, and esophageal stricture [12]. While tragic, these early publications were part of what spurned later innovation, in a century-long drive toward safer operative approaches.

The first innovation, which became the most widely accepted in the early twentieth century was a two-stage approach, introduced by Goldmann in 1909, and practiced and promoted by Charles Mayo and Frank Lahey [12, 17]. In the first stage, a lateral neck incision was made over the anterior border of the sternocleidomastoid, and the diverticulum completely dissected from its surrounding attachments, but not divided. The mobilized diverticulum was then temporarily suspended within the deeper layers of the surgical wound, which was then closed. Patients remained in the hospital for 7–10 days, until the second stage operation was performed 7–10 days later. The same incision was reopened and the neck of the diverticulum ligated and divided, and the esophagus closed. The proposed advantage of this technique was that fascial planes contiguous between the neck and the mediastinum would be obliterated at the time of the second operation, preventing mediastinitis as a consequence of esophageal leak, relegating it rather to the surgical space in the neck where drainage was simpler and complications were decreased [16, 18]. A single stage transcervical approach to hypopharyngeal diverticulectomy was popularized later especially after publications by Sweet in 1956 [19, 20] and Payne [21] in that showed a similar profile of complications compared to the two stage diverticulectomy [17]. However, it should be noted that these series with single stage diverticulectomy were largely performed in the era where antibiotics were more readily available, arming the surgeon with more than scalpel and a drain to treat mediastinal sepsis, and leading to better outcomes [16]. Open, transcervical diverticulectomy continues to be a viable option for operative management of symptomatic hypopharyngeal diverticula, though typically when other approaches are nonfeasible.

Open Hypopharyngeal Diverticulopexy

Schmid proposed diverticulopexy alone as a treatment option in 1912. In this technique, the diverticulum was approached from an identical left lateral neck incision. After complete dissection of the diverticulum, permanent sutures secured the fundus to the prevertebral fascia, inverting the diverticulum, and positioning the fundus cephalad to diverticular neck. This configuration both allows dependent drainage of any accumulated food and inhibits accumulation of new debris [17]. Importantly, diverticulopexy avoided violation of the mucosa and resultant esophageal leak [16]. However, in some patients this leads to a caudally extending diverticulum [16, 17]. Diverticulopexy was later incorporated into combination procedures, but is no longer acceptable as a standalone surgical therapy.

Open Hypopharyngeal Diverticular Invagination

Invagination of a hypopharyngeal diverticulum was reported in 1896 by Girard [16, 17]. In this technique, the diverticulum was approached trough a lateral neck incision and completely dissection. To avoid violation of the mucosa, the fundus of the diverticulum was pushed though the diverticular neck and inverted into the esophageal lumen. The muscular defect was then oversewn. A high recurrence rate made this therapy nonviable, and it is rarely used in clinical practice.

Open Cricopharyngeal Myotomy

Better understanding of role that the cricopharyngeal muscle, including both spasm and impaired relaxation, has in the development of hypopharyngeal diverticula led to a new phase in open surgical management and helped to lay the surgical framework that later supported endoscopic approaches. Cricopharyngeal myotomy was first reported in 1958 by Harrison [17, 22]. Sutherland followed this report in 1962, with an accompanying proposal that myotomy alone may be effective therapy for small diverticula and that resection or inversion of the diverticulum was not necessary [17, 23]. Belsey demonstrated complete radiographic resolution of small diverticula after cricopharyngeal myotomy alone [24]. Several other series that mainly included small hypopharyngeal diverticula noted that cricopharyngeal myotomy was efficacious in reducing symptoms, without addressing the diverticulum itself. Cricopharyngeal myotomy was performed through a lateral neck incision as well, but, because it avoids the extensive dissection that leads to the more severe complications (recurrent laryngeal nerve injury, esophageal leak), there was significantly less morbidity compared to diverticulectomy. However, in a series that included patients with larger pouches, cricopharyngeal myotomy alone failed to resolve symptoms, likely because some of the symptoms were directly derived from the presence of a large pouch and not the underlying dysmotility. Later studies evaluated the influence of the myotomy length on efficacy and duration of symptomatic relief. Lerut *et al* advocated a 5 cm myotomy based on histologic analysis suggesting muscular abnormalities extended beyond the cricopharyngeus to the esophagus itself among patients with hypopharyngeal diverticula [25]. Using intraoperative manometry, Pera and colleagues demonstrated that esophageal pressurization was significantly reduced after cricopharyngeal myotomy. They additionally demonstrated that extending the myotomy 2 cm further into the hypopharyngeus led to an even greater reduction in esophageal pressurization [26].

Open Combination Procedures: Cricopharyngeal Myotomy with Other Open Techniques

Current understanding supports the notion that symptoms may arise from either the pouch or from the pharyngeal constriction and pressurization from a hypertonic or dysfunctional cricopharyngeus muscle. Simultaneously addressing both the cricopharyngeus and the pouch had guided surgical thought for the past six decades. Reports of both cricopharyngeal myotomy in combination with both diverticulectomy and diverticulopexy were published from several centers beginning in the 1960s. Interestingly, the addition of cricopharyngeal myotomy to transcervical diverticulectomy actually reduced complications, likely because the decreased pressurization of the pharynx did not promote esophageal leaks [16].

There is little comparative literature with regard to open techniques to treat hypopharyngeal diverticula and no randomized trails. However, taken altogether, the literature best supports myotomy alone from pouches <1 cm. Moderate-sized pouches may be treated with combination of cricopharyngeal myotomy and diverticulopexy, while large pouches are best suited with cricopharyngeal myotomy and diverticulectomy if an open technique is pursued [16]. For patients with large pouches, but significant comorbid disease, cricopharyngeal myotomy, and diverticulopexy may be entertained as an option as it may avoid mucosal breach and resultant risk of complications related to diverticulectomy [17]. However, as discussed below, there are currently other, less invasive options that exist, provided the surgeon has experience with these techniques.

Transoral Surgical Approaches for Hypopharyngeal Diverticula

Primarily in an attempt to reduce morbidity and mortality associated with open approaches, surgeons have sought less invasive therapeutic options. Literature published regarding these techniques is highly varied, and suffers from a terminology that has co-evolved with technology. The term endoscopic is frequently used; however, this may refer to an esophagoscope, a rigid diverticuloscope (Weerda-scope), or a flexible endoscope, among others. We have chosen to refer to all these techniques collectively as transoral approaches and divide between rigid and flexible devices. Rigid or fixed devices are traditionally used to position the head and neck and/or provide a conduit to visualize the hypopharynx or diverticulum directly. Flexible endoscopic approaches use a flexible bronchoscope or endoscope more typically used for gastrointestinal endoscopy, where the effector end of the scope is manipulated by hand controls, and the device integrates a channel or channels through which instruments may be introduced. The majority of literature on transoral techniques is retrospective series typically of single centers. Where comparative literature does exist, it is in comparison to open surgical approaches. Comparisons between two or more transoral techniques are generally lacking.

Transoral Hypopharyngeal Diverticulotomy

The first report of a transoral therapy for a hypopharyngeal diverticulum was made in 1917 by Mosher [27]. Using esophagoscopic visualization, he described dividing the common wall between the esophagus and the diverticulum using a scissor punch [12]. However, as the base of the divided wall was unable to be sealed, the risk of leak increased. Unfortunately leaks almost certainly lead to mediastinitis, which proved to be a fatal complication in one of his first patients. As a result, he abandoned the technique. The technique of dividing the common wall, almost certainly accomplished a cricopharyngeal myotomy, a fact that was only recognized in hindsight as the cricopharyngeal myotomy was developed and studied in the open technique.

Before discussing further transoral therapies, we would be remiss to not mention the contributions of Chevalier Jackson on this field. His report in 1915 was the first use of an esophagoscope to aid in diverticulopexy [28, 29]. While his manuscripts did more to support a one-stage approach to transcervical diverticulectomy, he was one of the first surgeons to utilize an endoscope intra-operatively as a tool to facilitate identification of anatomy and to complete an open operation. He used an endoscope to first visualize the diverticulum, then to clear the pouch of its food debris. Advancing the esophagoscope into the pouch, he capitalized on transillumination of the pouch to identify the pouch externally. Then, following resection the endoscope was advanced into the esophageal lumen and the closure performed around the endoscope to ensure the lumen was not narrowed [12]. While it would be difficult to confirm whether this was the first instance of endoscopic assistance for open surgery, it is worth noted that this technique elegantly mirrors contemporary use of a flexible endoscope to perform multiple intraoperative functions.

Transoral Hypopharyngeal Diverticulotomy with Thermal Devices

The next major advance in transoral therapy for hypopharyngeal diverticula was in 1960, by Dohlman and Mattsson. In a report of 100 patients, they described using a modified rigid esophagoscope (Weerda-scope®, Karl Storz, Fig. 15.4) to visualize a hypopharyngeal diverticulum and the common wall, similar to that described by Chevalier Jackson). Dohlman's advance in terms of technique over that of Mosher was the use of electrocautery to complete the division of the common wall [30]. Based on his own prior radiographic studies, this work both described the importance of the cricopharyngeus muscle and properly described the endoscopic division of this muscle. The series described the "endoscopic esophagodiverticulostomy" included no cases of mediastinitis and a recurrence rate of 7%, which was noteworthy for the time. Additionally, the assertion was made that in the setting of a recurrent diverticulum previously treated with a transoral approach, a transoral reoperation was likely to be considerably easier than repeating an open surgical approach, where natural planes would be obscured [10, 12].

In the subsequent three decades, a number of authors offered improvements on the Dohlman diverticulotomy technique, using a variety of instruments and new thermal technologies to divide the common wall shared between the diverticulum and esophagus, with division of the cricopharyngeus muscle. This included additional centers reporting us of laparoscopy scissors connected to an electrosurgical unit [31, 32]. In the late 1990s, Lippert introduced a microendoscopic approach using a CO_2 laser to divide the mucosa and the cricopharyngeus muscle contained within the common wall [33, 34]. Results were similar; however, electrocautery was still needed often to seal the distal dissection flaps or any mediastinal opening.

Fig. 15.4 Rigid distracting diverticuloscope, without attached stabilization arm (Weerda® scope, Karl Storz). (Reproduced from Kroh and Reavis [134]; Fig. 18.3)

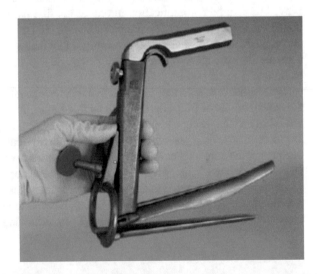

Another laser (KTP/532 nm) was also adapted in a similar technique by other authors [35]. Taken together, each of these authors used a thermal energy device to expose and divide the diverticular septum and seal the exposed edges. These reports were generally associated with short hospital stays, more rapid resumption of diet, and similar efficacy to trans-cervical surgery. There were more risks of mediastinitis using thermal devices for transoral diverticulotomy, though this was typically less severe than mediastinitis associated with open approaches likely because the defects were small. Mediastinitis after these transoral approaches more often responded to medical therapy alone. Moreover, the risk of recurrent laryngeal nerve injury is decreased with transoral approaches over that of transcervical approaches. The lack of widespread use of laser technology in general limited more general use of those techniques. There was also a general sense among most surgeons treating hypopharyngeal diverticula that the lack of mechanical device to seal the edges increased the risk of mediastinitis and thus "suture-less endoscopic esophagodiverticulostomy" fell out of favor [10].

Transoral Stapled Hypopharyngeal Diverticulotomy

The next major advance in transoral approach to hypopharyngeal diverticula was the use of a stapling device to both divide and seal the common wall between the diverticulum and the esophagus, in conjunction with the cricopharyngeus muscle contained therein. The first of these reports was by Collard and colleagues in 1993 [36], in a contemporary patient cohort to those advocating microendoscopic laser-based approaches. Collard and colleagues modified a rigid transoral diverticuloscope to have narrower lips. They introduced a 12 mm diameter laparoscopic gastrointestinal stapler (30 mm cartridge length) through the diverticuloscope and then use a 5 mm endoscopic camera to verify position prior to firing the stapler (see Fig. 15.5) [36]. They also point out that the divided cricopharyngeus muscle, since it is sealed by the overlying stapled mucosa, provides lateral retraction to the cut edges, creating a wide opening between the diverticulum and the esophagus [36]. Their report included 6 patients, 5 of who had complete resolution of dysphagia and

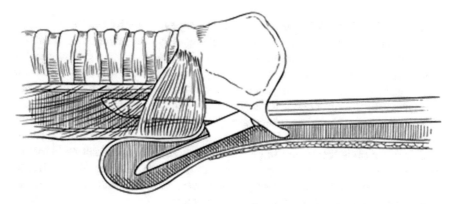

Fig. 15.5 Position of laparoscopic linear stapler/cutter in trans-oral stapled diverticulotomy. Image shown without the accompanying rigid diverticuloscope. (Reproduced from Fisichella and Patti [135]; Fig. 11.5)

the last was improved. Numerous additional publications replicated these results using very similar techniques [37–52]. One of the challenges of this technique is that the stapling devices have a small portion at the tip, beyond the cut line, which results in a small residual septum. To overcome this, some authors modify the stapler by filing down the end of the anvil to ensure the staple line reaches as far into the diverticulum as possible [36]. Several authors also report placement of temporary traction sutures at either end of the septum to aid in pulling the septum into the stapler jaw and positioning it appropriately. The largest study included a total of 585 patients who were culled from previously published literature between 1995 and 2010 (534 patients) and 51 patients retrospectively identified at the study center (1999–2011) [53]. There were 92.3% of attempted transoral stapling procedures completed, in a mean 22 minutes. Of those with completed operations, 91% reported improved symptoms. Most aborted procedures were due to small diverticula (<3 cm), or inability to adequately extend the neck to position the diverticuloscope. Complications occurred in a total of 9.6% of patients, though most were minor [53]. The most common complication was iatrogenic perforation ($n = 26$, 4.8%), and most complications were managed with medical therapy alone. There was one death included in that study (0.2%). Recurrence of symptoms was estimated to be 12.8% [53]. However, they stated that restapling with a transoral approach for recurrence can be accomplished with little additional risk compared to index stapling procedures [16, 54]. Similar results to this study were noted in a in a recent systematic review [55]. Transoral stapling may be difficult in patients with diverticula that are small (<2 cm) as the stapler may not be able to engage the short septum, or very large diverticulum, where the stapler may not be able to reach the furthest extent of the common septum [16]. For larger diverticula, more than one staple cartridge may be necessary and are allowable [43]. Patient satisfaction is noted to be higher among patients undergoing transoral stapled diverticulotomy compared to open techniques, though this is likely related to decreased pain, shorter hospitalization and generally shorter convalescent period [16]. Overall, transoral stapled diverticulotomy is likely the most widely practiced transoral technique to treat hypopharyngeal diverticula and is likely the first-line operation practiced at most centers.

Transoral Flexible Endoscopic Hypopharyngeal Diverticulotomy

A major limitation to the rigid transoral techniques is that they are dependent on using a rigid device to visualize the diverticulum and septum. The rigid diverticuloscope functions in a linear fashion, demanding that the neck be extended, to allow a direct line of visualization to the junction between the hypopharynx and the esophagus. Osteoarthritis, prior cervical disk fusion, or kyphosis, which is common in the population among whom hypopharyngeal diverticula are more prevalent, may limit neck extension such that a rigid scope cannot be properly positioned. Advances in flexible endoscopic techniques in general, largely afforded by advances in instrumentation, have led to new approaches to treat hypopharyngeal diverticula. Figure 15.6 depicts barium esophagograms obtained before and after a flexible endoscopic transoral hypopharyngeal diverticulotomy.

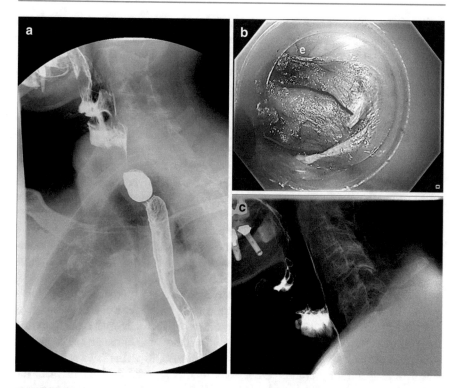

Fig. 15.6 (**a**) A lateral view of the neck obtained from a barium esophagram demonstrating a hypopharyngeal diverticulum filling with contrast. This image was obtained prior to a flexible endoscopic transoral diverticulotomy. (**b**) An endoscopic view of the cricopharyngeus muscle from a submucosal tunnel. The red line outlines the edges of the muscle, "e" marks the true lumen of the esophagus. (**c**) Lateral view of the neck obtained from a barium esophagram after a flexible endoscopic transoral diverticulotomy demonstrates that contrast enters the persistent pouch but is still able to empty freely into the esophagus

While the first description of a flexible endoscopic approach to treatment of hypopharyngeal diverticulum was made in 1982 [56], the first case series with follow-up data available were not made until 1995, with reports from two centers using similar techniques [57, 58]. Ishioka and colleagues utilized a needle knife to perform mucosal incision and myotomy, while Mulder and colleagues reported using monopolar coagulation forceps. Both techniques utilize an electrosurgical instrument to both divide and seal the common wall shared between the esophagus and the diverticulum, as well as the underlying cricopharyngeus muscle [57, 58]. In these series, complications were rare and success rates were high in terms of short-term symptomatic relief. However, there were patients included in those (and subsequent) series that needed multiple endoscopic sessions, wherein partial division was accomplished, and then symptoms evaluated. If symptoms persisted, a subsequent endoscopic session was scheduled for further division, separated by at least 1 day [57–59]. While there may be some theoretical advantage in titrating the extent of division to the minimum possible to produce symptomatic relief, this is likely offset by the need for multiple rounds of sedation/anesthesia and its associated risks. These early reports were followed by other series utilizing other endoscopic devices, including argon plasma coagulation [59, 60], hook knife [61, 62], and more recently knifes that were developed for endoscopic mucosal resection and endoscopic submucosal dissection, including the Dualknife™ [63], insulated tip knife [64], and the stag beetle knife [65, 66]. Various assistive devices have been reported as well, including endoscopic caps [61, 67, 68] and endoscopic clips to seal mucosal edges, or the inferior extent of resection. However, the most commonly mentioned device is a flexible diverticuloscope (see Fig. 15.7) [63–66, 69, 70]. Most studies that utilize a flexible diverticuloscope originate from centers in Europe, where commercial devices are more readily available [71]. Other centers have reported modifying the end of endoscopic overtubes to resemble a flexible diverticuloscope. The purpose of the flexible diverticuloscope, which is introduced over the endoscope, is to isolate and stabilize the septum during division. A summary of early manuscripts, endoscopic devices, complications, and reported outcomes is given in Table 15.2.

One of the reported advantages of flexible endoscopic approaches to hypopharyngeal diverticula is that they may be performed without general anesthesia. As is well stated in an anecdote in an editorial by Sakai, "...open surgery has been advised for patients at excessive surgical risk...[however] the same rationale has been used to suggest the opposite, namely flexible endoscopy" [56]. That is to say, patients with severe respiratory comorbidities, such that it may be difficult to wean the patient from intraprocedural mechanical ventilation, may be better suited to a flexible endoscopic approach. This is an inversion of conventional thought, where open

Fig. 15.7 (**a**) This part depicts a flexible diverticuloscope (ZD Overtuube, Cook Endoscopy); (**b**) The septum or common wall of a hypopharyngeal diverticulum and the esophagus, visualized and stabilized by a flexible diverticuloscope. (Reproduced [136] from Kroh and Reavis [134]; Fig. 18.5)

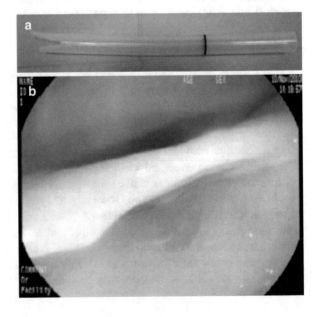

Table 15.2 Summary of nontunneled flexible endoscopic procedures for hypopharyngeal diverticula

Authors; country	Publication year	Study subjects	Age in years, (range, if reported)	Device for myotomy; accessory devices	Size of diverticulum	Single/multiple procedures	Adverse events	Symptom resolution	Follow-up duration (range if reported)	Recurrences
Ishioka et al.; [57] Brazil	1995	42	Mean 68.4 (46–102)	Needle knife	NR	Multiple (1–5)	2 (4.8%): 1 subcutaneous emphysema; 1 hemorrhage	100%	38 months	7.1%
Mulder et al.; [58] The Netherlands	1995	20	Mean 82.3 (64–88)	Coagulation forceps	5.65 cm (1–12)	Multiple (1–12)	0 (0%)	100%	Mean 6.7 months (1–18)	0%
Hashiba et al.; [72] Brazil	1999	47	(51–81)	Needle knife	Mean 4.1 cm (2–7)	Multiple (1–4)	7 (14.8%) 1 hemorrhage; 5 limited subcutaneous emphysema; 1 conspicuous subcutaneous emphysema	96%	(0–12)	NR
Mulder; [59] The Netherlands	1999	125	Median 77 (41–100	Argon plasma coagulation	Mean 4.5 cm (1–12)	Multiple (1–12)	24 (19.2%): 17 subcutaneous emphysema; 5 mediastinal emphysema; 2 bleeding	NR	NR	NR
Sakai et al.; [73] Brazil	2001	10	(67–87)	Needle knife Endoscopic cap	NR	Single	None	100%	(2–12)	0%

(continued)

Table 15.2 (continued)

Authors; country	Publication year	Study subjects	Age in years, (range, if reported)	Device for myotomy; accessory devices	Size of diverticulum	Single/ multiple procedures	Adverse events	Symptom resolution	Follow-up duration (range if reported)	Recurrences
Christiaens et al.; [74] Belgium	2007	21	Mean 77.5 ± 9.7)	Coagulation forceps Endoscopic cap	NR	Multiple (1–2)	1 (4.7%) cervical emphysema	100%	Median 22.6 months	0%
Evrard et al.; [75] Belgium	2003	30	Median 78 (57–93)	Needle knife Diverticuloscope	4 cm (2–6)	Single	4 (13.3%); 3 minor bleeding; 2 pneumonia; 1 subcutaneous emphysema; 1 perforation with mediastinitis and sepsis	96%	Median 12.5 months (3–34)	1 (3.3%)
Rabenstein et al.; [60] Germany	2006	41	Mean 73 ± 11	Argon plasma coagulator Endoscopic cap	NR	Multiple (1–3)	8 (19.5%): 7 fever; 1 perforation with mediastinitis	95.1%	Mean 16 months (6–43)	14.7%
Costamagna et al. (a); [67] Italy	2007	28	Median 66 (47–86)	Needle knife Endoscopic cap	4 cm (2–8 cm)	Single	9 (32%) overall: 9 (32%) cap assisted; 4 bleeding, 2 microscopic perforations, 3 macroscopic perforations	43%	Mean 39 months (9–60)	14%
Costamagna et al. (b); [7] Italy	2007	11	Median 70 (63–84)	Needle knife Diverticuloscope	NR	NR	0	91%	mean 6.5 months (3–15)	9%

Vogelsang et al.; [68] Germany	2006	31	Median 69 (52–92)	Needle knife Endoscopic cap	3.7 ± 1.3 cm	Multiple (1–3)	7 (22.6%); 1 moderate bleeding; 7 mediastinal/ cervical emphysema	84%	Mean 26 months (14–29)	NR
Al-Kadi et al.; [76] Canada	2010	18	Mean 80 (68–91)	Needle knife	NR	Single	4 (22.2%) 1 perforation; 3 minor bleeding	87.5%	Mean 27.5 months (0.5–84)	11.1%
Case and Baron; [77] USA[7]	2010	22	Median 84.5 (59–96)	Needle knife	NR	Single	8 (36.4%); 5 bleeding; 6 perforation	100%	Mean 12.7 months	31.8%
Repici et al.; [61] Italy	2010	32	74.8 (58–92)	Hook knife Endoscopic cap	NR	Single	2 (6.2%): 1 bleeding; 1 mediastinal emphysema	28 (87.5%)	Mean 23.9 months (12–48)	6.2%
Huberty et al.; [69] Belgium	2012	150	73 (42–94)	Needle knife Diverticuloscope, endoscopic clips	Median 3 cm (range 1–8)	Single	4 (2.2%) 3 fever; 1 pneumonia	90.3%	Median 43 months (13–121)	23.1%
Manno et al.; [64] Italy	2014	19	median 74 (46–84)	Insulated tip knife Diverticuloscope	Median 4.2 cm (range 3.0–5.5)	Single	0	100%	Median 27 months (3–48)	10.5%
Laquière et al.; [63] France	2014	42	Mean 74.5	Hybrid knife /dual knife Diverticuloscope	Median 3.5 cm	Multiple (1–3)	8 (19%) 5 bleeding; 3 fever	88.1%	16 months for all patients	14.2%
Battaglia et al.; [65] Italy	2015	31	Median 71 (52–85)	Stag beetle knife, endoscopic snare; diverticuloscope; endoscopic clips	3 cm (1–8)	Multiple	1 (3.2%); 1 late onset bleeding	90.3%	Median 7 months (2–18)	6.5%

(continued)

Table 15.2 (continued)

Authors; country	Publication year	Study subjects	Age in years, (range, if reported)	Device for myotomy; accessory devices	Size of diverticulum	Single/multiple procedures	Adverse events	Symptom resolution	Follow-up duration (range if reported)	Recurrences
Antonello et al., (a) [66] Italy	2015	34 treatment naïve patients	Median 71 (48–88)	Needle knife/hook knife/stag beetle knife; diverticuloscope, endoscopic clips	2 cm (1.0–5.4);	Multiple	3; (8.8%): 1 perforation, 2 moderate bleeding	82.3%	Median 18 months (6–50)	14.7%
Antonello et al., (b) [66] Italy	2015	25 relapsing patients	Median 68 (48–85)	Needle knife/hook knife/stag beetle knife; diverticuloscope, endoscopic clips	2.2 cm (1.0–4.4)	Multiple	2 (8%): 1 microperforation, 1 bleeding	84%	Median 18 (6–58)	24%
Costamagna et al.; [70] Italy	2016	89	Mean 70 ± 10	Needle knife Diverticuloscope	NR	Single	3 (3.3%): 1 bleeding, 2 perforations	71 (85.5%)	Median 32 months (1–98)	15%
Halland et al., [78] USA	2016	52	median 77 (34–97)	Needle knife/hook knife	Mean 2.8 cm (1–5)	Single	11 (21%) 10 microperforation; 1 perforation needing stent 1 neck abscess	100%	Median 21 months (0.5–68)	26.9%
Pescarus et al.; [79] Canada	2016	26	Mean 74.9 (47.3–96.7)	Needle knife/hook knife	2.8 cm (1–5)	Single	1 (3.8%): 1 perforation	100%	Median 21 months (1–68.2)	0
Rouquette et al.; [62]	2017	24	Median 77 (44–90)	Hook knife Diverticuloscope	Mena 3.0 cm (2–8)	Multiple (1–3)	2 (8.3%)	91.7%	Median 19.5 months (6–53)	12.5%

Adapted and modified from [55, 80, 81]

Abbreviations: *NR* not reported, *cm* centimeter

transcervical approaches were the most conservative, and reserved for higher risk individuals. Many of the early reports of flexible endoscopic approaches reported use of conscious sedation [57, 58, 60, 72, 74]. This was likely largely driven by provider comfort, in that most authors were endoscopists and were comfortable performing similar procedures under conscious sedation. However, later series used intubation and general anesthesia, and or allowed for selective use of general anesthesia. Procedure times are on the order of 15–25 minutes in most series reporting outcome of flexible endoscopic approaches.

Most published techniques, including all those in the Table 15.2, employ a single incision technique, in which a single liner cut is made from the septum toward the base of the diverticulum. This maneuver replicates the division accomplished via rigid transoral endoscopic stapling. There have been recent publications that have advanced that approach to a two-incision approach, where two parallel incisions are made 1 cm apart and continued to the base of the diverticulum, with the distal extent taken by an endoscopic snare [82, 83]. The resultant wedge-shaped resection does remove a larger portion of tissue and may result in less frequent recurrence, but data are lacking long term [84].

The extent of resection with flexible endoscopic approaches to hypopharyngeal diverticula is also a matter of debate. While few would argue that complete division of the septum is most likely to resolve symptoms and reduce recurrence [70], when facing a screen and deciding which will be the last fibers to cut is another matter entirely. One of the justifications of the step-wise, multisession approach in early publications was likely fear to free perforation into the mediastinum and resultant mediastinitis; however, this leads to a similar problem noted with transoral stapling, where residual septa can contribute to persistent symptoms. Over time, accumulated evidence demonstrates that even when perforations occur, they are generally small and can be managed with endoscopic clips and do not often need surgery. Some even advocate that the dissection can be readily advanced into the neck, up to a centimeter beyond the base of the diverticulum to extend the myotomy onto the esophagus [85]. They note a reduction in postprocedure dysphagia rates when the myotomy is extended [79].

One of the implications of the introduction of the flexible endoscopic platform to treat hypopharyngeal diverticula was a shift in the medical providers that were providing therapy. Transcervical and most rigid transoral techniques were developed by surgeons with specialization in general surgery, otolaryngology, or thoracic surgery. On the other hand, many of the authors of papers involving flexible endoscopy arose from gastroenterology. Gastroenterologists, while facile with endoscope and therapeutic devices that can be introduced through them, are not typically trained in principles of surgical practice. These complementary specializations have a history of collaboration and co-evolution as organized under the auspices of Natural Orifice Trans-Endoscopic Surgery (NOTES). There are some gastroenterologists that remain trepid regarding their specialties' role in treating hypopharyngeal diverticula [71]. However, as is noted in the next section, the most recent advances in the treatment of hypopharyngeal diverticula, from within the submucosal plane, would have likely not been possible without this history of cross-specialty collaboration.

Transoral Flexible Endoscopic Submucosal Approach Hypopharyngeal Diverticula

As submucosal tunneling technique has become more prevalent for the treatment of various malignant and benign conditions of the gastrointestinal tract, including early stage colon, rectal and gastric cancers, leiomyomas, gastroparesis, and achalasia, submucosal treatment of hypopharyngeal diverticula has begun to be explored as well. In this technique, the cricopharyngeus is approached with a submucosal tunnel [85–89]. The endoscope is oriented such that the septum is vertical, as opposed to horizontal. A mucosal incision is made roughly 3 cm proximal to the septum and extended longitudinally to accommodate the endoscope. A tunnel is made to the septum and then developed on either side of the muscle. The muscle fibers are then divided. This myotomy may be extended as distally as desired, even beyond the base of the diverticula if needed. The mucosal incision is then closed with clips. While currently limited to only select centers which have broad experience with submucosal tunneling, this is an emerging area of application to hypopharyngeal diverticula.

Preoperative Assessment

The diagnosis of hypopharyngeal diverticulum is confirmed using the methods described above. It is often helpful for the surgeon performing the procedure to perform their own endoscopic inspection for operative planning, and is typically best accomplished with a flexible endoscopy. This may also reveal evidence of concomitant disease, including reflux associated esophagitis that may be comorbid in these patients. Physical examination should include an evaluation of active next extension and inspection of the mouth opening. A review of comorbidities, especially cardiac and pulmonary conditions, will guide the provider toward an anesthetic approach; however, we most often prefer general anesthesia.

Postoperative Care

A wide variety of protocols exist regarding postoperative care, without any comparative studies to suggest superiority of one over another. The time to resumption of diet, content of diet, duration of antibiotics if they are used at all, and radiographic esophageal imaging are all variable. We typically use a transoral flexible endoscopic approach, performed in the operating room, under general anesthesia. Our typical approach is to keep patients with only sips of clear liquids on the day of the procedure. On the following day, a contrast esophagram is obtained both to verify no leak and to establish a new baseline should symptoms recur in the future. If there is no leak or perforation and the patient is able to perform the study without bothersome dysphagia, then they are advanced to a thick liquid diet. This diet is continued for 1–2 weeks thereafter to allow healing of the mucosa and to reduce mechanical insult to the tissue. Hospitalization is typically only the night of surgery in our practice.

Contemporary Surgical Techniques to Hypopharyngeal Diverticula: Open Approach to Hypopharyngeal Diverticula

The patient is positioned supine on the operating room table, often with a shoulder roll to facilitate neck extension. In some practices, a preincision flexible endoscopy is performed and the diverticulum packed with gauze to aid in identification of the diverticulum. A nasogastric tube and/or esophageal dilator may also be passed to aid in identification of the true esophageal lumen. An incision is made over the anterior border of the sternocleidomastoid muscle ipsilateral to the diverticulum, typically the left side. Alternately a transverse incision is made in a skin crease between the hyoid and the clavicle. Subplatysmal flaps are developed. Posterolateral retraction of the sternocleidomastoid is performed. As the posterior pharynx is identified, the recurrent laryngeal nerve is identified, as well as the thyroidal vessels. These may need to be ligated depending on the size and position of the diverticulum. The diverticulum is then identified and freed from the surrounding attachments. Once this is completed, the diverticular sac may be resected or suspended. A cricopharyngeal myotomy is nearly always performed as well. Numerous studies have demonstrated that leaving the cricopharyngeus intact leads to frequent recurrence. For small diverticula, cricopharyngeal myotomy may be a sufficient treatment alone.

In early descriptions, the need for multiple interventions and the lack of antibiotics contributed to a high rate of morbidity and even mortality. In contemporary series, open techniques for hypopharyngeal diverticula have an aggregate mortality rate of around 1.5% and morbidity of around 11.5%. Complications include fistula formation, recurrence, recurrent laryngeal nerve injury, mediastinitis, and esophageal strictures [90].

Rigid Transoral Approach to Hypopharyngeal Diverticula

The patient is positioned supine on the operating room table, often with a shoulder roll to facilitate neck extension. General anesthesia is induced and the patient is intubated. A bivalve diverticuloscope is positioned, with the anterior (upper) blade within the esophageal lumen and the posterior (lower) blade within the diverticulum. A telescope is used to visualize the septum and the diverticuloscope is suspended. Temporary traction sutures may be placed at the lateral aspect if desired. Any bezoar is removed from the diverticulum. The endoscopic stapler is then introduced. The stapler cartridge (the hammer portion) of the stapler is often easier to position in the diverticulum, as this is often a larger orifice in this view, and the anvil is positioned in the esophageal lumen. Once the stapler has been fired, the septum is divided and a common opening (diverticulo-esophagostomy) is created in the posterior wall of the esophagus. The edges of this divided tissue included both mucosal edges, and the underlying muscle is sealed by the staple rows. Multiple firings may be necessary depending on the size of the stapler cartridges used and the size of the diverticulum. Because the anvil of the stapler always extends beyond the cutting blade, there may be a small remnant septum.

There are descriptions of division of this remaining septum using ultrasonic shears or monopolar forceps. Limitations to this technique include inability to extend neck or position the diverticuloscope due to small mouth opening or prominent dentition. Small diverticula (<3 cm) are difficult to treat using this technique. For both reasons, up to 30% of eligible patients will be not be able to be managed with this approach, and an alternative approach should be sought.

Flexible Endoscopic Approach to Hypopharyngeal Diverticula

The patient is positioned supine on the operating room table, often with a shoulder roll to facilitate neck extension. Numerous publications report performed flexible endoscopic treatment of hypopharyngeal diverticulum under conscious sedation or monitored anesthesia care/deep sedation. While this in an option, we prefer intubation and general anesthesia, in case an open approach is needed. Moreover, as scope stability is the most challenging aspect of this approach, general anesthesia, and resultant minimal patient movement may make the procedure more facile. We would recommend a general anesthetic approach in particular for providers that have less experience with the flexible endoscopic techniques, as prolonged procedure times may not be well tolerated by less sedate patients. A standard gastroscope is used, fitted with a transparent cap, which helps to maintain visualization of the tissue. A diagnostic endoscopy is performed first. We typically place a nasogastric tube into the true esophageal lumen under endoscopic guidance; a guidewire may be used for the same purpose. This helps to maintain orientation and may aid in scope stability as well. While there are numerous reports of using a flexible diverticuloscope, or modified overtube, we do not prefer this approach. The main benefit of the flexible diverticuloscope is scope stabilization, but we often find the resultant limitation in scope mobility to be detrimental. Any bezoar is removed from the diverticulum. We prefer to use a triangular tip knife for the procedure. A cut current is used to divide the mucosa and a coagulation current thereafter. The triangular tip knife is larger than most other endoscopic knives, so caution must be exercised as thermal spread can also be greater. However, the increased surface area allows the knife to be used to push fibers or edges away, and the corners may be used to pull fibers as well; the multiple ways to use the knife may be advantageous in the small space.

There are two approaches we use the first is a cutting only technique. The mucosa overlying the central part of the septum is divided, orthogonal to the long axis of the septum. This is carried distally toward the base of the diverticulum. The pressure applied from the cap will tend to spread the mucosal edges apart and the underlying muscle and connective tissue will appear as a V. If areolar fibers are visualized with no muscle beyond, the mediastinum has been reached. Clips should be placed at the base to help reduce the risk of leak into the mediastinum in case an unnoticed iatrogenic peroration has occurred.

The alternative approach is a submucosal tunneling technique, which exposes the underlying cricopharyngeus muscle while maintaining musical flaps to later close. In this case, the mucosotomy is along the long axis of the septum, long enough to accommodate the endoscopic cap. The loose connective tissue of the submucosal is then carefully teased away to separate the mucosa from the underlying muscle on both sides of the septum. The cricopharyngeus can then be completely divided once its fibers are exposed. The mucosotomy can then be closed with endoscopic clips. In this technique, there may be a partial persistent septum; however, the complete cricopharyngeal myotomy that is accomplished will still produce durable symptomatic relief.

Non-Zenker's Diverticula of the Esophagus

Mid-esophageal and epiphrenic diverticula occur within the general population, though with less commonality compared to hypopharyngeal diverticulae. Given their more distal location, management differs from hypopharyngeal diverticula, and given their relative rarity, evidence to guide treatment is more limited.

Mid-Esophageal Diverticula

Mid-esophageal diverticula occur in an area with 5 cm above or below the carina and make up roughly 10–17% of all esophageal diverticula [5, 91]. While these anatomic limits are somewhat arbitrary, diverticula in this region are unique, in that they have traditionally demanded transthoracic procedures for treatment. Mid-esophageal diverticula are often related to underlying conditions, in particular conditions leading to paraesophageal inflammation. Early studies linked many mid-esophageal diverticula to tuberculosis-related lymphadenitis, or histoplasmosis. The inflammation of peri-bronchial lymph nodes results in a true traction diverticulum, where all layers of the esophageal wall are pulled into an outpouching. Most often diverticula occurring by this mechanism form on the right side of the esophagus, just below the carina, as the subcarinal lymph nodes lie nearest the esophagus in this position [5]. More contemporary studies have demonstrated that pulsion diverticula may also occur, and may be related to neuromuscular dysfunction of the esophagus [5, 92]. Specifically, hypertonicity or hyperactivity of the distal esophagus may lead to an area of hyperpressurization at the proximal aspect of the abnormal segment [92]. However, it should be noted that most studies that have established hyperpressurization as a causitive factor were performed prior to the availability of high-resolution manometry, which has resulted in substantial changes in classification of some subsets of esophageal motility disorders. There may also be congenital attachments that act as traction lead points in the mid-esophagus and contribution to enlargement of pulsion diverticula [5]. An alternative explanation is that mid-esophageal pulsion diverticula form through a weakness in the esophageal wall where a congenital foregut cyst is present. This also fits with observed patterns of pulsion diverticula occurring primarily on the left side of esophagus [5].

Symptoms of Mid-Esophageal Diverticula

Small mid-esophageal diverticula may be asymptomatic, as they were often small and wide mouthed. This appearance was typical of diverticula associated with tuberculosis. However, complications including hemorrhage, and/or fistulous connections to the aerobronchial or central vasculature have been reported [5]. The association between mid-esophageal diverticula and neuromuscular or motility disorders of the esophagus, may make it difficult to ascertain what if any symptoms arise from the diverticulum as opposed to the underlying motility disorder.

Diagnosis of Mid-Esophageal Diverticula

Diagnosis of mid-esophageal diverticula is typically made radiographically. An esophagram is the best for diagnosis and characterization of mid-esophageal diverticula. Similar to hypopharyngeal diverticula, some mid-esophageal diverticula are discovered incidentally as the use of cross-sectional imaging continues to be more common. Endoscopy may be useful in evaluating complications of diverticula, but it is of little additional diagnostic yield. Manometric analysis may be useful in determining etiology. Manometric catheters may be difficult to place when large diverticula are present, as the catheter may preferential course into the diverticulum; endoscopic guidance may be necessary to ensure passage into the esophageal lumen.

Surgical Treatment of Mid-Esophageal Diverticula

Indications for treatment of mid-esophageal diverticula are symptoms or complications. Traction type diverticula of the mid-esophagus may be treated by diverticulectomy. Traditionally, this was performed via a right-sided thoracotomy, with the assistance of an esophageal bougie to avoid narrowing the esophageal lumen. Myotomy is traditionally performed on the opposite side of the esophagus in this approach, and is associated with a significant decrease in leak rates [93]. The defects were closed in with absorbable sutures in two layers and often buttressed with the pleuropericardial fat pad, or pleura [5]. Alternatives include diverticulopexy with suspension to the prevertebral fascia [5]. Where this is an associated motility disorder, myotomy alone may be sufficient to relieve symptoms. Thoracoscopic approaches are possible, but are likely best performed by surgeons in centers with significant experience with minimally invasive esophageal surgery [91, 94]. Robot-assisted approaches have also been reported. There are also increasing reports of using submucosal tunneled approaches to perform myotomies for mid-esophageal diverticula similar to those discussed above with hypopharyngeal diverticula [86, 95]. Given the likely association with motility disorders for some mid-esophageal diverticula, this therapy is intriguing; however, long-term data are lacking.

Intramural Pseudodiverticula of the Esophagus

Intramural pseudodiverticula appear on barium esophagram. Multiple small (usually <5 mm) cystic structures appear in the esophagus, perpendicular to the esophageal wall [96]. Patients presenting with intramural pseudodiverticula often do not have associated endoscopic abnormalities. However, intramural psuedodiverticula are typically associated with a distal stricture, and may not resolve with treatment of the distal stricture. They do not warrant surgical intervention.

Epiphrenic Diverticula of the Esophagus

Epiphrenic diverticula are pulsion type diverticula that form in the distal portion of the esophagus, typically in the distal 10 cm. They are quite uncommon, with an estimate incidence of 1 in 500,000 per year [97]. Typically epiphrenic diverticula occur on the right side of the esophagus [98]. The first description is attributed Hoxie in 1804 based on anatomical studies, and then radiographically by Zeitstein in 1898 [6]. Mondiere described symptoms attributed to epiphrenic diverticula and was the first to postulate in 1833 that intraluminal pressure played a role in the development epiphrenic diverticula [99]. Current understanding is the epiphrenic diverticula are pulsion-type diverticula that result from herniation of the mucosa and submucosa through an intrinsic weakness in the esophageal wall. Similar to hypopharyngeal diverticula, most epiphrenic diverticula are related to an underlying motility disorder that results in a functional distal obstruction and hyper-pressurization of the esophageal lumen [24, 99, 100]. One group was able to perform barium videoesophagography, upper gastrointestinal endoscopy, and esophageal manometric in patients with symptomatic epiphrenic diverticula [98]. By performing this complement of studies, they were able to demonstrate that all of the patients had a concomitant motor abnormality, and were distributed across five separate diseases: achalasia, diffuse esophageal spasm, hypertensive lower esophageal sphincter, nutcracker esophagus, and vigorous achalasia [98]. However, even in the absence of a diagnosed esophageal motility disorder, patients with epiphrenic diverticula will have alterations in the myenteric plexus leading to poor coordination of muscular contraction [101].

Symptoms of Epiphrenic Diverticula

As with other esophageal diverticula, the association with motility disorders can make it difficult to ascertain what symptoms may be due to an epiphrenic diverticulum. Dysphagia and reflux are the most common symptoms experienced by patients [102]. Regurgitation, chest pain, epigastric pain, reflux, and aspiration pneumonia have been additionally reported. Severity of symptoms and size do not appear to be correlated [102].

Diagnosis of Epiphrenic Diverticula

Most epiphrenic diverticula are diagnosed on barium esophagram. An upper endoscopy should be pursued as well, to rule out associated malignancy or dysplasia. The frequency with which esophageal motility disorders are co-morbid also warrants esophageal manometry. Mobile esophageal monitoring may be necessary and/or illuminating in some patient who only experience symptoms intermittently or with food [98]. Manometry catheters may need to be placed under endoscopic guidance if diverticula significantly distort the distal esophagus. Esophageal manometry is particularly helpful to aid in operative planning regarding the length of myotomy required and whether a simultaneous antireflux procedure should be performed.

Surgical Treatment of Epiphrenic Diverticula

While there is general consensus that surgery should be reserved only for symptomatic patients, even this is not without controversy. While some authors have used a size criteria for indication for operation for epiphrenic diverticula [103], both the poor correlation between size and symptoms and better understanding of the underlying pathophysiology have removed this an indication alone [104]. Additionally, while some authors advocate all patients with a known epiphrenic diverticulum should be operated upon [105], this must be balanced against the significant risk of morbidity, and a mortality rate as high as 11.1% in published series [106]. Moreover, many patients with minimal symptoms do not progress, or at least progress slowly over time [107]. Perhaps the best summary statement was crafted by Orringer, "masterful inactivity is generally the best approach" in describing annual surveillance for patients with minimal symptoms from epiphrenic diverticula [6, 108]. When surgical intervention becomes necessary, frequently diverticulectomy and esophageal myotomy are performed [93, 109].

Surgical approach is also a matter for debate. Classically, the distal esophagus was best accessed from a left thoracotomy, and was the preferred approach, despite the more frequent right-sided location of epiphrenic diverticula. Over the past several decades, there has been a progression toward minimally invasive approaches in published literature, either thoracoscopic, laparoscopic, or both [93, 109, 110]. It is worth noting that even in centers that perform high volumes of minimally invasive esophageal surgery, complications of surgical procedures to address epiphrenic diverticula are substantial [104].

Given that esophageal motility disorders underlie the development of epiphrenic diverticula, myotomy has been advocated as part of the surgical treatment. Myotomy is now considered routine, and is performed in the majority of cases (85.5%) in the reported literature, and is selectively employed without intervention on the epiphrenic diverticulum itself [93]. Myotomy is intended to relief the high pressure zone, similar to cricopharyngeal myotomy for hypopharyngeal diverticula; failure to eliminate the high pressure zone is associated with increased risk of perioperative leak, and recurrence of an epiphrenic diverticula [110]. Accordingly, extension of the myotomy of onto the stomach has been advocated [104, 110, 111]. However, this puts patients at risk for postoperative reflux. Thus, selective myotomy or limited myotomy is employed in some centers, guided by the esophageal manometry results from preoperative testing [98, 112].

An antireflux procedure performed in conjunction with epiphrenic diverticulectomy and myotomy was introduced as an option in the open surgical era [107]. Among published studies, less than 70% of patients have undergone concomitant antireflux operations [93]. Some feel that there is limited risk of reflux, if the lower esophageal sphincter is not divided, which generally implies a transthoracic approach with a limited myotomy [6, 109]. What emerges from the literature is that nonobstructing antireflux procedures are preferred over a full fundoplication. The most common antireflux operations and Dor type (anterior, 180° wrap) or a Belsey-Mark IV (anterior 220–240° wrap with diaphragmatic plication) [93]. Overall, a recent meta-analysis of surgical options for epiphrenic diverticulum concludes that diverticulectomy with myotomy is likely the best operation in most circumstances, with our without an antireflux procedure [93]. Given that open and minimally invasive approaches had similar outcomes in terms of morbidity and mortality, the approach is best left to the discretion of the surgeon, and which approach they are most comfortable Table 15.3.

Table 15.3 Summary of studies of surgical treatment of epiphrenic diverticulum

Author	Year	Patients	Mean age (years)	Approach	Esophageal myotomy (%)	Antireflux (%)	Diverticulectomy (%)	Leak (%)	Morbidity (%)	Reoperation (%)	Mortality (%)	Follow-up	Recurrence
Fekete and Vonns [106] France	1992	27	63	Open	55.6	51.9	85.2	8.7	18.5	37.0	11.1	6	2 (7.4)
Streitz et al. [112] USA	1992	16	62	Open	81.3	0.0	100.0	63.0	37.5	0.0	0.0	84	0
Altorki et al. [105] USA	1993	17	65	Open	100.0	100.0	82.4	7.1	5.9	0.0	5.9	84	0
Benacci et al. [107] USA	1993	33	65	Open	69.7	18.2	97.0	18.8	33.3	6.1	9.1	83	0
Hudspeth et al. [115] USA	1993	9	62	Open	66.7	0.0	100.0	11.1	11.1	11.1	0.0	36	0
Castrucci et al. [116] Italy	1998	27	55	Open	81.5	63.0	63.0	11.8	11.1	7.4	7.4	47	0
Jordan and Kinner [117] USA	1999	19	59	Open	68.4	21.1	84.2	63.0	5.3	0.0	0.0	NR	0
van der Peet et al. [118] The Netherlands	2001	5	58	Laparoscopy/thoracoscopy	40.0	0.0	100.0	20.0	20.0	20.0	0.0	NR	1 (20.0)
Nehra et al. [98] USA	2002	18	66	Open	94.4	94.4	77.8	71.0	16.7	11.1	9.1	24	0

(continued)

Table 15.3 (continued)

Author	Year	Patients	Mean age (years)	Approach	Esophageal myotomy (%)	Antireflux (%)	Diverticulectomy (%)	Leak (%)	Morbidity (%)	Reoperation (%)	Mortality (%)	Follow-up	Recurrence
Klaus et al. [111] USA	2003	11	68	Laparoscopy/thoracoscopy	90.9	90.9	54.5	16.7	18.2	9.1	0.0	26	0
Matthews et al. [119] USA	2003	5	64	Laparoscopy/thoracoscopy	100.0	80.0	100.0	0.0	0.0	0.0	0.0	16	0
Tedesco et al. [120] USA	2005	7	73	Laparoscopy	100.0	100.0	100.0	14.3	14.3	14.3	0.0	60	0
Varghese et al. [104] USA	2007	35	71	Open	94.3	97.1	94.3	6.1	14.3	2.9	2.9	45	NR
D'Journo et al. [121] Canada	2009	23	58	Open	100.0	95.7	56.5	0.0	8.7	0.0	0.0	61	0
Melman et al. [122] USA	2009	13	67	Laparoscopy	100.0	92.3	100.0	7.7	15.4	7.7	0.0	14	0
Soares et al. [123] USA	2011	23	57	Both	91.3	100.0	100.0	4.3	21.7	4.3	4.3	34	0
Fumagalli et al. [124] Italy	2012	30	62	Laparoscopy	100.0	100.0	100.0	3.3	6.7	33.0	0.0	52	0
Zaninotto et al. [125] Italy	2012	24	61	Laparoscopy	87.5	100.0	100.0	16.7	25.0	0.0	0.0	96	NR
Rossetti et al. [126] Italy	2013	21	59	Laparoscopy	100.0	100.0	100.0	23.8	28.6	0.0	4.8	78	0

Study	Year			Approach									
Bagheri et al. [127] Iran	2014	17	39	Open	70.6	0.0	76.5	7.7	17.6	0.0	0.0	12	0
Gonzalez-Calatayud et al. [128] Spain	2014	6	64	Laparoscopy/thoracoscopy	100.0	100.0	100.0	33.3	33.3	0.0	0.0	62	0
Hauge et al. [129] Norway	2014	11	60	Open/laparoscopic	27.3	27.3	81.2	33.3	27.3	18.2	0.0	27	0
Allaix et al. [130] USA	2015	13	65	Laparoscopy	100.0	100.0	46.2	15.7	7.7	0.0	0.0	24	0
Bowman et al. [131] USA	2015	44	70	Laparoscopy	100.0	100.0	100.0	18.2	75.0	0.0	0.0	39	0
Macke et al. [132] USA	2015	57	71	Laparoscopy/thoracoscopy	82.5	42.1	100.0	7.0	31.6	7.0	1.8	21	0
Kao et al. [110]	2018	27	62	Laparoscopic/thoracoscopic	88.9	85.2	100.0	0.0	29.6	0.0	0.0	35.8	0
Brandeis et al. [133]	2018	27	67	Laparoscopic/thoracoscopic	100.0	92.6	96.0	3.7	11.1	0.0	0.0	33.1	0
Tapias et al. [109]	2018	31	65	Open	90.3	19.4	90.3	3.1	35.5	0.0	0.0	34	NR

Notes: Adapted, modified, and expanded from [93]

Emerging Transoral Endoscopic Treatment of Epiphrenic Diverticula
Given the development of the per-oral esophago-myotomy (POEM) procedure
[113] as a treatment for achalasia and other esophageal motility disorders, and that
these same motility disorders occur in conjunction with epiphrenic diverticula, it is
perhaps not surprising that POEM and submucosal tunneling have been applied to
epiphrenic diverticula. There are scattered case reports of this technique and single
multicenter study that includes three patients [86, 114]. Initial technical success has
been good, with symptomatic relief noted in the short term [86]. We expect there to
be more reports similar to this in the coming years, and eagerly look to studies
describing selection criteria, correlation with high-resolution manometry pre- and
postprocedure, as well as longer term outcomes.

Conclusions

Surgeons evaluating published literature reports results of operative management of
esophageal diverticula are left wanting for comparative literature. The rarity of
esophageal diverticula and diversity of presentation likely render randomized controlled trials impossible. The heterogeneity of techniques and nonstandardized
reporting of symptoms and success rates make direct comparison difficult. No standard set of criteria for preoperative currently exist that comprise symptoms (dysphagia, odynophagia, aspiration, reflux, regurgitation), assessment of symptom severity
(dysphagia scoring), indications for operation (size vs symptoms vs comorbidities),
definition of clinical success (elimination or symptoms, improvement of symptoms)
recurrence (after multiple or single procedures) or time-frame for follow-up (early
vs late). There is no way for us to recommend substantial superiority of one procedure in comparison to another. Moreover, operative approaches offered to symptomatic patients are increasingly likely to be a function of the specialty training of
the provider. However, given that the majority of the procedures described here have
a high degree of efficacy, and fairly low risk of complications, the best approaches
are likely best left to the surgeon or endoscopist to determine the best approach
based upon their training, experience, and most importantly the patient sitting in
front of them.

References

1. Law R, Katzka DA, Baron TH. Zenker's Diverticulum. Clin Gastroenterol Hepatol.
   2014;12:1773–82; quiz e111-112.
2. Ferreira LEVVC, Simmons DT, Baron TH. Zenker's diverticula: pathophysiology, clinical
   presentation, and flexible endoscopic management. Dis Esophagus. 2008;21:1–8.
3. Laing MR, Murthy P, Ah-See KW, Cockburn JS. Surgery for pharyngeal pouch: audit of
   management with short- and long-term follow-up. J R Coll Surg Edinb. 1995;40:315–8.
4. van Overbeek JJ. Meditation on the pathogenesis of hypopharyngeal (Zenker's) diverticulum and a report of endoscopic treatment in 545 patients. Ann Otol Rhinol Laryngol.
   1994;103:178–85.

5. Rice TW, Baker ME. Midthoracic esophageal diverticula. Semin Thorac Cardiovasc Surg. 1999;11:352–7.
6. Allen MS. Treatment of epiphrenic diverticula. Semin Thorac Cardiovasc Surg. 1999;11:358–62.
7. Scher RL, Puscas L. Chapter 71: Zenker diverticulum. In: Cummings Otolaryngology. 6th ed. Philadelphia: Saunders Elsevier; 2015. p. 1025–34.
8. Zaninotto G, Costantini M. Chapter 11: Cricopharyngeal dysfunction and Zenker diverticulum. In: Shackelfords surgery alimentary tract. 8th ed. Philadelphia: Elsevier; 2019. p. 157–72.
9. Cook IJ, Gabb M, Panagopoulos V, Jamieson GG, Dodds WJ, Dent J, Shearman DJ. Pharyngeal (Zenker's) diverticulum is a disorder of upper esophageal sphincter opening. Gastroenterology. 1992;103:1229–35.
10. Veenker EA, Andersen PE, Cohen JI. Cricopharyngeal spasm and Zenker's diverticulum. Head Neck. 2003;25:681–94.
11. Zainabadi K, Courcoulas AP, Awais O, Raftopoulos I. Laparoscopic revision of Nissen fundoplication to Roux-en-Y gastric bypass in morbidly obese patients. Surg Endosc. 2008;22:2737–40.
12. Hillel AT, Flint PW. Evolution of endoscopic surgical therapy for Zenker's diverticulum. Laryngoscope. 2009;119:39–44.
13. Regan J, Walshe M, Timon C, McMahon BP. Endoflip® evaluation of pharyngo-oesophageal segment tone and swallowing in a clinical population: a total laryngectomy case series. Clin Otolaryngol. 2015;40:121–9.
14. Regan J, Walshe M, Rommel N, Tack J, McMahon BP. New measures of upper esophageal sphincter distensibility and opening patterns during swallowing in healthy subjects using EndoFLIP®. Neurogastroenterol Motil. 2013;25:e25–34.
15. Pomerri F, Costantini M, Dal Bosco C, Battaglia G, Bottin R, Zanatta L, Ancona E, Muzzio PC. Comparison of preoperative and surgical measurements of Zenker's diverticulum. Surg Endosc. 2012;26:2010–5.
16. Aly A, Devitt PG, Jamieson GG. Evolution of surgical treatment for pharyngeal pouch. Br J Surg. 2004;91:657–64.
17. Stewart K, Sen P. Pharyngeal pouch management: an historical review. J Laryngol Otol. 2016;130:116–20.
18. Lahey FH. Pharyngo-esophageal diverticulum: its management and complications. Ann Surg. 1946;124:617–36.
19. Sweet RH. Pulsion diverticulum of the pharyngo-esophageal junction: technic of the one-stage operation: a preliminary report. Ann Surg. 1947;125:41–8.
20. Sweet RH. Excision of diverticulum of the pharyngo-esophageal junction and lower esophagus by means of the one stage procedure; a subsequent report. Ann Surg. 1956;143:433–8.
21. Payne WS. The treatment of pharyngoesophageal diverticulum: the simple and complex. Hepato-Gastroenterology. 1992;39:109–14.
22. Harrison MS. The aetiology, diagnosis and surgical treatment of pharyngeal diverticula. J Laryngol Otol. 1958;72:523–34.
23. Sutherland HD. Cricopharyngeal achalasia. J Thorac Cardiovasc Surg. 1962;43:114–26.
24. Belsey R. Functional disease of the esophagus. J Thorac Cardiovasc Surg. 1966;52:164–88.
25. Lerut T, van Raemdonck D, Guelinckx P, Dom R, Geboes K. Zenker's diverticulum: is a myotomy of the cricopharyngeus useful? How long should it be? Hepato-Gastroenterology. 1992;39:127–31.
26. Pera M, Yamada A, Hiebert CA, Duranceau A. Sleeve recording of upper esophageal sphincter resting pressures during cricopharyngeal myotomy. Ann Surg. 1997;225:229–34.
27. Mosher H. Webs and pouches of the oesophagus, their diagnosis and tratment. Surg Gynecol Obstet. 1917;25:175.
28. Gaub O, Jackson C. Pulsion diverticulum of the esophagus: a new operatoin for its cure. Surg Gynecol Obstet. 1915;21:52.

29. Jackson C, Shallow TA. Diverticula of the oesophagus, pulsion, traction, malignant and congenital. Ann Surg. 1926;83:1–19.
30. Dohlman G, Mattsson O. The endoscopic operation for hypopharyngeal diverticula: a roentgencinematographic study. AMA Arch Otolaryngol. 1960;71:744–52.
31. Von Doersten PG, Byl FM. Endoscopic Zenker's diverticulotomy (Dohlman procedure): forty cases reviewed. Otolaryngol Head Neck Surg. 1997;116:209–12.
32. Wayman DM, Byl FM, Adour KK. Endoscopic diverticulotomy for the treatment of Zenker's diverticulum. Otolaryngol Head Neck Surg. 1991;104:448–52.
33. Lippert BM, Folz BJ, Rudert HH, Werner JA. Management of Zenker's diverticulum and postlaryngectomy pseudodiverticulum with the CO2 laser. Otolaryngol Head Neck Surg. 1999;121:809–14.
34. Lippert BM, Folz BJ, Gottschlich S, Werner JA. Microendoscopic treatment of the hypopharyngeal diverticulum with the CO2 laser. Lasers Surg Med. 1997;20:394–401.
35. Kuhn FA, Bent JP. Zenker's diverticulotomy using the KTP/532 laser. Laryngoscope. 1992;102:946–50.
36. Collard JM, Otte JB, Kestens PJ. Endoscopic stapling technique of esophagodiverticulostomy for Zenker's diverticulum. Ann Thorac Surg. 1993;56:573–6.
37. Scher RL, Richtsmeier WJ. Long-term experience with endoscopic staple-assisted esophagodiverticulostomy for Zenker's diverticulum. Laryngoscope. 1998;108:200–5.
38. Thaler ER, Weber RS, Goldberg AN, Weinstein GS. Feasibility and outcome of endoscopic staple-assisted esophagodiverticulostomy for Zenker's diverticulum. Laryngoscope. 2001;111:1506–8.
39. Cook RD, Huang PC, Richtsmeier WJ, Scher RL. Endoscopic staple-assisted esophagodiverticulostomy: an excellent treatment of choice for Zenker's diverticulum. Laryngoscope. 2000;110:2020–5.
40. Lüscher MS, Johansen LV. Zenker's diverticulum treated by the endoscopic stapling technique. Acta Otolaryngol Suppl. 2000;543:235–8.
41. Baldwin DL, Toma AG. Endoscopic stapled diverticulotomy: a real advance in the treatment of hypopharyngeal diverticulum. Clin Otolaryngol Allied Sci. 1998;23:244–7.
42. Philippsen LP, Weisberger EC, Whiteman TS, Schmidt JL. Endoscopic stapled diverticulotomy: treatment of choice for Zenker's diverticulum. Laryngoscope. 2000;110:1283–6.
43. Narne S, Cutrone C, Bonavina L, Chella B, Peracchia A. Endoscopic diverticulotomy for the treatment of Zenker's diverticulum: results in 102 patients with staple-assisted endoscopy. Ann Otol Rhinol Laryngol. 1999;108:810–5.
44. Omote K, Feussner H, Stein HJ, Ungeheuer A, Siewert JR. Endoscopic stapling diverticulostomy for Zenker's diverticulum. Surg Endosc. 1999;13:535–8.
45. Koay CB, Bates GJ. Endoscopic stapling diverticulotomy for pharyngeal pouch. Clin Otolaryngol Allied Sci. 1996;21:371–6.
46. Peracchia A, Bonavina L, Narne S, Segalin A, Antoniazzi L, Marotta G. Minimally invasive surgery for Zenker diverticulum: analysis of results in 95 consecutive patients. Arch Surg. 1998;133:695–700.
47. Raut VV, Primrose WJ. Long-term results of endoscopic stapling diverticulotomy for pharyngeal pouches. Otolaryngol Head Neck Surg. 2002;127:225–9.
48. Stoeckli SJ, Schmid S. Endoscopic stapler-assisted diverticuloesophagostomy for Zenker's diverticulum: patient satisfaction and subjective relief of symptoms. Surgery. 2002;131:158–62.
49. Bonavina L, Aiolfi A, Scolari F, Bona D, Lovece A, Asti E. Long-term outcome and quality of life after transoral stapling for Zenker diverticulum. World J Gastroenterol. 2015;21:1167–72.
50. Wasserzug O, Zikk D, Raziel A, Cavel O, Fleece D, Szold A. Endoscopically stapled diverticulostomy for Zenker's diverticulum: results of a multidisciplinary team approach. Surg Endosc. 2010;24:637–41.
51. Jaramillo MJ, McLay KA, McAteer D. Long-term clinico-radiological assessment of endoscopic stapling of pharyngeal pouch: a series of cases. J Laryngol Otol. 2001;115:462–6.

52. Morse CR, Fernando HC, Ferson PF, Landreneau RJ, Luketich JD. Preliminary experience by a thoracic service with endoscopic transoral stapling of cervical (Zenker's) diverticulum. J Gastrointest Surg. 2007;11:1091–4.
53. Leong SC, Wilkie MD, Webb CJ. Endoscopic stapling of Zenker's diverticulum: establishing national baselines for auditing clinical outcomes in the United Kingdom. Eur Arch Otorhinolaryngol. 2012;269:1877–84.
54. Koay CB, Commins D, Bates GJ. The role of endoscopic stapling diverticulotomy in recurrent pharyngeal pouch. J Laryngol Otol. 1998;112:954–5.
55. Verdonck J, Morton RP. Systematic review on treatment of Zenker's diverticulum. Eur Arch Otorhinolaryngol. 2015;272:3095–107.
56. Sakai P. Endoscopic myotomy of Zenker's diverticulum: lessons from 3 decades of experience. Gastrointest Endosc. 2016;83:774–5.
57. Ishioka S, Sakai P, Maluf Filho F, Melo JM. Endoscopic incision of Zenker's diverticula. Endoscopy. 1995;27:433–7.
58. Mulder CJ, den Hartog G, Robijn RJ, Thies JE. Flexible endoscopic treatment of Zenker's diverticulum: a new approach. Endoscopy. 1995;27:438–42.
59. Mulder CJ. Zapping Zenker's diverticulum: gastroscopic treatment. Can J Gastroenterol. 1999;13:405–7.
60. Rabenstein T, May A, Michel J, Manner H, Pech O, Gossner L, Ell C. Argon plasma coagulation for flexible endoscopic Zenker's diverticulotomy. Endoscopy. 2007;39:141–5.
61. Repici A, Pagano N, Romeo F, Danese S, Arosio M, Rando G, Strangio G, Carlino A, Malesci A. Endoscopic flexible treatment of Zenker's diverticulum: a modification of the needle-knife technique. Endoscopy. 2010;42:532–5.
62. Rouquette O, Abergel A, Mulliez A, Poincloux L. Usefulness of the Hook knife in flexible endoscopic myotomy for Zenker's diverticulum. World J Gastrointest Endosc. 2017;9:411–6.
63. Laquière A, Grandval P, Arpurt JP, Boulant J, Belon S, Aboukheir S, Laugier R, Penaranda G, Curel L, Boustière C. Interest of submucosal dissection knife for endoscopic treatment of Zenker's diverticulum. Surg Endosc. 2015;29:2802–10.
64. Manno M, Manta R, Caruso A, Bertani H, Mirante VG, Osja E, Bassotti G, Conigliaro R. Alternative endoscopic treatment of Zenker's diverticulum: a case series (with video). Gastrointest Endosc. 2014;79:168–70.
65. Battaglia G, Antonello A, Realdon S, Cesarotto M, Zanatta L, Ishaq S. Flexible endoscopic treatment for Zenker's diverticulum with the SB Knife. Preliminary results from a single-center experience. Dig Endosc. 2015;27:728–33.
66. Antonello A, Ishaq S, Zanatta L, Cesarotto M, Costantini M, Battaglia G. The role of flexible endotherapy for the treatment of recurrent Zenker's diverticula after surgery and endoscopic stapling. Surg Endosc. 2016;30:2351–7.
67. Costamagna G, Iacopini F, Tringali A, Marchese M, Spada C, Familiari P, Mutignani M, Bella A. Flexible endoscopic Zenker's diverticulotomy: cap-assisted technique vs. diverticuloscope-assisted technique. Endoscopy. 2007;39:146–52.
68. Vogelsang A, Preiss C, Neuhaus H, Schumacher B. Endotherapy of Zenker's diverticulum using the needle-knife technique: long-term follow-up. Endoscopy. 2007;39:131–6.
69. Huberty V, El Bacha S, Blero D, Le Moine O, Hassid S, Devière J. Endoscopic treatment for Zenker's diverticulum: long-term results (with video). Gastrointest Endosc. 2013;77:701–7.
70. Costamagna G, Iacopini F, Bizzotto A, Familiari P, Tringali A, Perri V, Bella A. Prognostic variables for the clinical success of flexible endoscopic septotomy of Zenker's diverticulum. Gastrointest Endosc. 2016;83:765–73.
71. Katzka DA, Baron TH. Transoral flexible endoscopic therapy of Zenker's diverticulum: is it time for gastroenterologists to stick their necks out? Gastrointest Endosc. 2013;77:708–10.
72. Hashiba K, de Paula AL, da Silva JG, Cappellanes CA, Moribe D, Castillo CF, Brasil HA. Endoscopic treatment of Zenker's diverticulum. Gastrointest Endosc. 1999;49:93–7.
73. Sakai P, Ishioka S, Maluf-Filho F, Chaves D, Moura EG. Endoscopic treatment of Zenker's diverticulum with an oblique-end hood attached to the endoscope. Gastrointest Endosc. 2001;54:760–3.

74. Christiaens P, De Roock W, Van Olmen A, Moons V, D'Haens G. Treatment of Zenker's diverticulum through a flexible endoscope with a transparent oblique-end hood attached to the tip and a monopolar forceps. Endoscopy. 2007;39:137–40.
75. Evrard S, Le Moine O, Hassid S, Devière J. Zenker's diverticulum: a new endoscopic treatment with a soft diverticuloscope. Gastrointest Endosc. 2003;58:116–20.
76. Al-Kadi AS, Maghrabi AA, Thomson D, Gillman LM, Dhalla S. Endoscopic treatment of Zenker diverticulum: results of a 7-year experience. J Am Coll Surg. 2010;211:239–43.
77. Case DJ, Baron TH. Flexible endoscopic management of Zenker diverticulum: the Mayo Clinic experience. Mayo Clin Proc. 2010;85:719–22.
78. Halland M, Grooteman KV, Baron TH. Flexible endoscopic management of Zenker's diverticulum: characteristics and outcomes of 52 cases at a tertiary referral center. Dis Esophagus. 2016;29:273–7.
79. Pescarus R, Shlomovitz E, Sharata AM, Cassera MA, Reavis KM, Dunst CM, Swanström LL. Trans-oral cricomyotomy using a flexible endoscope: technique and clinical outcomes. Surg Endosc. 2016;30:1784–9.
80. Perbtani Y, Suarez A, Wagh MS. Techniques and efficacy of flexible endoscopic therapy of Zenker's diverticulum. World J Gastrointest Endosc. 2015;7:206–12.
81. Ishaq S, Hassan C, Antonello A, et al. Flexible endoscopic treatment for Zenker's diverticulum: a systematic review and meta-analysis. Gastrointest Endosc. 2016;83:1076–1089.e5.
82. Gölder SK, Brueckner J, Ebigbo A, Messmann H. Double incision and snare resection in symptomatic Zenker's diverticulum: a modification of the stag beetle knife technique. Endoscopy. 2018;50:137–41.
83. Pang M, Koop A, Brahmbhatt B, Bartel MJ, Woodward TA. Comparison of flexible endoscopic cricopharyngeal myectomy and myotomy approaches for Zenker diverticulum repair. Gastrointest Endosc. 2019;89:880–6.
84. Ishaq S, Sultan H, Siau K, Kuwai T, Mulder CJ, Neumann H. New and emerging techniques for endoscopic treatment of Zenker's diverticulum: State-of-the-art review. Dig Endosc. 2018;30:449–60.
85. Beard K, Swanström LL. Zenker's diverticulum: flexible versus rigid repair. J Thorac Dis. 2017;9:S154–62.
86. Yang J, Zeng X, Yuan X, et al. An international study on the use of peroral endoscopic myotomy (POEM) in the management of esophageal diverticula: the first multicenter D-POEM experience. Endoscopy. 2019;51:346–9.
87. Li Q-L, Chen W-F, Zhang X-C, Cai M-Y, Zhang Y-Q, Hu J-W, He M-J, Yao L-Q, Zhou P-H, Xu M-D. Submucosal tunneling endoscopic septum division: a novel technique for treating Zenker's diverticulum. Gastroenterology. 2016;151:1071–4.
88. Brieau B, Leblanc S, Bordacahar B, Barret M, Coriat R, Prat F, Chaussade S. Submucosal tunneling endoscopic septum division for Zenker's diverticulum: a reproducible procedure for endoscopists who perform peroral endoscopic myotomy. Endoscopy. 2017;49:613–4.
89. Hernández Mondragón OV, Solórzano Pineda MO, Blancas Valencia JM. Zenker's diverticulum: submucosal tunneling endoscopic septum division (Z-POEM). Dig Endosc. 2018;30:124.
90. Chang CY, Payyapilli RJ, Scher RL. Endoscopic staple diverticulostomy for Zenker's diverticulum: review of literature and experience in 159 consecutive cases. Laryngoscope. 2003;113:957–65.
91. Palanivelu C, Rangarajan M, Senthilkumar R, Velusamy M. Combined thoracoscopic and endoscopic management of mid-esophageal benign lesions: use of the prone patient position : Thoracoscopic surgery for mid-esophageal benign tumors and diverticula. Surg Endosc. 2008;22:250–4.
92. Cross FS, Johnson GF, Gerein AN. Esophageal diverticula. Associated neuromuscular changes in the esophagus. Arch Surg. 1961;83:525–33.
93. Chan DSY, Foliaki A, Lewis WG, Clark GWB, Blackshaw GRJC. Systematic review and meta-analysis of surgicaltreatment of Non-Zenker's Oesophageal diverticula. J Gastrointest Surg. 2017;21:1067–75.

94. Fernando HC, Luketich JD, Samphire J, Alvelo-Rivera M, Christie NA, Buenaventura PO, Landreneau RJ. Minimally invasive operation for esophageal diverticula. Ann Thorac Surg. 2005;80:2076–80.

95. Mou Y, Zeng H, Wang Q, Yi H, Liu W, Wen D, Tang C, Hu B. Giant mid-esophageal diverticula successfully treated by per-oral endoscopic myotomy. Surg Endosc. 2016;30:335–8.

96. Baker ME, Zuccaro G, Achkar E, Rice TW. Esophageal diverticula: patient assessment. Semin Thorac Cardiovasc Surg. 1999;11:326–36.

97. Abdollahimohammad A, Masinaeinezhad N, Firouzkouhi M. Epiphrenic esophageal diverticula. J Res Med Sci. 2014;19:795–7.

98. Nehra D, Lord RV, DeMeester TR, Theisen J, Peters JH, Crookes PF, Bremner CG. Physiologic basis for the treatment of epiphrenic diverticulum. Ann Surg. 2002;235:346–54.

99. Soares R, Herbella FA, Prachand VN, Ferguson MK, Patti MG. Epiphrenic diverticulum of the esophagus. From pathophysiology to treatment. J Gastrointest Surg. 2010;14:2009–15.

100. Effler DB, Barr D, Groves LK. Epiphrenic diverticulum of the esophagus: surgical treatment. Arch Surg. 1959;79:459–67.

101. Rice TW, Goldblum JR, Yearsley MM, Shay SS, Reznik SI, Murthy SC, Mason DP, Blackstone EH. Myenteric plexus abnormalities associated with epiphrenic diverticula. Eur J Cardiothorac Surg. 2009;35:22–7; discussion 27.

102. Fasano NC, Levine MS, Rubesin SE, Redfern RO, Laufer I. Epiphrenic diverticulum: clinical and radiographic findings in 27 patients. Dysphagia. 2003;18:9–15.

103. Debas HT, Payne WS, Cameron AJ, Carlson HC. Physiopathology of lower esophageal diverticulum and its implications for treatment. Surg Gynecol Obstet. 1980;151:593–600.

104. Varghese TK, Marshall B, Chang AC, Pickens A, Lau CL, Orringer MB. Surgical treatment of epiphrenic diverticula: a 30-year experience. Ann Thorac Surg. 2007;84:1801–9; discussion 1801-1809.

105. Altorki NK, Sunagawa M, Skinner DB. Thoracic esophageal diverticula. Why is operation necessary? J Thorac Cardiovasc Surg. 1993;105:260–4.

106. Fékéte F, Vonns C. Surgical management of esophageal thoracic diverticula. Hepato-Gastroenterology. 1992;39:97–9.

107. Benacci JC, Deschamps C, Trastek VF, Allen MS, Daly RC, Pairolero PC. Epiphrenic diverticulum: results of surgical treatment. Ann Thorac Surg. 1993;55:1109–13; discussion 1114.

108. Orringer MB. Epiphrenic diverticula: fact and fable. Ann Thorac Surg. 1993;55:1067–8.

109. Tapias LF, Morse CR, Mathisen DJ, Gaissert HA, Wright CD, Allan JS, Lanuti M. Surgical management of esophageal epiphrenic diverticula: a transthoracic approach over four decades. Ann Thorac Surg. 2017;104:1123–30.

110. Kao AM, Arnold MR, Schlosser KA, Siddiqui SL, Prasad T, Colavita PD, Heniford BT. Epiphrenic diverticulum: 20-year single-institution experience. Am Surg. 2018;84:1159–63.

111. Klaus A, Hinder RA, Swain J, Achem SR. Management of epiphrenic diverticula. J Gastrointest Surg. 2003;7:906–11.

112. Streitz JM, Glick ME, Ellis FH. Selective use of myotomy for treatment of epiphrenic diverticula. Manometric and clinical analysis. Arch Surg. 1992;127:585–7; discussion 587–88.

113. Inoue H, Minami H, Kobayashi Y, Sato Y, Kaga M, Suzuki M, Satodate H, Odaka N, Itoh H, Kudo S. Peroral endoscopic myotomy (POEM) for esophageal achalasia. Endoscopy. 2010;42:265–71.

114. Demeter M, Bánovčin P, Ďuriček M, Kunda R, Hyrdel R. Peroral endoscopic myotomy in achalasia and large epiphrenic diverticulum. Dig Endosc. 2018;30:260–2.

115. Hudspeth DA, Thorne MT, Conroy R, Pennell TC. Management of epiphrenic esophageal diverticula. A fifteen-year experience. Am Surg. 1993;59:40–2.

116. Castrucci G, Porziella V, Granone PL, Picciocchi A. Tailored surgery for esophageal body diverticula. Eur J Cardiothorac Surg. 1998;14:380–7.

117. Jordan PH, Kinner BM. New look at epiphrenic diverticula. World J Surg. 1999;23:147–52.

118. van der Peet DL, Klinkenberg-Knol EC, Berends FJ, Cuesta MA. Epiphrenic diverticula: minimal invasive approach and repair in five patients. Dis Esophagus. 2001;14:60–2.

119. Matthews BD, Nelms CD, Lohr CE, Harold KL, Kercher KW, Heniford BT. Minimally invasive management of epiphrenic esophageal diverticula. Am Surg. 2003;69:465–70; discussion 470.
120. Tedesco P, Fisichella PM, Way LW, Patti MG. Cause and treatment of epiphrenic diverticula. Am J Surg. 2005;190:891–4.
121. D'Journo XB, Ferraro P, Martin J, Chen L-Q, Duranceau A. Lower oesophageal sphincter dysfunction is part of the functional abnormality in epiphrenic diverticulum. Br J Surg. 2009;96:892–900.
122. Melman L, Quinlan J, Robertson B, Brunt LM, Halpin VJ, Eagon JC, Frisella MM, Matthews BD. Esophageal manometric characteristics and outcomes for laparoscopic esophageal diverticulectomy, myotomy, and partial fundoplication for epiphrenic diverticula. Surg Endosc. 2009;23:1337–41.
123. Soares RV, Montenovo M, Pellegrini CA, Oelschlager BK. Laparoscopy as the initial approach for epiphrenic diverticula. Surg Endosc. 2011;25:3740–6.
124. Fumagalli Romario U, Ceolin M, Porta M, Rosati R. Laparoscopic repair of epiphrenic diverticulum. Semin Thorac Cardiovasc Surg. 2012;24:213–7.
125. Zaninotto G, Parise P, Salvador R, Costantini M, Zanatta L, Rella A, Ancona E. Laparoscopic repair of epiphrenic diverticulum. Semin Thorac Cardiovasc Surg. 2012;24:218–22.
126. Rossetti G, Fei L, del Genio G, et al. Epiphrenic diverticula mini-invasive surgery: a challenge for expert surgeons--personal experience and review of the literature. Scand J Surg. 2013;102:129–35.
127. Bagheri R, Maddah G, Mashhadi MR, Haghi SZ, Tavassoli A, Ghamari MJ, Sheibani S. Esophageal diverticula: analysis of 25 cases. Asian Cardiovasc Thorac Ann. 2014;22:583–7.
128. Gonzalez-Calatayud M, Targarona EM, Balague C, Rodriguez-Luppi C, Martin AB, Trias M. Minimally invasive therapy for epiphrenic diverticula: systematic review of literature and report of six cases. J Minim Access Surg. 2014;10:169–74.
129. Hauge T, Johnson E, Sandstad O, Johannessen H-O, Trondsen E. Surgical treatment of epiphrenic oesophageal diverticulum. Tidsskr Nor Laegeforen. 2014;134:1047–50.
130. Allaix ME, Borraez Segura BA, Herbella FA, Fisichella PM, Patti MG. Is resection of an esophageal epiphrenic diverticulum always necessary in the setting of achalasia? World J Surg. 2015;39:203–7.
131. Bowman TA, Sadowitz BD, Ross SB, Boland A, Luberice K, Rosemurgy AS. Heller myotomy with esophageal diverticulectomy: an operation in need of improvement. Surg Endosc. 2016;30:3279–88.
132. Macke RA, Luketich JD, Pennathur A, Bianco V, Awais O, Gooding WE, Christie NA, Schuchert MJ, Nason KS, Levy RM. Thoracic esophageal diverticula: a 15-year experience of minimally invasive surgical management. Ann Thorac Surg. 2015;100:1795–802.
133. Brandeis AE, Singhal S, Lee TH, Mittal SK. Surgical management of epiphrenic diverticulum: a single-center experience and brief review of literature. Am J Surg. 2018;216:280–5.
134. Kroh M, Reavis KM, editors. Chap. 18: Endoscopic interventions for the thoracic esophagus: Zenker's and other diverticula. In: The SAGES manual: operating through the endoscope. Cham: Springer; 2016. https://doi.org/10.1007/978-3-319-24,145-6_18.
135. Conigliaro R, Frazzoni M, editors. Chap. 11: Endoscopic and surgical management of Zenker's diverticulum: new approaches. In: Diagnosis and endoscopic management of digestive diseases. Cham: Springer; 2017. https://doi.org/10.1007/978-3-319-42,358-6_11.
136. Fisichella P, Patti M, editors. Chap. 11: Operations for Zenker's diverticulum. In: Atlas of esophageal surgery. Cham: Springer; 2015.

Surgical Techniques for Lower Esophageal Diverticula

16

Francesca M. Dimou and Alfons Pomp

Introduction

An esophageal epiphrenic diverticulum is defined as an outpouching in the distal 10 cm of the esophagus, which consists of esophageal mucosa and submucosa. It is not necessarily an anatomic abnormality, but likely secondary to an outflow obstruction at the level of the gastroesophageal (GE) junction. There is a spectrum of esophageal motility disorders that typically result in an epiphrenic diverticulum, but one common example is in patients with achalasia [1–3].

Patients with an epiphrenic diverticulum may present with dysphagia, epigastric pain, reflux, regurgitation, aspiration pneumonia, or persistent cough [4]. Others may be asymptomatic and diagnosed when being evaluated for an esophageal motility disorder. Preoperative workup in these patients should include an upper endoscopy, barium esophagram, and manometry.

Surgery is considered the standard of care when treating patients with an epiphrenic diverticulum, but the optimal surgical approach remains controversial. In this chapter, we discuss the different minimally invasive approaches when treating patients with an epiphrenic diverticulum.

Surgical Treatment

Regardless of the operative approach, there are three main goals when treating a patient with an epiphrenic diverticulum: diverticulectomy, a concomitant myotomy, and a partial fundoplication. Three surgical approaches that will be described in this chapter are laparoscopic, thoracoscopic, and robotic.

F. M. Dimou · A. Pomp (✉)
Department of Surgery, Weill Cornell Medicine/New York Presbyterian Hospital, New York, NY, USA
e-mail: alfons.pomp.chum@ssss.gouv.qc.ca

© Springer Nature Switzerland AG 2021
N. Zundel et al. (eds.), *Benign Esophageal Disease*,
https://doi.org/10.1007/978-3-030-51489-1_16

Laparoscopic Approach

A laparoscopic approach is the most common technique undertaken when treating an epiphrenic diverticulum. The laparoscopic operative details may vary depending on surgeon preference; this includes patient positioning, suturing techniques, and port placement. Here we describe our specific technique when doing an epiphrenic diverticulectomy.

(a) Patient Position

The patient is placed in the supine position. It is our preference to have patients with arms and legs extended and abducted; this position allows the surgeon to stand between the legs. It is important to ensure the arms and legs are secured, and footboards are placed as the patient will be placed in steep reverse Trendelenburg.

(b) Port Placement

If there is no history of previous abdominal operations, the abdominal cavity can be entered using a 5 mm optical trocar with a 30 degree laparoscope at Palmer's point in the left upper quadrant. Once the abdominal cavity is entered, the abdomen is inspected for any injuries or adhesions. A 5 mm supraumbilical port is then inserted under direct visualization. The camera is now placed in this port and a 5 mm epigastric incision is made with placement of a Nathanson liver retractor. An additional 5 mm trocar is placed in the right upper quadrant and a 5 mm trocar is inserted in the left abdomen. Once all ports are placed, the patient is placed in reverse Trendelenburg.

(c) Key Laparoscopic Techniques

The distal esophagus must first be mobilized by taking down the gastrohepatic ligament. We prefer to use a 5 mm Harmonic scalpel as an energy device. Dissection is carried toward the right crus and anteriorly along the esophagus with care not to damage the anterior branch of the vagus nerve. Next, the posterior esophagus is dissected and the posterior vagus nerve is protected. Continue with circumferential dissection of the posterior esophagus until there is identification of the left crus. A Penrose drain is placed around the esophagus to help with further retraction and mobilization.

Dissection is carried proximal into the mediastinum where the diverticulum is identified and dissected off of the pleura. It is important to fully dissect the diverticulum including the neck to allow for complete resection.

A tapered-tip bougie should be carefully inserted into the esophagus to aid in stenting and preventing stenosis; a 54–58 Fr is adequate. Next, the 5 mm entry trocar is upsized to a 12 mm trocar in order to accommodate a laparoscopic stapler for transection. The laparoscopic stapler is inserted and the neck of the diverticulum is transected. The staple line is imbricated with an interrupted layer of silk sutures intracorporeally.

A myotomy on the contralateral aspect of the esophagus is created. This is performed to alleviate the distal obstruction; a combination of blunt dissection, hook cautery, and Harmonic scalpel may be used to divide the muscle fibers. The myotomy should extend far enough to ensure the obstruction is relieved; in the setting of achalasia, we commonly do a 6–7 cm myotomy on the esophagus and extend distally 2–3 cm onto the stomach. If there is any concern regarding potential perforation during this dissection, an intraoperative EGD should be done.

The last step should include hiatal closure and a partial fundoplication to reduce the likelihood of postoperative reflux. It is recommended to close the hiatus without tension and permanent suture. We typically use interrupted silk suture. Most commonly we recommend a Dor fundoplication. This requires division of the short gastric vessels. The fundoplication is created by suturing the gastric fundus to the myotomy and apex of the right crus. The fundus is also sutured to the diaphragmatic hiatus anteriorly and the left crus. This is done with 3-0 silk sutures tied intracorporeally (Figs. 16.1 and 16.2; Table 16.1).

Fig. 16.1 Laparoscopic Port Placement. (**A**) is Palmer's point - the intial trocar placement site, (**B**) 5mm supraumbilical port, (**C**) is the high epigastric site for the Nathanson liver retractor, (**D**) 5mm rigth upper quadrant port, (**E**) 5mm left abdomen port

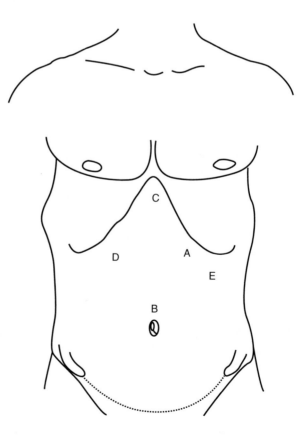

Fig. 16.2 Robotic Port Placement. (**A**) Palmer's point, (**B**) is the intial reference point, (**C**) is the site for Arm 3, (**D**) is for Arm 4, (**E**) is for Arm 1 and (**F**) is the site for the Nathanson liver retractor

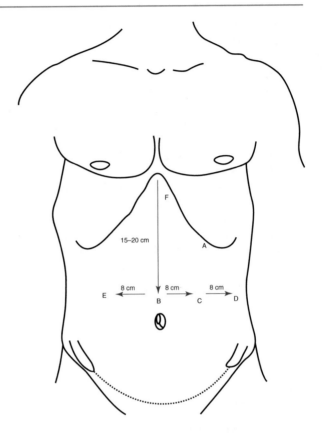

Table 16.1 Key technical points and potential pitfalls

Key technical points	Potential pitfalls
Esophageal mobilization	Placing ports too low may result in inability to reach diverticular neck for transection
Complete exposure of diverticular neck	Inadequate myotomy
Esophageal stenting	Iatrogenic perforation using cautery
Myotomy	Splenic injury taking down short gastric vessels
Partial fundoplication	

Thoracoscopic Approach

In those patients who have an epiphrenic diverticulum that is located more proximal and an abdominal approach is not feasible, a thoracoscopic approach is preferred. These patients will require a double-lumen endotracheal tube to allow single-lung ventilation.

(a) Patient Position

The patient is placed in lateral decubitus; the specific side is dependent on the side of the diverticulum. For example, those with a right-sided diverticulum should be placed in left lateral decubitus. Care is taken to alleviate pressure points and to flex the bed to open the rib space and accommodate trocar placement.

(b) Trocar Placement

First, a 5 mm trocar is placed for the laparoscope at the level of the seventh intercostal space in the posterior axillary line. Another 5 mm trocar is placed at the level of the fifth intercostal space in the anterior axillary line. The last 5 mm trocar is placed posteriorly just below the tip of the scapula. An anterior incision at the level of the fourth intercostal space should be made for access of the stapler and specimen removal.

(c) Key Thoracoscopic Techniques.

The inferior pulmonary ligament is taken down. The esophagus is identified, mobilized, and the diverticulum dissected out. Care is taken not to injure the vagus nerves. A Penrose drain is again used to facilitate retraction. Once the diverticulum is dissected free, the same principles apply for resection as in the laparoscopic approach including placement of a tapered bougie. To complete the fundoplication and myotomy, a laparoscopic approach should also be undertaken.

Robotic Approach

The indications for a robotic approach in these patients are not well studied, although it does provide an alternative minimally invasive technique. The advantages of robotic surgery include 3D visualization, improvement ergonomics, and the potential of accessing the proximal esophagus via the abdominal cavity. With our experience, we have utilized robotic technology in foregut surgery and primarily using the DaVinci Xi™ robotic platform.

(a) Patient Position

In the robotic approach, patients are placed in the supine position with both arms abducted and a footboard. Once the patient is prepped and draped, the patient should be placed in reverse Trendelenburg and left side up. Pneumoperitoneum is achieved with placement of a Veress needle at Palmer's point. The patient is then placed in the supine position for trocar placement.

(b) Port Placement

The abdomen is marked in the following manner: a reference point is marked approximately 13–15 cm inferior from the xiphoid process in the midline. Two centimeters left of this reference point, an 8 mm trocar is inserted under direct visualization (Arm 2). The abdomen is inspected for any injury and the Veress needle is removed. Next, another 12 mm trocar is placed 8 cm to the patient's left (Arm 3; this will allow for firing of the stapler), and another mark 8 cm left from that (Arm 4). The last port is marked 8 cm right lateral from the reference point (Arm 1).

Once all ports are placed, the patient is placed in reverse Trendelenberg. A 5 mm epigastric incision is made with placement of a Nathanson liver retractor. We typically place the retractor on the right side of the patient and adjust the holder of the liver retractor to be as close to the patient as possible in order to prevent collisions with the robot arms. The robot is then docked (this can be done on the right or left side of the patient). Arm 2 will be used as the camera port; Arms 1 and 4 will be used for traction using small grasping retractors. Arm 3 will utilize a Vessel Sealer for dissection of the greater curvature of the stomach, the esophagus, hiatus, and mediastinum.

Most dissection is done with the Vessel Sealer and once the diverticulum is dissected free, we use the Robotic SureForm™ stapler for our diverticulectomy. After this has been completed and the myotomy is performed, a robotic hook cautery or Maryland Bipolar grasper is used for fine dissection of the muscle fibers. We also do a partial fundoplication when undertaking a robotic approach, specifically a Dor fundoplication. Again, silk sutures are used to secure the wrap and to pexy it to the hiatus.

Postoperative Care

Patients are admitted overnight and started on a clear liquid diet; they are advanced to a full liquid diet the following morning. Given a minimally invasive approach, patients are discharged on postoperative day one and require limited narcotics. We do not routinely obtain a postoperative contrast study unless there is concern for the patient's clinical status.

Conclusion

Regardless of the surgical approach for excision of an epiphrenic diverticulum, the technical principles remain the same. It is important to not only resect the diverticulum but relieve the distal obstruction with a myotomy. Not one approach is necessarily superior to the other; however, it is dependent on the surgeon's skillset and learning curve with each minimally invasive technique. Most importantly, taking a minimally invasive strategy when treating these patients results in excellent long-term outcomes.

References

1. Herbella FAM, Patti MG. Modern pathophysiology and treatment of esophageal diverticula. Langenbeck's Arch Surg. 2012;397(1):29–35. https://doi.org/10.1007/s00423-011-0843-2.
2. Nehra D, Lord RV, DeMeester TR, et al. Physiologic basis for the treatment of epiphrenic diverticulum. Ann Surg. 2002;235(3):346–54. https://doi.org/10.1097/00000658-200203000-00006.
3. Melman L, Quinlan J, Robertson B, et al. Esophageal manometric characteristics and outcomes for laparoscopic esophageal diverticulectomy, myotomy, and partial fundoplication for epiphrenic diverticula. Surg Endosc. 2009;23(6):1337–41. https://doi.org/10.1007/s00464-008-0165-9.
4. Andrási L, Paszt A, Simonka Z, Ábrahám S, Rosztóczy A, Lázár G. Laparoscopic surgery for epiphrenic esophageal diverticulum. JSLS. 2018;22(2):e2017.00093. https://doi.org/10.4293/JSLS.2017.00093.

Medical Evaluation of Barrett's Esophagus

17

Brian Hodgens, Reid Sakamoto, and Dean Mikami

Introduction

Barrett's esophagus (BE) is a pathologic condition of the esophagus caused by excessive and chronic inflammation and irritation of the esophageal mucosa. This long-standing inflammation leads to epithelial metaplasia that transforms normal stratified squamous epithelium into abnormal columnar epithelium with goblet cells. Over time, ongoing metaplasia can give rise to dysplasia that predisposes an individual to the development of esophageal adenocarcinoma (EAC). The cause of Barrett's esophagus (BE) is exposure to acid and bile in gastroesophageal reflux disease (GERD), which causes chronic inflammation of the esophageal mucosa. GERD in itself is a very common condition, and several risk factors have been identified to diagnose which patients are at higher risk for development of BE. What remains unclear, however, is whether or not enrolling these high-risk patients (and others diagnosed with BE) in a rigorous screening and surveillance program confers a survival benefit. While the logic behind monitoring this premalignant condition is sound, the methods to do so are invasive, time consuming, anxiety provoking, and may not actually improve mortality from esophageal cancer [1, 2].

B. Hodgens (✉)
Department of Surgery, University of Hawaii, Honolulu, HI, USA
e-mail: bhodgens@hawaii.edu

R. Sakamoto
Department of Surgery, John A. Burns School of Medicine, Honolulu, HI, USA

D. Mikami
Department of Surgery, The Queen's Medical Center, Honolulu, HI, USA

Definition

GERD has been steadily increasing since the 1990s. The prevalence of GERD is estimated to be 18.1–27.8% in North America [3], and it is likely that more people are affected than are truly diagnosed. Patients with GERD have a 10–15% risk of developing BE, which is defined as at least 1 cm or more of metaplastic change from normal stratified squamous epithelium to columnar epithelium in the distal esophagus [4]. In the United States, the prevalence of Barrett's esophagus is 5.6% [5], and development of esophageal adenocarcinoma (EAC) secondary to Barrett's has become the most common cause of esophageal cancer [6].

While intestinal metaplasia is considered pathologic in the esophagus and stomach, the risk of developing dysplasia is directly related to the length of mucosa involved. Less than 1 cm of metaplastic change in the esophagogastric junction is simply classified intestinal metaplasia and confers a low risk of progression to EAC. BE can be further broken down into short-segment BE (1–3 cm of metaplasia) and long-segment BE (greater than 3 cm of metaplasia). There are several key differences between these two diagnoses that can influence management decisions. It is worth noting as well that since these categories of disease are broken down by the distance from the GEJ, it is critically important that endoscopists diagnosing and surveying patients with Barrett's be very precise about locating the Z-line, the GEJ, identifying hiatal hernias, and tracking metaplasia proximally.

Metaplasia at the GEJ can be either cardiac-type mucosa or intestinal type and it is traditionally defined as being present at and just proximal to the GEJ. In a study by Dresner et al. in 2003, subtotal esophagectomy patients who underwent serial endoscopy displayed a pattern of metaplasia from normal to cardiac to intestinal-type mucosa over 27 months in response to severe reflux [7]. These findings help demonstrate the spectrum of change that occurs in the distal esophagus in response to reflux but also help to confirm that the presence of non-stratified squamous mucosa at the GEJ is abnormal, no matter what the type. Nonetheless, available studies show that risk of progression from this ultra-short segment of metaplasia to EAC is minimal and there are no current guidelines on their management.

Short- and long-segment BE differs in length of mucosa affected, prevalence, the severity of symptoms, and risk of progression to EAC. Short-segment BE is found in about 6.4% of patients with GERD whereas long-segment BE is found in 1.5% [8]. Patients with short-segment BE tend to have less severe reflux and often no GERD symptoms while long-segment patients tend to have both supine and upright reflux as well as more frequent GERD symptoms. Short-segment patients also tend to have higher LES pressures and stronger peristalsis compared to long-segment patients [9]. Finally, the risk of progression to dysplasia and cancer is directly related to the length of mucosa involved. Several studies comparing the incidence of dysplasia and cancer in short- versus long-segment BE highlight a nearly three times higher incidence of dysplasia and EAC in long-segment BE [8, 10].

Risk Factors

Several risk factors for the development of BE have been identified. These include chronic GERD (>5 years), the presence of a hiatal hernia, central obesity, male gender, age >50 years, Caucasian race, smoking, and a history of BE or ECA in a first-degree relative [4, 11–13]. Several case-control studies have demonstrated a direct relationship between frequency of GERD symptoms and development of ECA [14]; however, it is also noted that up to 40% of ECA patients studied had no symptoms of GERD. Based on these data and other studies correlating risk factors with ECA, it is unclear which combination of these factors are most concerning and therefore which patients would benefit most from screening.

Medical Treatment and Surveillance

Patients with BE are recommended to have indefinite treatment with a proton pump inhibitor (PPI). The use of long-term (2–3 years) PPI after diagnosis of BE has been associated with a 71% reduction in EAC or BE with high-grade dysplasia (OR 0.29; 95% CI = 0.12–0.71) [15]. PPIs are the preferred acid-reducing therapy as the use of histamine receptor antagonist has not shown a protective effect against progression to EAC (HR 0.83; 95% CI = 0.11–6.03) [16].

Patients who participate in surveillance programs for BE are diagnosed with EAC at an earlier stage, which is associated with an overall mortality benefit. Kalstelein and colleagues showed that the 5-year survival for patients with EAC in a surveillance program was 74% (CI = 60–87%) versus just 17% in the general population [17]. Just 4% of patients undergoing surveillance died from EAC with the majority of mortalities being from cardiovascular disease or other malignancies. Furthermore, patients who developed EAC while participating in a surveillance program were noted to have a lower tumor stage at diagnosis (stage I versus IV; HR = 0.19; 95% CI = 0.16–0.23) [18]. While there is an ongoing debate about the optimal patient population and frequency of surveillance, it continues to be an important aspect of the early identification and treatment of EAC.

The identification of BE and early diagnosis of EAC have shown to improve overall mortality; however, the cost-effectiveness of surveillance is unproven [17, 18]. As many as 43.7% of patients with BE do not have previous reflux symptoms, therefore screening based upon GERD symptoms alone may not be reliable [19]. Instead, screening is recommended in patients with chronic (>5 years) and frequent (weekly or more) symptoms of GERD with two or more risk factors for BE [4]. Screening of females is generally not recommended and must be individualized to those who have multiple risk factors. Screening in the general population is not recommended.

For appropriate individuals, high-definition/high-resolution white light esophagogastroduodenoscopy (EGD) is considered the gold standard for the identification of BE and EAC. Endoscopic evaluation should include four quadrant biopsies at every 2 cm intervals in patients without dysplasia and every 1 cm in those with prior evidence of dysplasia. If initial endoscopy is negative for BE, further evaluation is not recommended. However, if esophagitis is identified on initial endoscopy, treatment with PPI should be initiated with repeat endoscopy in 8–12 weeks. In those patients where BE is identified without dysplasia, standard surveillance should be performed every 3–5 years.

If dysplasia is identified on initial endoscopy, acid suppression should be optimized using a PPI for 3–6 months. Repeat endoscopy should be performed at 3 months and should not be delayed for >6 months. If low-grade dysplasia is identified on repeat exam, endoscopic intervention is preferred; however, surveillance with endoscopy every 12 months is acceptable. If high-grade dysplasia or intramucosal carcinoma without evidence of submucosal invasion is identified, endoscopic treatment is recommended. All pathology should be reviewed by at least two pathologists and one should have specialization in gastrointestinal pathology.

Endoscopy should be performed methodically and described according to the Prague C & M criteria. Endoscopic reports should include the circumferential (C) extent of metaplasia as well as the maximal (M) extent of metaplasia above the GEJ [20]. For example, a C4M7 lesion would describe 4 cm of circumferential metaplasia with the longest tongue of metaplasia reaching 7 cm. Furthermore, endoscopic inspection time should be longer than 1 minute per centimeter for improved identification of suspicious lesions, HGD, and EAC [21].

Unsedated transnasal endoscopy (uTNE) is a safe and well-tolerated alternative to white light endoscopy (WLE), which has shown efficacy in the evaluation of Barrett's esophagus. uTNE has been shown to be better tolerated by patients as the camera is small (less than 6 mm) and may be preferred to traditional white light EGD by patients. Transnasal endoscopy (TNE) does not touch the root of the tongue, thus reducing the gag reflux and decreasing need for sedation [22]. uTNE has been noted to have a 100% sensitivity and specificity for the endoscopic identification of BE as confirmed by standard endoscopy. However, histologic diagnosis demonstrated a sensitivity of 66.7% and specificity of 100% for BE likely secondary to the small biopsy forceps that are used for TNE [23]. The American College of Gastroenterology has recommended uTNE as an acceptable alternative to conventional endoscopy for the screening of BE [4].

Several other modalities exist for endoscopic and histologic evaluations of BE. Capsule endoscopy is a method by which a tethered wireless capsule endoscope is passed into the esophagus. Images are obtained during transit for the evaluation of BE. Capsule endoscopy is well tolerated by patients; however, it is inadequately specific or sensitive to be recommended for screening [4, 23, 24].

The Cytosponge is a gelatin-coated, self-expanding sponge that is passed into the stomach and then retrieved for the collection of cytologic samples of the distal esophagus. Samples are then stained for the protein Trefoil Factor 3 (TTF3), which is able to distinguish BE cells from the rest of the alimentary tract. Cytosponge showed a sensitivity of 73% and a specificity of 94% when combined with immunohistochemical staining [25]. The Cytosponge may provide an inexpensive and convenient screening modality for BE with randomized controlled trials starting for the validation for this new technology [26].

Chromoendoscopy with methylene blue and indigo carmine have not shown an increased diagnostic yield in comparison to WLE alone [22]. Acetic acid chromoendoscopy has demonstrated increased diagnostic yield and improved detection of neoplasia in comparison to standard endoscopy and biopsies. Acetic acid will color nondysplastic Barrett's tissue white; while dysplastic BE tissue will have rapid loss of acetowhitening [22, 27, 28]. Image enhancement techniques, however, have yet to be routinely recommended for the screening of BE.

Conclusion

With the rise of GERD, the increasing incidence of esophageal adenocarcinoma, and the advancement in diagnostic and therapeutic endoscopies, the diagnosis, surveillance, and management of Barrett's esophagus continue to be an important topic for surgeons and gastroenterologists. The benefit of diagnosing dysplasia and EAC at an early stage is clear; however, finding the right population to survey and monitor remains a topic of debate. Serial endoscopy and biopsy carry their own risk and still have been shown to miss developing cancers. Moving forward, newer technologies may offer a less invasive and more sensitive test to detect dysplasia, which could marginalize some of the current risks of frequent endoscopy.

References

1. Corley DA, Mehtani K, Quesenberry C, et al. Impact of endoscopic surveillance on mortality from Barrett's esophagus-associated esophageal adenocarcinomas. Gastroenterology. 2013;145:312–9.
2. Garside R, Pitt M, Somerville M, et al. Surveillance of Barrett's oesophagus: exploring the uncertainty through systematic review, expert workshop and economic modeling. Health Technol Assess. 2006;10:1–6.
3. El-Serag HB, Sweet S, Winchester CC, et al. Update on the epidemiology of gastro-oesophageal reflux disease: a systematic review. Gut. 2014;63:871–80.
4. Shaheen NJ, Falk GW, Iyer PG, et al. ACG clinical guideline: diagnosis and management of Barrett's esophagus. Am J Gastroenterol. 2016;111:30–50.
5. Hayeck TJ, Kong CY, Spechler SJ, et al. The prevalence of Barrett's esophagus in the US: estimates from a simulation model confirmed by SEER data. Dis Esophagus. 2010;23:451–7.
6. Barret M, Prat F. Diagnosis and treatment of superficial esophageal cancer. Ann Gastroenterol. 2018;31:256–65.
7. Dresner SM, Griffin SM, Waymn J, et al. Human model of duodenogastro-oesophageal reflux in the development of Barrett's metaplasia. Br J Surg. 2003;90:1120–8.
8. Hirota WK, Loughney TM, Lazas DJ, et al. Specialized intestinal metaplasia, dysplasia, cancer of the esophagus and esophagogastric junction: prevalence and clinical data. Gastroenterology. 1999;116:277.
9. Loughney T, Maydonovitch CL, Wong RK. Esophageal manometry and ambulatory 24-hour pH monitoring in patients with short and long segment Barrett's esophagus. Am J Gastroenterol. 1998;93:916.
10. Weston AP, Krmpotich PT, Cherian R, et al. Prospective long-term endoscopic and historical follow-up of short segment Barrett's esophagus: comparison with traditional long segment Barrett's esophagus. Am J Gastroenterol. 1997;92:407.

11. Cook MB, Wild CP, Forman D. A systematic review and meta-analysis of the sex ratio for Barrett's esophagus, erosive reflux disease, and nonerosive reflux disease. Am J Epidemiol. 2005;162:1050–61.

12. Thrift AP, Kramer JR, Qureshi Z, et al. Age at onset of GERD symptoms predicts risk of Barrett's esophagus. Am J Gastroenterol. 2013;108:915–22.

13. Spechler SJ, Sharma P, Souza RF, et al. American Gastroenterological Association technical review on the management of Barrett's esophagus. Gastroenterology. 2011;140:18.

14. Rubenstein JH, Taylor JB. Meta-analysis: the association of oesophageal adenocarcinoma with symptoms of gastro-oesophageal reflux. Aliment Pharmacol Ther. 2010;32:1222.

15. Singh S, Garg SK, Singh PP, et al. Acid-suppressive medications and risk of oesophageal adenocarcinoma in patients with Barrett's oesophagus: a systematic review and meta-analysis. Gut. 2014;63:1229–37.

16. Kastelein F, Spaander MCW, Steyerberg EW, et al. Proton pump inhibitors reduce the risk of neoplastic progression in patients with Barrett's esophagus. Clin Gastroenterol Hepatol. 2013;11:382–8.

17. Kastelein F, van Olphen SH, Steyerberg EW, et al. Impact of surveillance for Barrett's oesohagus on tumor stage and survival of patients with neoplastic progression. Gut. 2016;65:548–54.

18. Verbeek RE, Leenders M, ten Kate FJW, et al. Surveillance of Barrett's esophagus and mortality from esophageal adenocarcinoma: a population-based cohort study. Am J Gastroenterol. 2014;109:1215–22.

19. Ronkainen J, Aro P, Storskrubb T, et al. Prevalence of Barrett's esophagus in the general population: an endoscopic study. Gastroenterology. 2005;129:1825–31.

20. Sharma P, Dent J, Armstrong D, et al. The development and validation of an endoscopic grading system for Barrett's esophagus: the Prague C&M criteria. Gastroenterology. 2006;131:1392–9.

21. Gupta N, Gaddam S, Wani SB, et al. Longer inspection time is associated with increased detection of high-grade dysplasia and esophageal adenocarcinoma in Barrett's esophagus. Gastrointest Endosc. 2012;76:531–8.

22. di Pietro M, Canto MI, Fitzgerald RC. Clinical endoscopic management of early adenocarcinoma and squamous cell carcinoma of the esophagus (screening, diagnosis and therapy). Gastroenterology. 2018;154:421–36.

23. Shariff MK, Varghese S, O'Donovan M, et al. Pilot randomized cross-over study comparing the efficacy of transnasal disposable endosheath to standard endoscopy to detect Barrett's oesophagus. Endoscopy. 2016;48:110–6.

24. Bhardwaj A, Hollenbeak CS, Pooran N, et al. A meta-analysis of the diagnostic accuracy of esophageal capsule endoscopy for Barrett's esophagus in patients with gastroesophageal reflux disease. Am J Gastroenterol. 2009;104:1533–9.

25. Ross-Innes CS, Debiram-Beecham I, O'Donnovan M, et al. Evaluation of a minimally invasive cell sampling device coupled with assessment of trefoil factor 3 expression for diagnosing Barrett's esophagus: a multi-center case-control study. PLoS Med. 2015;12:1–19.

26. Offman J, Muldrew B, O'Donovan M, et al. Barrett's oESophagus trial 3 (BEST3): study protocol for a randomized controlled trial comparing the Cytosponge-TFF3 test with usual care to facilitate the diagnosis of oesophageal pre-cancer in primary care patients with chronic acid reflux. BMC Cancer. 2018;18:784.

27. Thorloor S, Bhattacharyya R, Tsagkournis O, et al. Acetic acid chromoendoscopy in Barrett's esophagus surveillance is superior to the standardized random biopsy protocol: results from a large cohort study (with video). Gastrointest Endosc. 2014;80:417–24.

28. Longcroft-Wheaton G, Duku M, Mead R, et al. Acetic acid spray is an effective tool for the endoscopic detection of neoplasia in patients with Barrett's esophagus. Clin Gastroenterol Hepatol. 2010;8:843–7.

Ablative Therapies in Barrett's Esophagus

18

Audrey C. Pendleton and W. Scott Melvin

Introduction

Barrett's esophagus (BE) is a condition in which the stratified squamous epithelium that normally lines the distal esophagus lumen is replaced by metaplastic columnar epithelium that has both gastric and intestinal features. It is usually caused by persistent damage to the esophageal mucosa due to long-standing gastroesophageal reflux disease (GERD) and predisposes patients to esophageal adenocarcinoma (EAC), a cancer with a significantly increasing incidence over the past 40 years. While there are several risk factors for EAC, including smoking and obesity, GERD is the most significant one. Patients with BE have an estimated 30–125-fold greater chance of developing EAC compared to the general population [1]. The prevalence of BE has been estimated at 1–2% in all patients undergoing endoscopy for any indication and anywhere from 5% to 15% in patients receiving endoscopy for GERD symptoms [2]. While the incidence of EAC is higher in patients with BE, only a small fraction of patients with BE develop cancer with an annual risk of 0.1–0.5% [3, 4].

Epidemiology of Barrett's Esophagus

Barrett's esophagus most commonly affects older adults in developed countries, with a Caucasian male predominance [5]. The age at diagnosis varies widely but the majority of patients are diagnosed in the sixth or seventh decade of life [6]. The true prevalence is challenging to determine because many individuals with BE are

A. C. Pendleton (✉) · W. Scott Melvin
Department of Surgery, Montefiore Medical Center, Bronx, NY, USA

© Springer Nature Switzerland AG 2021
N. Zundel et al. (eds.), *Benign Esophageal Disease*,
https://doi.org/10.1007/978-3-030-51489-1_18

asymptomatic and are not diagnosed. In fact, one of the first estimates of BE was through an autopsy study. Cameron and colleagues estimated that the prevalence of long-segment BE (LSBE) was approximately 0.4% and that only a small fraction of cases was clinically evident [7]. Studies out of tertiary endoscopy centers have attempted to quantify the true prevalence of BE. In one study, investigators performed upper endoscopy on 961 patients undergoing routine screening colonoscopies and found BE in 65 patients, which translates to an overall prevalence of 6.8%, with 1.2% having LSBE. In patients with symptomatic heartburn, the prevalence was higher at 8.3% but most patients with BE on endoscopy were asymptomatic [8].

Risk Factors

Gastroesophageal Reflux Disease

GERD is the major risk factor for the development of BE. Several case-control studies demonstrate that patients with GERD are six to eight times more likely to have BE. Additionally, it has been shown that longer duration of symptoms is associated with an increased risk of developing BE [9–11]. A systematic review found no association between reflux symptoms and short-segment BE (SSBE) but found increased odds of LSBE in patients with reflux symptoms [12]. Patients with BE have been found to have significant evidence of abnormal acid exposure, such as longer periods of acid exposure, lower pH, weaker peristaltic contractions, and lower esophageal sphincter (LES) tone [13, 14]. While some data exist that suggest that the use of proton pump inhibitors (PPI) may decrease the risk of developing cancer, the effects that these medications have on the development of BE is unclear [15].

Management

The goal of treatment of BE is to prevent the progression to high-grade dysplasia (HGD) and ultimately EAC, which carries a dismal prognosis. Management has traditionally focused on mitigating insult to the esophagus by treating the GERD symptoms, preventing erosive injury, and performing surveillance endoscopy to monitor for evidence of dysplasia [16–18]. Studies have demonstrated that non-dysplastic BE has the potential to progress to HGD and to EAC, with the rate of progression 0.9% and 0.5%, respectively [19–26].

Endoscopic Ablative Therapies

The treatment of BE has evolved over the last decade. Historically, patients with BE, specifically those with dysplasia, were treated with an esophagectomy, a procedure that is associated with significant morbidity and mortality. However, endoscopic therapies have gained acceptance and have replaced esophagectomy as the mainstay of treatment. Patients with non-dysplastic BE are managed with surveillance endoscopy with biopsies to look for dysplasia and adenocarcinoma [27]. Endoscopic procedures fall into two main categories: endoscopic mucosal resection (EMR), which will be discussed in the next chapter, and ablation techniques, such as radiofrequency ablation (RFA), argon plasma coagulation (APC), or cryotherapy [28].

Radiofrequency Ablation

RFA involves using radiofrequency energy and applying it directly to the Barrett's epithelium. 350–500 kHz is typically used and the high-frequency energy is thought to limit the damage to the mucosa and does not involve the submucosa or muscularis propria, which decreases the subsequent risk of stricture formation. The energy is delivered either circumferentially using a balloon-based 360 degree catheter or focally using an endoscopic-mounted probe [29]. One study, which compared these two techniques, found that treatment with the focal device resulted in a greater reduction in length of the BE segment compared to the balloon device [30].

The efficacy of RFA has been studied comprehensively. The seminal study addressing this topic is the Ablation of Intestinal Metaplasia (AIM) trial. This landmark study was the first randomized controlled trial to examine RFA as the treatment for dysplastic BE. In this trial, 127 patients with BE dysplasia, divided evenly between HGD and LGD, were randomized to receive either RFA or a sham procedure. The results demonstrated that in the LGD and HGD groups, there was eradication of the neoplasia in 90.5% and 81%, respectively, compared to 22.7% and 19%, respectively, in the sham arm. Additionally, 77.4% had complete eradication of intestinal metaplasia (CE-IM) compared to 2.3% in the sham group [31]. Other studies followed this landmark trial and reinforced the efficacy of RFA. A retrospective analysis looked at 244 patients with BE-related neoplasia who were treated with RFA and found that 80% achieved CE-IM and 87% achieved complete eradication of dysplasia (CE-D). Four patients progressed to cancer despite RFA [32]. A large meta-analysis reinforced these results. This analysis consisted of 18 studies in the USA, the UK, and Europe with over 3000 patients and demonstrated CE-IM in 78% of patients and CE-D in 91% of patients treated with RFA [33].

After these initial landmark studies were conducted and showed promising results, the next step was to demonstrate durability and examine long-term outcomes. The AIM trial conducted a 3 year follow-up and found that of the patients available for follow-up, 98% had CE-D and 91% had CE-IM [34]. Orman et al. reported data from 262 patients with 155 patient-years who had received RFA and found on follow-up that the recurrence rate was 5.2%/year with a progression rate of 1.9%/year [33]. In a series of 592 patients over 8 years, Gupta et al. showed that 33% of patients who achieved successful eradication experienced a recurrence after 2 years [35]. In evaluating the UK RFA registry, the recurrence rate of intestinal metaplasia was 5.1%, 19 months after treatment [36]. This elaborate collection of data demonstrates that while RFA provides high short-term success rates, there is still a risk of recurrence and surveillance must continue following treatment.

RFA is not without complications. A large meta-analysis examined 37 studies with over 9000 patients and demonstrated an adverse event rate of 8.8%, the most common being stricture formation at 5.6%, followed by less common issues such as bleeding at 1% and a very low rate of perforation at 0.6%. Risk factors for complications include increasing BE length and RFA performed in conjunction with endoscopic mucosal resection [37].

Cryotherapy

This technique involves using extremely cold temperature to destroy the aberrant tissue. The two main cryogens used are liquid nitrogen and carbon dioxide [28].

The efficacy of cryotherapy has been examined in several studies. One multicenter prospective registry reported that in patients with LGD, rates of CE-D and CE-IM were 81% and 65%, respectively, and in patients with HGD, CE-D and CE-IM rates were 81% and 65%, respectively. This study also examined short-segment BE and demonstrated that in these patients, CE-D was accomplished in 97% and CE-IM in 77% of patients [38]. A retrospective, non-randomized study looked at patients who received cryotherapy as a salvage treatment following failed RFA. At 1 year, the response rate was 77% for cancer, 89% for dysplasia, and 94% for HGD [39].

A single-center retrospective study evaluated the recurrence rates at 3 and 5 years. The recurrence rates per person-year follow-up of intestinal metaplasia, dysplasia, and HGD were 12.2%, 4%, and 1.4%, respectively. Adenocarcinoma was very uncommon and most recurrences were successfully managed [40].

Cryotherapy has a reasonable safety profile. Complications are minimal and the procedure appears to be well tolerated. When the national cryospray registry was examined, the results showed that none of the patients had a perforation and there were no mortalities. Only one patient developed a stricture, but it did not require dilatation [41].

Argon Plasma Coagulation (APC)

APC uses a non-contact thermal energy to ablate tissue. A probe is used to ionize argon gas and an electric current is conducted through the jet of ionized argon, which coagulates the tissue. In order to mitigate the risk of stricture, hybrid APC is used and consists of injecting saline in the submucosa, which protects the deeper esophageal layers during the procedure [28].

The efficacy of APC has been examined in several studies. The APE trial was a randomized study that compared APC with surveillance after EMR of neoplastic BE lesions. It included 63 patients and showed a significant decrease in secondary lesions in the APC-treatment arm, 3% versus 36.7%, respectively ($p = 0.005$) [42].

Studies that examined the long-term outcomes of APC have showed variable results. One of the first studies, which was done by Kahaleh et al., had a median follow-up of 36 months and showed that over 50% of the 39 patients who underwent

APC had a relapse on either endoscopy or histological analysis [43]. However, in another small study of 19 patients treated with APC, 70% had complete reversal of BE at 2 years [44]. These studies are small and more research is needed to evaluate the long-term outcomes and durability of APC. Additionally, long-term outcomes for hybrid APC have not been examined to date.

Conclusion

Endoscopic ablative therapies have replaced esophagectomies for dysplastic BE and have become the standard of care. However, it is an evolving and dynamic field and more long-term data are needed. While EMR is the most utilized method for visible nodular dysplastic lesions in BE, ablative therapies have emerged as the standard treatment for flat BE mucosa. Among these therapies, RFA is the most extensively studied with its high-efficacy data that has been demonstrated in several large studies. While cryotherapy has been shown to be promising and has an excellent safety profile, the data are limited and many patients receive it as a salvage treatment after failing RFA. APC is also promising but is most safe when used with the hybrid technology, and long-term data on the efficacy of this combined technique are lacking at this time. Regardless of which ablative technique is used, it is paramount that surveillance endoscopy continues to be used as follow-up since recurrence remains a possibility.

References

1. Cameron AJ, Ott BJ, Payne WS. The incidence of adenocarcinoma in columnar-lined (Barrett's) esophagus. N Engl J Med. 1985;313(14):857–9.
2. Shaheen NJ, Richter JE. Barrett's oesophagus. Lancet. 2009;373:850–61.
3. Lund O, et al. Risk stratification and long-term results after surgical treatment of carcinomas of the thoracic esophagus and cardia. A 25-year retrospective study. J Thorac Cardiovasc Surg. 1990;99(2):200–9.
4. Siegel R, Naishadham D, Jemal A. Cancer statistics, 2013. CA Cancer J Clin. 2013;63(1):11–30.
5. Spechler SJ. Barrett's esophagus and esophageal adenocarcinoma: pathogenesis, diagnosis, and therapy. Med Clin North Am. 2002;86(6):1423–45.
6. van Blankenstein M, et al. Age and sex distribution of the prevalence of Barrett's esophagus found in a primary referral endoscopy center. Am J Gastroenterol. 2005;100(3):568–76.
7. Cameron AJ, et al. Prevalence of columnar-lined (Barrett's) esophagus. Gastroenterology. 1990;99(4):918–22.
8. Rex DK, et al. Screening for Barrett's esophagus in colonoscopy patients with and without heartburn. Gastroenterology. 2003;125(6):1670–7.
9. Conio M, et al. Risk factors for Barrett's esophagus: a case-control study. Int J Cancer. 2002;97(2):225–9.
10. Johansson J, et al. Risk factors for Barrett's oesophagus: a population-based approach. Scand J Gastroenterol. 2007;42(2):148–56.
11. Anderson LA, et al. Risk factors for Barrett's oesophagus and oesophageal adenocarcinoma: results from the FINBAR study. World J Gastroenterol. 2007;13(10):1585.
12. Taylor JB, Rubenstein JH. Meta-analyses of the effect of symptoms of gastroesophageal reflux on the risk of Barrett's esophagus. Am J Gastroenterol. 2010;105(8):1730–7.

13. Brandt MG, Darling GE, Miller L. Symptoms, acid exposure and motility in patients with Barrett's esophagus. Can J Surg. 2004;47(1):47.
14. Singh P, Taylor RH, Colin-Jones DG. Esophageal motor dysfunction and acid exposure in reflux esophagitis are more severe if Barrett's metaplasia is present. Am J Gastroenterol. 1994;89(3):349–56.
15. El-Serag HB, et al. Proton pump inhibitors are associated with reduced incidence of dysplasia in Barrett's esophagus. Am J Gastroenterol. 2004;99(10):1877–83.
16. Shaheen N, Ransohoff DR. Gastroesophageal reflux, Barrett's esophagus and esophageal cancer. JAMA. 2002;287:1972–81.
17. Provenzale D, Kemp JA, Arora S, et al. A guide for surveillance of patients with Barrett's esophagus. Am J Gastroenterol. 1994;89:670–80.
18. Sampliner RE. Updated guidelines for the diagnosis, surveillance, and therapy of Barrett's esophagus. Am J Gastroenterol. 2002;97:1888–95.
19. Shaheen NJ, Crosby MA, Bozymski EM, et al. Is there a publication bias in reporting cancer risk in Barrett's esophagus? Gastroenterology. 2000;119:333–8.
20. Sharma P, Falk GW, Weston AP, et al. Dysplasia and cancer in a large multicenter cohort of patients with Barrett's esophagus. Clin Gastroenterol Hepatol. 2006;4:566–72.
21. Drewitz DJ, Sampliner RE, Garewal HS. The incidence of adenocarcinoma in Barrett's esophagus: a prospective study of 170 patients followed 4.8 years. Am J Gastroenterol. 1997;92:212–5.
22. Rudolph RE, Vaughan TL, Storer BE, et al. Effect of segment length on risk for neoplastic progression in patients with Barrett's esophagus. Ann Intern Med. 2000;132:612–20.
23. O'Connor JB, Falk GW, Richter JE. The incidence of adenocarcinoma and dysplasia in Barrett's esophagus: report on the Cleveland Clinic Barrett's Esophagus Registry. Am J Gastroenterol. 1999;94:2037–42.
24. Robertson CS, Mayberry JF, Nicholson DA, et al. Value of endoscopic surveillance in the detection of neoplastic change in Barrett's esophagus. Br J Surg. 1988;75:760–3.
25. Hameeteman W, Tytgat GN, Houthoff HJ, et al. Barrett's esophagus: development of dysplasia and adenocarcinoma. Gastroenterology. 1989;96:1249–56.
26. Vaughan TL, Dong LM, Blount PL, et al. Non-steroidal anti-inflammatory drugs and risk of neoplastic progression in Barrett's oesophagus: a prospective study. Lancet Oncol. 2005;6:945–52.
27. Triadafilopoulos G. Radiofrequency ablation for dysplastic and nondysplastic Barrett esophagus. Gastroenterol Hepatol (N Y). 2016;12(9):576–8.
28. Hamade N, Sharma P. Ablation therapy for Barrett's esophagus: new rules for changing times. Curr Gastroenterol Rep. 2017;19:48.
29. Visrodia K, et al. Radiofrequency ablation of Barrett's esophagus: efficacy, complications, and durability. Gastrointest Endosc Clin N Am. 2017;27(3):491–501.
30. Brown J, Alsop B, Gupta N, Buckles DC, Olyaee MS, Vennalaganti P, et al. Effectiveness of focal vs. balloon radiofrequency ablation devices in the treatment of Barrett's esophagus. United European Gastroenterol J. 2016;4(2):236–41.
31. Shaheen NJ, Sharma P, Overholt BF, Wolfsen HC, Sampliner RE, Wang KK, et al. Radiofrequency ablation in Barrett's esophagus with dysplasia. N Engl J Med. 2009;360(22):2277–88.
32. Bulsiewicz WJ, Kim HP, Dellon ES, Cotton CC, Pasricha S, Madanick RD, et al. Safety and efficacy of endoscopic mucosal therapy with radiofrequency ablation for patients with neoplastic Barrett's esophagus. Clin Gastroenterol Hepatol. 2013;11(6):636–42.
33. Orman ES, Li N, Shaheen NJ. Efficacy and durability of radiofrequency ablation for Barrett's esophagus: systematic review and meta-analysis. Clin Gastroenterol Hepatol. 2013;11(10):1245–55.
34. Shaheen NJ, Overholt BF, Sampliner RE, et al. Durability of radiofrequency ablation in Barrett's esophagus with dysplasia. Gastroenterology 2011;141(2):460–8.
35. Gupta M, Iyer PG, Lutzke L, Gorospe EC, Abrams JA, Falk GW, et al. Recurrence of esophageal intestinal metaplasia after endoscopic mucosal resection and radiofrequency abla-

tion of Barrett's esophagus: results from a US Multicenter consortium. Gastroenterology. 2013;145(1):79–86.e1.

36. Haidry RJ, Dunn JM, Butt MA, Burnell MG, Gupta A, Green S, et al. Radiofrequency ablation and endoscopic mucosal resection for dysplastic Barrett's esophagus and early esophageal adenocarcinoma: outcomes of the UK National Halo RFA Registry. Gastroenterology. 2013;145(1):87–95.

37. Qumseya BJ, Wani S, Desai M, Qumseya A, Bain P, Sharma P, et al. Adverse events after radiofrequency ablation in patients with Barrett's esophagus: a systematic review and meta-analysis. Clin Gastroenterol Hepatol. 2016;14(8):1086–95.e6.

38. Ghorbani S, Tsai FC, Greenwald BD, Jang S, Dumot JA, McKinley MJ, et al. Safety and efficacy of endoscopic spray cryotherapy for Barrett's dysplasia: results of the National Cryospray Registry. Dis Esophagus. 2016;29(3):241–7.

39. Sengupta N, Ketwaroo GA, Bak DM, Kedar V, Chuttani R, Berzin TM, et al. Salvage cryotherapy after failed radiofrequency ablation for Barrett's esophagus-related dysplasia is safe and effective. Gastrointest Endosc. 2015;82(3):443–8.

40. Ramay FH, Cui Q, Greenwald BD. Outcomes after liquid nitrogenspray cryotherapy in Barrett's esophagus-associated high-grade dysplasia and intra mucosal adenocarcinoma: 5-year follow-up. Gastrointest Endosc. 2017;86(4):626–32.

41. Desai M, Saligram S, Gupta N, Vennalaganti P, Bansal A, Choudhary A, et al. Efficacy and safety outcomes of multi-modal endoscopic eradication therapy in Barrett's esophagus-related neoplasia: a systematic review and pooled analysis. Gastrointest Endosc. 2017;85(3):482–95.

42. Manner H, Rabenstein T, Pech O, Braun K, May A, Pohl J, et al. Ablation of residual Barrett's epithelium after endoscopic resection: a randomized long-term follow-up study of argon plasma coagulation vs. surveillance (APE study). Endoscopy. 2014;46(1):6–12.

43. Kahaleh M, Van Laethem JL, Nagy N, Cremer M, Deviere J. Long-term follow-up and factors predictive of recurrence in Barrett's esophagus treated by argon plasma coagulation and acid suppression. Endoscopy. 2002;34(12):950–5.

44. Sharma P, Wani S, Weston AP, Bansal A, Hall M, Mathur S, et al. A randomised controlled trial of ablation of Barrett's oesophagus with multipolar electrocoagulation versus argon plasma coagulation in combination with acid suppression: long term results. Gut. 2006;55(9):1233–9.

Endoscopic Mucosal Resection

19

Terence Jackson, David Faugno-Fusci, Aric Wogsland,
and Jeffrey Marks

Background

An injection-based endoscopic submucosal resection (EMR) was first studied in 1955 using in-vitro models in the human sigmoid colon. It was demonstrated that injecting saline to create a submucosal wheal had a protective effect from the complications of thermal cautery [1]. The first live endoscopic mucosal resection with submucosal injection using a loop diathermy was described in 1973 by Deyhle et al., who reported seven resections of sessile polyps from the colon without any complications [2]. This method was then later pioneered by Soetikno in Japan for the management of early gastric cancer [3] in 1974. Since that time, endoscopic submucosal resection utilization has expanded to Barrett's esophagus (BE), esophageal dysplasia, and early esophageal cancer.

With increasing use of endoscopy for surveillance, we now frequently identify esophageal lesions that are amenable to endoscopic treatment. The progression of BE to esophageal cancer is directly related to the degree of dysplasia. The incidence of esophageal cancer in patients with BE without dysplasia is 0.12–0.5% [4, 5]. EMR offers a minimally invasive technique to ameliorate this risk by directed removal of benign and early malignant superficial lesions. It can be used not only as a curative tool, but also for diagnosis by providing adequate tissue for accurate staging.

In combination with ablative technologies like radiofrequency ablation (RFA) and cryotherapy, EMR has significantly decreased the incidence of metachronous and recurrent lesions in BE with high-risk pathologic features. This is also evidenced by several national guidelines that recommend EMR combined with

T. Jackson · D. Faugno-Fusci · A. Wogsland · J. Marks (✉)
Department of General Surgery, University Hospitals of Cleveland, Cleveland, OH, USA
e-mail: jeffrey.marks@uhhospitals.org

© Springer Nature Switzerland AG 2021
N. Zundel et al. (eds.), *Benign Esophageal Disease*,
https://doi.org/10.1007/978-3-030-51489-1_19

ablation of all remaining BE if high-grade dysplasia (HGD) and intramucosal carcinoma (imCa) are found [5, 6]. In combination with a multidisciplinary approach in dedicated BE units [7], the efficacy and safety of endoscopic therapy in the management of HGD and early esophageal cancer have been reported as comparable to performing esophagectomies [8–10]. This has led to endoscopic therapy becoming standard of care for management of dysplastic BE and early esophageal adenocarcinoma [11, 12].

Indications

In the evaluation of esophageal lesions, EMR is used for diagnostic and therapeutic purposes. Therapeutically, it is indicated in all nodular, focal, short-segment, and circumferential lesions of BE; short-segment dysplastic BE; and early superficial esophageal adenocarcinoma (T1a) without any signs of lymph node or distant metastasis. The Japanese Society of Gastroenterology published the following criteria for lesions suitable for EMR [13].

1. Lesions less than or equal to 2 cm in diameter.
2. Lesions involving less than one-third of the circumference of esophagus.
3. Intramucosal carcinoma of the esophagus (ImCa).

By providing adequate tissue, EMR allows for definitive staging and is a final diagnostic tool in endoscopic evaluation of HGD and esophageal adenocarcinoma in BE. Low-risk lesions (T1a/T1sm1) are considered appropriate for endoscopic therapy [14]. EMR can also be curative when an R0 resection is achieved, providing 95% remission at 5 years [15]. However, assessment of the depth of the lesion is key prior to consideration of EMR. Depth can be assessed using an endoscopic ultrasound or by looking for the "non-lifting" sign on injection.

If the evaluation of depth shows a T1b lesion, an endoscopic resection would not be indicated given the high (30%) risk of lymph node metastasis. However, a T1a lesion would have less than 5% risk [14, 16]. EMR can also assess for high-risk features such as depth of invasion of tumor to the submucosa or deeper, tumor diameter of >3 cm, lymphovascular invasion, and poorly differentiated pathology [17]. In the presence of these findings, an esophagectomy would be recommended. Thus, it is imperative that a clear differentiation between T1a and T1b lesions is made. Endoscopic resections safely allow us to make this differentiation.

Pre-procedural Preparation

An informed consent must be obtained from the patient. Indications for the procedure, anticipated benefits, and risks (bleeding, perforation, and strictures) must be discussed well ahead of time as well. This procedure is performed in a monitored setting under moderate sedation or general anesthesia. The latter is used for patients with higher cardiopulmonary risk, those who are difficult to sedate, and when a prolonged procedure is expected.

In addition to an endoscope (Fig. 19.1) equipped with high-definition white-light examination with electronic chromoendoscopy (e.g., narrow-band imaging), additional equipment like injection needles (Fig. 19.2), distal attachment (Fig. 19.3), coagulation forceps, thermal electrocautery snares (Fig. 19.4), and endoclips for closure of mucosotomy and hemostasis must be available.

Fig. 19.1 Endoscope

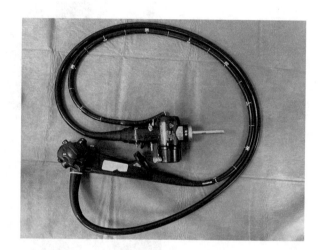

Fig. 19.2 Olympus single-use injector

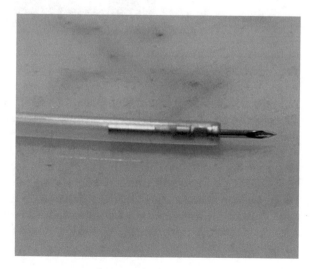

Fig. 19.3 Olympus
disposable distal
attachment

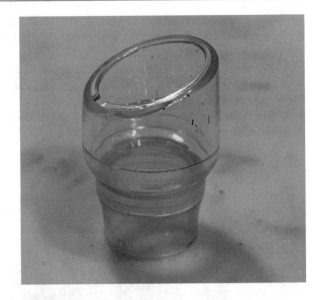

Fig. 19.4 Olympus
disposable
electrosurgical snare

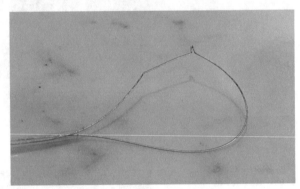

Techniques

A thorough examination of the lesion planned for resection must first be completed.
Visualization adjuncts like chromoendoscopy, near focus visualization, and image
magnification is used to delineate the edges of the lesion. Cautery devices are used
to mark the 2–5 mm clean outer margin. After the margins of resection are identified, a number of different methods can be used for resection. EMR is typically very
successful for lesions smaller than 10 mm, allowing the highest chance for a successful en bloc resection. EMR has been described in lesions as large as 20 mm in
animal models [18]; however, piecemeal resections do not allow for confirmation of
negative margins. A broad classification of the various described techniques is provided in Table 19.1.

Table 19.1 Classification of endoscopic mucosal resection (EMR) techniques

Ligation-assisted EMR: "Suck and cut"	Injection-assisted EMR: "Lift and cut"
Single-band EMR	Traditional lift and cut
Multiband mucosectomy	Cap-assisted EMR
Complete eradication EMR	Strip biopsy

Ligation-Assisted EMR

1. *Single-band EMR*: These were the initial versions of the endoscopic banding devices and have now been phased out by the multiband devices. This involved the use of a variceal ligator without any submucosal injections. Once the lesion to be resected is identified, it is sucked into the banding device and a band is applied at its base, thus creating a pseudopolyp. The endoscope then has to be withdrawn to remove the banding apparatus. It is then reintroduced with a traditional snare. This pseudopolyp is then resected using an electrocautery snare and the specimen is retrieved.

2. *Multiband mucosectomy*: This method uses a modified version of the banding device (Duette Multi-band Mucosectomy Device: Wilson-Cook, Winston-Salem, NC) that contains six bands and a dedicated hexagonal 7 French snare that passes through the endoscope working channel. This device fits endoscopes of varying outer diameters ranging from 9.5 to 14 mm. This device is able to fire multiple bands and perform resections during the same session without needing to remove the endoscope out of the patient. This method has been shown to be significantly faster compared to cap-assisted resections, with a median procedure duration of 37 minutes vs 50 minutes and medical time per resection of 6 minutes vs 12 minutes [19]. The resection specimens were also significantly larger in the multiband mucosectomy group. It has also been shown that even though no submucosal injections are used, this procedure can be performed with a very low risk of perforation [20].

   The true advantage of multiband mucosectomy lies in the fact that it does not require the endoscope to be removed from the patient between resections and thus is a faster, more convenient process with few complications. It also does not require a cap or injections. However, in the setting of larger lesions where a piecemeal resection is required, an incomplete resection is always a possibility. Ablative therapies may need to avoid incomplete resections and minimize recurrent or positive margins.

3. *Complete eradication EMR/circumferential EMR*: This technique uses a larger 30 × 50 mm Erlangen-type polypectomy snare and resections are performed using pure cutting electrocautery. This is performed circumferentially with a few millimeters of overlap between resection sites if neoplastic changes were noted at the previous margins. The maximum size of resection at one session was 30–40 mm in length and encompassed three-fourths of the circumference. This

process is repeated every 3–4 weeks to ensure eradication of BE [21]. This has also been described without the use of a cap or overtube [22]. This technique has been used with success but is associated with an increased risk of stenosis [23–25]. Using this technique, complete eradication of 95% at 32 months was achieved [26].

Injection-Assisted EMR

1. *Traditional lift and cut*: This technique uses an injecting solution into the submucosal space to create a layer of separation between the mucosal lesion and the submucosa, minimizing the risk of cautery damage to the deeper layers. By creating a cushion, it also facilitates mucosectomy. A snare polypectomy is then performed around the elevated cushion.

   There are many options for injecting solutions available. An ideal injecting solution must have the following characteristics.
   (i)   Neutral to surrounding tissue. It must not react or biochemically change the surrounding tissue.
   (ii) Must not get absorbed too quickly. It must remain in the submucosal cushion long enough for the procedure to be completed.
   (iii) Must help with hemostasis and prevent deeper tissue injury.
         Many different solutions have been studied and used at various institutions [27]. Normal saline is the most commonly used injection, but it dissipates very quickly. Other options include: 50% dextrose, sodium hyaluronate, 4% succinylated gelatin, hydroxypropyl methyl cellulose, and fibrinogen solution. Dilute epinephrine is another agent that can be added to the solution to decrease blood flow to the area, subsequently decreasing dissipation and bleeding.

2. *Cap-assisted EMR*: A clear cap is fitted at the tip of the endoscope, which is then advanced to the lesion. This method also uses a submucosal injection to raise the target lesion. A dedicated hexagonal snare is then passed through the endoscope and seated in a notch in the cap. The lesion is then suctioned into the cap and resected using electrocautery [28]. Oblique caps are commonly used to compensate for the parallel positioning of the endoscope in relation to esophageal lesions.

   Using this method, resections of lesions up to 23 mm have been safely performed. Bleeding was encountered in 24% of cases, which were all endoscopically controlled. Two perforations were encountered and managed nonoperatively [29]. Cap-assisted EMR works better when there is scar tissue present around the lesion. This can be challenging, especially with adjustment of the snare in the cap. Multiple resections also require multiple injections and thus can be time consuming. This has been compared to band resections with no significant difference in outcomes [30].

3. *Strip biopsy*: This is a technique that uses a double-channel endoscope and a submucosal injection. Following resection, a forcep is passed through the second channel to grasp the specimen [31].

Advantages of EMR

The benefits of EMR lie in its simplicity. It provides a minimally invasive approach to a complex disease that otherwise has only much more morbid treatment options. EMR also offers a great option for obtaining pathologic samples for accurate staging. EMR is much less time consuming and less morbid compared to endoscopic submucosal dissection (ESD) [32].

Limitations of EMR

When compared to ESD, EMR has a higher recurrence rate and a lower percentage of en bloc resections, specifically when larger lesions are involved and piecemeal resections are needed. A major limitation for this procedure is the presence of multifocal neoplasia and the associated risk of developing synchronous and metachronous lesions.

Post-procedural Considerations

EMR is usually performed under moderate sedation or general anesthesia as an outpatient procedure. Sometimes admission for monitoring may be necessary for complications or if a larger area is resected. Proton pump inhibitors must be maintained at high doses throughout the peri-procedural period. Some authors advise restricting patients to clear liquid diet for the first day after resection and then advancing diet as tolerated. Anticoagulant needs in the peri-procedural period must be carefully balanced on a patient-to-patient basis.

Complications

Bleeding has been reported as the most common complication with up to 7–8% incidence [33]. A majority of bleeds are endoscopically managed using hemostatic clips, injection, and coagulation.

Perforations occur in endoscopic resections in 1–5% of cases [34–37]. The risk of a perforation is higher when a piecemeal resection is performed [3]. When compared to ESD, EMR has a lower incidence of perforations (1.34% vs 4%) [38]. Most small perforations are managed nonoperatively or endoscopically with excellent outcomes. Pneumomediastinum is commonly seen.

Strictures may also occur after endoscopic resections with an overall incidence of 1–4.6% [39, 40]. However, in cases of circumferential EMR, the incidence can be as high as 26–37% [21, 41, 42]. The risks of strictures are higher when longer segments or circumferential resections are performed [43], and are usually managed successfully with endoscopic dilation. Both the cap-assisted technique and the ligation-assisted methods appear to have no difference in incidences of complications [30].

Oncologic Efficacy

EMR provides excellent oncologic benefit in patients with BE with dysplasia and early esophageal cancer. It has been found to be safe and efficacious when compared to surgery, but with significantly lower morbidity [15, 39, 44–48]. In patients with low-risk features, EMR provides 95% eradication of neoplasia and 98% 5-year survival. In those with high-risk features, complete eradication is achieved in about 80% of cases [15, 34, 38, 45, 46, 49, 50]. There is an associated risk of metachronous and recurrent lesions in about 6–30% of patients. The factors associated with recurrence are larger lesions, longer BE segments, piecemeal resections, presence of multifocal lesions, and positive neoplastic margins. Most recurrences can be safely managed endoscopically [34]. Using ablative therapy like radiofrequency ablation in combination with EMR has shown similar eradication rates. It may be useful in cases with high-risk features or piecemeal resection. Ablation does reduce the risk of bleeding, perforation, and stricture formation when compared to standard EMR [51].

Conclusion

In summary, endoscopic mucosal resection is a minimally invasive tool for accurate staging and eradication of Barrett's esophagitis with dysplasia and early esophageal cancer. The low morbidity and excellent oncologic benefit make it a valuable tool in the management of esophageal dysplasia and early adenocarcinoma.

References

1. Rosenberg N. Submucosal saline wheal as safety factor in fulguration of rectal and sigmoid polyp. AMA Arch Surg. 1955;70:120–2.
2. Deyhle P, Jenny S, Fumagalli I. Endoskopische Polypektomie im proximalen Kolon. DMW Dtsch Med Wochenschr. 1973;98(05):219–20.
3. Soetikno RM, Gotoda T, Nakanishi Y, Soehendra N. Endoscopic mucosal resection. Gastrointest Endosc. 2003;57(4):567–78.
4. Hvid-Jensen F, Pedersen L, Drewes AM, Sørensen HT, Funch-Jensen P. Incidence of adenocarcinoma among patients with Barrett's esophagus. N Engl J Med. 2011;365(15):1375–83.
5. American Gastroenterological Association, Spechler SJ, Sharma P, Souza RF, Inadomi JM, Shaheen NJ. American Gastroenterological Association medical position statement on the management of Barrett's esophagus. Gastroenterology. 2011;140(3):1084–91.
6. Fitzgerald RC, et al. British Society of Gastroenterology guidelines on the diagnosis and management of Barrett's oesophagus. Gut. 2014;63:7–42.
7. Cameron GR, Hons M, Hons B, Macrae FA, Hons M, Desmond PV. Detection and staging of esophageal cancers within Barrett's esophagus is improved by assessment in specialized Barrett's units. Gastrointest Endosc. 2014;80(6):971–83.e1.
8. Pech O, et al. Long-term results and risk factor analysis for recurrence after curative endoscopic therapy in 349 patients with high-grade intraepithelial neoplasia and mucosal adenocarcinoma in Barrett's oesophagus. Gut. 2008;57:1200–6.
9. Nijhawan PK, Wang KK. Endoscopic mucosal resection for lesions with endoscopic features suggestive of malignancy and high- grade dysplasia within Barrett's esophagus. Gastrointest Endosc. 2000;52(3):328–32.

10. Galey KM, Wilshire CL, Watson TJ, Schneider MD. Endoscopic management of early esophageal neoplasia: an emerging standard. J Gastrointest Surg. 1728–1735;15:2011.
11. Evans JA, et al. The role of endoscopy in the assessment and treatment of esophageal cancer. Gastrointest Endosc. 2013;77(3):328–34.
12. Bennett C, et al. Consensus statements for management of Barrett's dysplasia and early-stage esophageal adenocarcinoma, based on a Delphi process. Gastroenterology. 2012;143(2):336–46.
13. Takeshita K, et al. Endoscopic treatment of early oesophageal or gastric cancer. Gut. 1997;40:123–7.
14. Manner H, et al. Early Barrett's carcinoma with low-risk submucosal invasion: long-term results of endoscopic resection with a curative intent. Am J Gastroenterol. 2008;103(10):2589–97.
15. Pech O, et al. Long-term results and risk factor analysis for recurrence after curative endoscopic therapy in 349 patients with high-grade intraepithelial neoplasia and mucosal adenocarcinoma in Barrett's oesophagus. Gut. 2008;57(9):1200–6.
16. Herrero LA, et al. Risk of lymph node metastasis associated with deeper invasion by early adenocarcinoma of the esophagus and cardia: study based on endoscopic resection specimens. Endoscopy. 2010;42:1030–6.
17. Buskens CJ, Westerterp M, Lagarde SM, Bergman JJGHM, Kate FJW, Van Lanschot JJB. Prediction of appropriateness of local endoscopic treatment for high-grade dysplasia and early adenocarcinoma by EUS and histopathologic features. Gastrointest Endosc. 2001;60(5):703–10.
18. Yamasaki M, Kume K, Yoshikawa I, Otsuki M. A novel method of endoscopic submucosal dissection with blunt abrasion by submucosal injection of sodium carboxymethylcellulose: an animal preliminary study. Gastrointest Endosc. Dec. 2006;64(6):958–65.
19. Peters FP, et al. Multiband mucosectomy for endoscopic resection of Barrett's esophagus: feasibility study with matched historical controls. Eur J Gastroenterol Hepatol. 2007;19(4):311–5.
20. Herrero LA, et al. Safety and efficacy of multiband mucosectomy in 1060 resections in Barrett's esophagus. Endoscopy. 2011;43:177–83.
21. Seewald S, et al. Circumferential EMR and complete removal of Barrett's epithelium: a new approach to management of Barrett's esophagus containing high-grade intraepithelial neoplasia and intramucosal carcinoma. Gastrointest Endosc. Jun. 2003;57(7):854–9.
22. Soehendra N, et al. Endoscopic snare mucosectomy in the esophagus without any additional equipment: a simple technique for resection of flat early cancer. Endoscopy. Jun. 1997;29(5):380–3.
23. Lopes CV, et al. Endoluminal/Transluminal circumferential endoscopic resection of Barrett Õ s esophagus with high-grade dysplasia or early adenocarcinoma. Surg Endosc. 2007;21:820–4.
24. Giovannini M, et al. Circumferential endoscopic mucosal resection in Barrett's esophagus with high-grade intraepithelial neoplasia or mucosal cancer. Preliminary results in 21 patients. Endoscopy. 2004;36(9):782–7.
25. Gerke H, Siddiqui J, Nasr I, Van Handel DM. Efficacy and safety of EMR to completely remove Barrett's esophagus: experience in 41 patients. YMGE. 2011;74(4):761–71.
26. Pouw RE, et al. Stepwise radical endoscopic resection for eradication of Barrett's oesophagus with early neoplasia in a cohort of 169 patients. Gut. 2010;59(9):1169–77.
27. Fujishiro M, et al. Comparison of various submucosal injection solutions for maintaining mucosal elevation during endoscopic mucosal resection. Endoscopy. 2004;36(7):579–83.
28. Inoue H, Endo M, Takeshita K, Yoshino K, Muraoka Y, Yoneshima H. A new simplified technique of endoscopic esophageal mucosal resection using a cap-fitted panendoscope (EMRC). Surg Endosc. 1992;6(5):264–5.
29. Peters FP, et al. Endoscopic cap resection for treatment of early Barrett's neoplasia is safe: a prospective analysis of acute and early complications in 216 procedures. Dis Esophagus. 2007;20:510–5.
30. May A, Gossner L, Behrens A, Kohnen R, Vieth M. A prospective randomized trial of two different endoscopic resection techniques for early stage cancer of the esophagus. Gastrointest Endosc. 2003;58(2):167–75.
31. Tada M, Murata M, Murakami F. Development of strip-off biopsy. Gastroenterol Endosc. 1984;26:833–9.

32. Oka S, Tanaka S, Kaneko I, Mouri R, Hirata M. Advantage of endoscopic submucosal dissection compared with EMR for early gastric cancer. Gastrointest Endosc. 2006;64(6):18–23.
33. Coda S, Lee S, Gotoda T. Endoscopic mucosal resection and endoscopic submucosal dissection as treatments for early gastrointestinal cancers in Western countries. Gut Liver. 2007;1(1):12–21.
34. Pech O, et al. Long-term efficacy and safety of endoscopic resection for patients. Gastroenterology. 2014;146(3):652–60.
35. Higuchi K, Tanabe S, Azuma M. Clinical endoscopy a phase II study of endoscopic submucosal dissection for superficial esophageal neoplasms (KDOG 0901). Gastrointest Endosc. 2013;78(5):704–10.
36. Oyama T, et al. Endoscopic submucosal dissection of early esophageal cancer. Clin Gastroenterol Hepatol. 2005;3:67–70.
37. Toyonaga T, James MM, Eisei EE, Wataru N. 1,635 endoscopic submucosal dissection cases in the esophagus, stomach, and colorectum: complication rates and long-term outcomes. Surg Endosc. 2013;27:1000–8.
38. Guo H, et al. Endoscopic submucosal dissection vs endoscopic mucosal resection for superficial esophageal cancer. World J Gastroenterol. 2014;20(18):5540–7.
39. Chennat J, et al. Complete Barrett's eradication endoscopic mucosal resection: an effective treatment modality for high-grade dysplasia and intramucosal carcinoma—an American Single-Center Experience. Am J Gastroenterol. 2009;104(11):2684–92.
40. Kim HP, et al. Focal endoscopic mucosal resection before radiofrequency ablation is equally effective and safe compared with radiofrequency ablation alone for the eradication of Barrett's esophagus with advanced neoplasia. Gastrointest Endosc. 2012;76(4):733–9.
41. Tomizawa Y, Iyer PG, Wong LM, Song K, Navtej S. Safety of endoscopic mucosal resection for Barrett's esophagus. Am J Gastroenterol. 2013;108(9):1–15.
42. Larghi A, Lightdale CJ, Memeo L, Bhagat G. EUS followed by EMR for staging of high-grade dysplasia and early cancer in Barrett's esophagus. Gastrointest Endosc. 2005;62(1):16–23.
43. Katada C, Muto M, Manabe T, Boku N, Ohtsu A. Esophageal stenosis after endoscopic mucosal resection of superficial esophageal lesions. Gastrointest Endosc. 2003;57(2):165–9.
44. Prasad G, et al. Endoscopic and surgical treatment of mucosal (T1a) esophageal adenocarcinoma in Barrett's esophagus ganapathy. Gastroenterol Endosc. 2009;137(3):1–18.
45. Ell C, et al. Endoscopic mucosal resection of early cancer and high-grade dysplasia in Barrett's esophagus. Gastroenterology. 2000;118(4):670–7.
46. Ell C, May A, Pech O, Gossner L, Guenter E. Curative endoscopic resection of early esophageal adenocarcinomas (Barrett's cancer). Gastrointest Endosc. 2007;65(1):3–10.
47. Pech O, Bollschweiler E, Manner H, Leers J, Ell C, Hölscher AH. Comparison between endoscopic and surgical resection of mucosal esophageal adenocarcinoma in Barrett's esophagus at two high-volume centers. Ann Surg. 2011;254(1):67–72.
48. Wu J, Pan Y, Wang T, Gao D, Hu B. Endotherapy versus surgery for early neoplasia in Barrett's esophagus: a meta-analysis. Gastrointest Endosc. 2014;79(2):233–41.e2.
49. Peters FP, Kara MA, Rosmolen WD, Aalders MCG. Endoscopic treatment of high-grade dysplasia and early stage cancer in Barrett's esophagus. Gastrointest Endosc. 2005;61(4):506–14.
50. Moss A, et al. Endoscopic resection for Barrett's high-grade dysplasia and early esophageal adenocarcinoma: an essential staging procedure with long-term therapeutic benefit. Am J Gastroenterol. Jun. 2010;105(6):1276–83.
51. Desai M, Saligram S, Gupta N, Vennalaganti P. Efficacy and safety outcomes of multimodal endoscopic eradication therapy in Barrett's esophagus-related neoplasia: a systematic review and pooled analysis. Gastrointest Endosc. 2017;85(3):482–95.e4.

Surgical Management of Esophageal Strictures After Caustic Ingestion

Derek Moore, Georgios Orthopoulos, and John R. Romanelli

Introduction

According to the annual report of the American Association of Poison Control, in the United States there were 195,715 cases (7.54%) of human exposure to cleaning substances (household) in 2016, which constitutes the second most common substance category that is involved in human poisoning. Twenty-nine of these cases resulted in death, whereas seventeen were suicide attempts. There is a bimodal distribution of the age of occurrence with the first peak presented in the pediatric ($\leq$5-year-old) age group and the second peak in the adolescent and young adult ($\geq$21-year-old) age group. More specifically, the vast majority of pediatric cases presenting with exposures to cleaning substances in the household was reported to reach 115,701 [1]. Children are more likely to ingest caustic substances accidentally, whereas adolescent/young adults frequently attempt intentional suicide that can result in more extensive injury [2].

Caustic substances can be alkaline or acidic in nature. Alkaline material is the most frequently ingested caustic substance in Western countries, since it can be found in a variety of household bleaches, toilet bowl cleaners, detergents, and dishwashing agents. On the other hand, acid-containing material that has been implicated in caustic ingestion can be found in anti-rust compounds, swimming pool cleaners, and toilet bowl cleaners.

Solutions with pH less than 2 or greater than 12 are very corrosive and can create severe damage in the upper gastrointestinal tract. Acidic and alkaline substances induce tissue damage using different pathophysiologic mechanisms. Alkaline agents are usually colorless and tasteless and for that reason the amount ingested tends to

D. Moore · G. Orthopoulos · J. R. Romanelli (✉)
University of Massachusetts Medical School – Baystate Medical Center,
Springfield, MA, USA
e-mail: john.romanelli@baystatehealth.org

© Springer Nature Switzerland AG 2021
N. Zundel et al. (eds.), *Benign Esophageal Disease*,
https://doi.org/10.1007/978-3-030-51489-1_20

Table 20.1 Endoscopic grading of corrosive esophageal injury (Zargar system)

Grade 0	Normal findings on endoscopy
Grade 1	Edema, hyperemia of mucosa
Grade 2a	Friability, blisters, hemorrhages, erosions, whitish membranes, exudates, and superficial ulcerations
Grade 2b	Grade 2a plus deep discrete or circumferential ulcerations
Grade 3a	Small scattered areas of multiple ulcerations and areas of necrosis (brown-black or grayish discoloration)
Grade 3b	Extensive necrosis

be increased. They produce liquefaction necrosis by reacting with proteins and fat-inducing transformation to proteinases and soaps. This can lead to deeper tissue penetration and greater possibility of transmural injury [2]. Acidic agents usually have a distinct odor and an unpleasant taste, so consumption of large amounts is usually limited. They induce coagulation necrosis with eschar formation; hence there is usually decreased transmural spreading, which results in decreased incidence of full-thickness injury. In general, tissue injury progresses rapidly within minutes after ingestion and it is characterized by thrombosis of small vessels. The tissue insult continues for several days and eventually mucosal sloughing occurs 4–7 days after the caustic ingestion. This is followed by bacterial invasion, inflammatory response, and development of granulation tissue. Collagen deposition usually begins 3 weeks after the ingestion and prior to that time the tensile strength of the healing tissue is the lowest. For that reason, avoidance of endoscopy between the 5th and the 15th day after caustic ingestion is advocated [3]. After that period, scar retraction occurs and continues for several months, which can eventually result in stricture formation, shortening of the involved segment of the esophagus, and alteration of the lower esophageal pressure. This eventually can lead to severe gastroesophageal reflux that further aggravates the existing mucosal injury and accelerates stricture formation [4].

A grading system has been developed based on the endoscopic findings after ingestion of corrosive materials (Table 20.1). A direct correlation between the degree of injury and the stricture formation has been noted. Almost 30% of patients with grade 2 burns may develop stenosis whereas more than 80% of patients with grade 3 injuries will develop strictures [5].

Clinical Presentation

Factors that can influence the degree of injury include the amount and concentration of the caustic agent, the length of time of tissue contact, as well as the pH and physical form of the agent. Crystals and solid materials can adhere to the oropharyngeal mucosa causing severe injury to these areas but result in limited injury to the esophagus. On the other hand, liquid caustic agents can be swallowed quicker and produce severe injury in the esophagus and stomach. The symptomatology upon presentation depends on the location of the damage.

Hoarseness and stridor are usually the presenting symptoms indicating a laryngeal or epiglottic involvement, whereas dysphagia and odynophagia is suggestive of esophageal injury. Due to the decreased collagen deposition in the first 2 weeks after the insult, perforation of the esophagus can occur at any time during this timeframe. For that reason, an acute deterioration of an initial stable condition with sudden onset of abdominal or chest pain should warrant immediate and thorough evaluation to rule out the possibility of a perforated viscus which can result in death [4].

Late sequelae of caustic ingestion include stricture formation, gastric outlet obstruction, and malignant transformation. Patients with esophageal stricture formation may become symptomatic within 3 months or even up to a year after the insult. Ingestion of liquid lye is usually associated with higher incidence and length of strictures compared to solid crystals. Symptoms usually include dysphagia and substernal pressure. Esophageal carcinoma is a well-known consequence of caustic ingestion, especially after alkaline agent consumption since the liquefactive necrosis causes deeper penetration of the injury.

Diagnosis

Ingestion of caustic substances is not usually associated with any major laboratory abnormalities unless they are associated with esophageal or gastric perforation. Different imaging modalities can be utilized in order to identify the extent of the diseased segment.

In the acute phase after injection, a plain chest radiograph may reveal air in the mediastinum or below the diaphragm suggesting esophageal or gastric perforation respectively. If there is a suspicion of perforation, then an upper gastrointestinal series study using water-soluble agent, like Gastrografin, should be utilized as it is less of an irritant to the mediastinum and peritoneal cavity compared to barium sulfate. Barium studies can be helpful as a follow-up measure for the evaluation of complications such as strictures, since it could reveal the extent of the strictured segment. Computer tomography (CT) scan has been widely accepted as the noninvasive imaging modality that can assess the extent of the esophageal injury, especially at an early stage. It can reveal the depth of necrosis and frequently the presence of transmural damage allowing clinicians to assess the degree of the injury. Other imaging studies such as endoscopic ultrasound and magnetic resonance imaging (MRI) appeared to provide less advantage in the assessment of caustic injury.

Besides the above-mentioned noninvasive diagnostic techniques, esophagogastroduodenoscopy (EGD) remains the most important diagnostic tool in the evaluation of early caustic injury especially during the first 48 hours of ingestion. As previously mentioned, endoscopy is generally not recommended 5–15 days after caustic ingestion due to tissue friability during the healing phase. Prior to initiating an endoscopic approach, the oropharynx needs to be examined. A third-degree burn of the hypopharynx is a contraindication for endoscopy, as well as hemodynamic instability, severe respiratory compromise, and suspected perforations [2]. There are no strict guidelines as to who needs endoscopic evaluation. However, it is strongly recommended in symptomatic patients who suffered intentional ingestion of large quantities of corrosives, taking into consideration that it should be avoided within the period 5–15 days following the ingestion [3]. Endoscopy is considered the ultimate tool to guide the management of the caustic ingestions since it can provide a grading system based on the mucosal appearance. The most commonly utilized classification system was created by Zargar et al. [5] (Table 20.1). Based on that system, grades 0, I, and IIA esophageal burns usually recover from their injuries without any adverse events, whereas the majority of grades IIb and III burns eventually develop major complications including strictures.

Initial Management of Corrosive Ingestion

The mainstay for management of caustic injuries includes airway and hemodynamic stabilization along with resuscitation. Intubation should be immediately considered since there is direct exposure of the upper respiratory tract to the caustic agent. Occasionally, intubation under fiberoptic laryngoscopy needs to be performed to avoid further trauma to the area, and also tracheostomy should be considered if there is significant edema in the epiglottis and larynx.

Neutralizing Agents

Consumption of neutralizing agents (weakly acidic or basic substances) had been considered one of the most important first steps in the management of caustic substances ingestion [6]. However, this practice has been aborted since administration of neutralizing agents can generate chemical reaction that can lead to increased thermal injury and overall tissue damage. Moreover, substances such as milk or charcoal can coat the esophageal mucosa and potentially obscure subsequent endoscopy.

Nasogastric Tube and Gastric Acid Suppression

Routine early insertion of nasogastric tube has been considered a necessary step in order to achieve evacuation of any remaining caustic material prior to endoscopic evaluation of the esophageal mucosa. However, this has been abandoned due to the possibility of inducing vomiting and further exposing the esophagus to caustic material. Also, the nasogastric tube can contribute to the development of long strictures or act as a nidus for infection, which may result in delayed mucosal healing [2].

Gastric acid suppression with liberal use of intravenous protein pump inhibitors should be utilized in order to allow faster mucosal healing and prevent stress ulcers [7]. Moreover, sucralfate is currently commonly used in the setting of caustic ingestion since it is said to promote mucosal healing by preventing exposure of the esophageal mucosa to the corrosive substance. Several small randomized controlled studies have also showed that sucralfate may result in decreased frequency of stricture formation following caustic material ingestion [2, 8].

Antibiotics

There are no concrete data regarding the use of antibiotics after caustic substance ingestion. Current practice advocates that patients treated with steroids should be concomitantly treated with antibiotics, but there are no controlled trials that have investigated this. Howell et al. performed a meta-analysis in 361 subjects from a total of 13 studies and concluded that there is a statistically significant difference between the strictures that occurred in patients not receiving corticosteroids and antibiotics compared to the ones who did (40% vs 19%). Although it is unclear if the observed difference could be attributed to the use of corticosteroids or antibiotics, the consensus appears to be that patients with caustic ingestion who are treated with corticosteroids should also be treated with antibiotics [9].

Triamcinolone and Mitomycin-C

Intralesional corticosteroid injection has been proposed as an adjunct to the management of strictures induced by caustic substance consumption. Kochhar et al. have recommended that intralesional injection of triamcinolone can result in decrease in the number of endoscopic dilations performed and subsequently lead to statistically significant improvement in the dysphagia score compared to patients who did not receive steroid injections [10, 11]. Mitomycin-C is another substance that has been utilized in the algorithm of esophageal stricture management following caustic injury. It has been proposed that topical application of mitomycin-C can result in improvement of long-segment esophageal strictures given its antifibroblastic activity. El-Asmar et al. evaluated the effect of topical mitomycin-C application after endoscopic esophageal dilatation in children in order to treat long-segment (>3 cm in length) esophageal strictures. The study revealed clinical, radiological, and endoscopic resolution of strictures in 85.7% of the study population without any short- or mid-term recurrences or complications [12].

Systemic Steroids

Studies regarding the use of steroids in the prevention of strictures after caustic ingestion in humans have been inconclusive. Most of them have been performed in pediatric population and they revealed conflicting results. Usta et al. concluded that administration of high doses of methylprednisolone (1 g/1.73 m^2/day for a total of 3 days) can lead to reduction in stricture formation in children who have suffered grade IIb esophageal burn [13]. Also, Bautista et al. showed that children who underwent administration of dexamethasone (1 mg/kg/day) resulted in stricture prevention and significantly decreased number of dilatations compared to children who received prednisolone (2 mg/kg/day) [14].

However, a prospective study conducted in 60 children over a period of 18 years concluded that there appeared to be no benefit from the use of steroids to treat children who have ingested a caustic substance [15]. Similar finding was noted in a systematic pooled analysis of a total of 328 patients who suffered grade II esophageal burns following caustic ingestion. This study revealed no additional benefit with the use of steroids in patients with caustic-induced grade II esophageal burns [16]. The use of corticosteroids remains a debatable issue; however, most practitioners agree that corticosteroids are not necessary in first-degree burns, but there might be an indication to use them in third-degree esophageal burns [3].

Endoscopy

Besides its use in the evaluation and diagnosis of caustic injury, EGD plays an important role in the subsequent management. In general, patients with Zargar grade I or IIA require in-hospital observation and gradual advancement in diet over a period of 24–48 hours. Patients with grade IIB or more severe esophageal burns will require close monitoring and possible endoscopically guided nasoenteric feeding tube placement to facilitate feeding distally to the area of necrosis [2].

One of the most common late complications following caustic substance ingestion is esophageal stricture. Katz et al. report that up to 70% of grade IIB and more than 90% of patients with grade III injuries will eventually develop esophageal strictures [17]. Management of esophageal strictures can be achieved endoscopically or surgically. Endoscopic measures that can be employed include mainly dilatation (with bougies or balloon dilators) and stent placement (self-expanding metal, plastic, or biodegradable stents), whereas surgical options include partial or total esophagectomy with gastric pullup or colonic interposition.

Endoscopic management has been described in a previous chapter. We are going to focus on the most commonly performed esophagectomy techniques.

Surgical Management of Esophageal Stricture

Esophageal stricture is a delayed sequela of caustic injury, and may require surgical management if it is of a long segment or refractory to dilation. Iatrogenic perforation during dilation is also an indication for acute surgical management. Given the nature of the extensive cellular injury and potential for malignant transformation caused by caustic ingestion, esophagectomy is the gold surgical standard. This is usually accompanied by a gastric conduit, although colon or jejunal interposition may also be used if the stomach is not a viable option for esophageal replacement. There are three common surgical approaches to esophagectomy: thoraco-abdominal Ivor Lewis, three-field McKeown, and transhiatal. Each has its own advantages, and consideration should be taken for the location of the caustic injury as well as surgeon comfort with the procedure.

Ivor Lewis Esophagectomy

This approach, first proposed in 1946 by Ivor Lewis [18] as a two-stage procedure, requires comfort operating in both the chest and the abdomen, and has the benefit of avoiding a cervical incision. Originally the abdominal portion was performed, followed by thoracotomy 10–15 days later. Currently performed in one setting, it is useful for mid and distal esophageal strictures, and utilizes an intrathoracic anastomosis. It may be performed open or minimally invasively using laparoscopy, thoracoscopy, or robotic techniques. The abdominal portion of the operation is performed first, with complete mobilization of the gastric conduit and distal esophagus. Feeding jejunostomy and surgical or chemical pyloroplasty are also performed in the abdomen at this time. The distal margin of specimen is divided, and proximal conduit is sutured to distal specimen. These are then placed through the hiatus, and the patient is repositioned into left lateral decubitus for the thoracic stage of the operation. In the right hemi-thorax, the remainder of the esophagus is mobilized, specimen is removed, and the gastric conduit is brought to length in the thorax and anastomosed to proximal intrathoracic esophagus, most commonly in an end-to-end fashion with an end-to-end anastomotic (EEA) stapler [19].

Procedure Steps: Minimally Invasive

Abdominal Portion

Step 1a. *Laparoscopic port placement:* A 10 or 12 mm port is placed under direct visualization approximately at two-thirds distance from xiphoid to umbilicus, slightly to the right of midline. This will be used as the operator's right-hand port. Four more ports are then placed under laparoscopic visualization. The first is a 5 mm right subcostal port for the operator's left hand, followed by another 5 mm left subcostal for the assistant's right hand. A 5 or 10 mm right lateral port is placed for the liver retractor, and a fourth 5 mm port is placed left of midline, just caudal to the original 10 mm port for the camera. (This port could be a 10 mm port if a 10 mm laparoscope is preferred.) The exact port placements may need to be modified based on patient's body habitus. The patient is then placed in steep reverse Trendelenburg position (Fig. 20.1).

Fig. 20.1 Laparoscopic
port placement

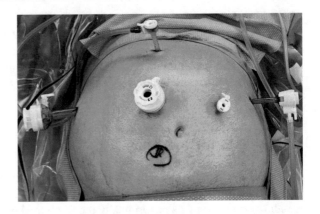

Step 1b. *Robotic port placement*: A 12 mm port is placed under direct visualization 18 cm below the xiphoid process. Two 8 mm ports should be placed to the patient's left at the same level, spaced approximately 9 cm between each port, and one 8 mm port spaced 9 cm to the right of the 12 mm camera port. A 5 mm port is placed for the liver retractor in the same manner as the laparoscopic procedure. A 12 mm assistant port is placed in the right lower quadrant to create a 9 cm equilateral triangle with the camera and robotic left arm working ports [20].

If the surgeon is not comfortable with laparoscopic surgery, then an upper midline laparotomy may be used for the abdominal portion of the operation.

Step 2. *Liver retraction:* A liver retractor is placed through right lateral port, and the left lobe of the liver is retracted cephalad.

Step 3. *Gastric mobilization:* The gastrohepatic ligament is divided and the right crus of the diaphragm is identified. The hiatus is then dissected out anteriorly from right to left until the left crus is identified. The greater curvature of the stomach is then mobilized by ligation of the short gastric vessels with an ultrasonic dissector or bipolar energy device. Afterward, any remaining gastrocolic ligamentous attachments and posterior gastric attachments are divided as the stomach is retracted anteriorly. Care should be taken to preserve the right gastroepiploic artery and its arcades during this dissection, as it will be the primary blood supply of the gastric conduit. The left gastric artery is then identified and stapled, which should be the final step in completely freeing the stomach.

Step 4. *Pyloroplasty:* After mobilizing any attachments of the pylorus, a Heineke-Mikulicz pyloroplasty [21] is then performed, with longitudinal myotomy, transverse interrupted closure, and omental buttress. Endoscopic Botox injection is a nonsurgical alternative to pyloroplasty, and has shown efficacy in small trials without additional complications [22].

Step 5. *Creation of gastric conduit:* With the fundus retracted cephalad, and the antrum retracted caudally, the stomach is divided with sequential staple loads along the lesser curvature to create a conduit approximately 5 cm in diameter (Fig. 20.2). The right gastric artery should be preserved if possible, but may be transected if necessary.

Step 6. *Jejunostomy tube creation:* A jejunostomy tube is then placed in Witzel fashion [23].

Step 7. *Conduit completion:* The specimen portion of the stomach is attached to the proximal gastric conduit with a stitch. The phrenoesophageal ligament is then divided, and the specimen and proximal conduit are then passed through the hiatus into the chest. In the absence of a pre-existing hiatal hernia, the hiatus may need to be surgically enlarged. If possible, an omental flap is also created and passed into the chest. Based on conduit size, a posterior crural closure stitch may be placed to prevent future herniation.

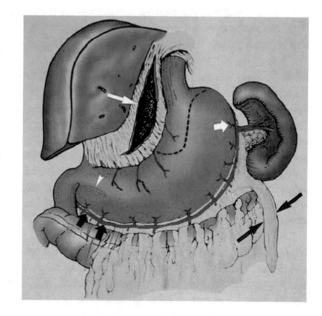

Fig. 20.2 Gastric conduit creation. The right gastroepiploic artery (short black arrows), possible omental flap (long black arrows), gastrohepatic ligament (long white arrow), site of pyloromyotomy (arrowhead), and the short gastric arteries (short white arrow) are illustrated. (Adapted with permission from Kim et al. [29])

Thoracic Portion

Step 8a. *Repositioning and thoracic port placement:* The patient is placed in left lateral decubitus position for the thoracic portion of the operation. Four thoracoscopic incisions are used for this phase. First, a 10 mm incision is made in the seventh intercostal space, mid-axillary line, for the camera. A second 10 mm is made in the eighth intercostal space, posterior axillary line, for the operator's right hand, followed by another 10 mm incision in the fourth intercostal space, anterior axillary line, to be used for anterior lung retraction. Lastly, a 5 mm incision is made posterior to the tip of the scapula for the operator's left hand. A traction stitch is placed through the central tendon of the diaphragm and brought through the chest wall using a laparoscopic suture passer through a small incision.

Step 8b. *Robotic thoracic port placement:* Patient is placed in left lateral decubitus position as with video-assisted thoracoscopic surgery (VATS). A trocar site for the right robotic arm is marked just below the hair line at the anterior axillary line. An 8 mm camera port is placed 9 cm inferior and slightly posterior to this marked future port site. The camera is then inserted to evaluate the pleural space for any adhesions. An 8 mm working port is then placed at the previously marked site (working right arm). A third 8 mm port is placed 9 cm inferior to the camera port and slightly posterior (working left arm 1). A 5 mm port is placed 10 cm posterior from the third port (working left arm 2), and a 12 mm assistant port is placed anteriorly to create a 9 cm equilateral triangle with the camera port and the third port [20].

If the surgeon is not comfortable with minimally invasive approaches, a right thoracotomy may be used.

Step 9. *Esophageal mobilization:* The inferior pulmonary ligament is divided using an ultrasonic dissector or bipolar energy device. The mediastinal pleura overlying the esophagus is divided up to the azygos vein, which is then divided using an endoscopic stapler containing a vascular staple load. The esophagus is then mobilized circumferentially. A Penrose drain may be placed around the esophagus to assist in maintaining tension for the dissection. The vagus nerves are divided bilaterally at the level of the azygos vein. The esophagus may then be divided above the level of injury/stricture. The eighth intercostal incision is enlarged at this time to allow for removal of specimen. The remainder of the conduit is brought into the chest, taking care to maintain proper orientation.

Step 10. *Intrathoracic anastomosis:* A 28 mm EEA anvil is placed into the proximal esophagus, secured by a two-layer purse-string stitch. A gastrotomy is made in the fundus, through which the EEA stapler is passed, and an end-to-end esophagogastric anastomosis is created. A nasogastric tube is placed under direct visualization. The gastrotomy is then closed using a laparoscopic linear gastrointestinal anastomotic (GIA) stapler, maintaining as much remaining conduit as possible, and an endoscopic leak test is performed using insufflation while the anastomosis is submerged in sterile saline. If available, an omental flap is placed over the anastomosis with suture, and a drain is placed posterior to the anastomosis. Finally, the conduit is anchored to right crus.

McKeown Esophagectomy

First described by Kenneth McKeown [24], the three-field esophagectomy utilizes abdominal, thoracic, and cervical techniques. It is useful for proximal esophageal strictures and its primary advantage over transhiatal esophagectomy is direct visualization of the intrathoracic mobilization of the esophagus. As with the Ivor Lewis approach, it requires comfort with minimally invasive or open thoracic surgery. For this approach, thoracic mobilization of the esophagus is performed first. Abdominal mobilization of the distal esophagus and conduit is performed next, followed by anastomosis through a left cervical incision [25].

Procedure Steps

Step 1. The thoracic portion of the surgery is performed first using the same technique as the Ivor Lewis esophagectomy, with the exception that the esophagus will be dissected into the thoracic inlet with care taken to spare the recurrent laryngeal nerves and thoracic duct. The esophagus is not divided in the chest, just dissected.

Step 2. The abdominal portion is performed in the same manner as the Ivor Lewis esophagectomy, again with the phrenoesophageal ligament division being the final step.

Step 3. A 4–6 cm transverse cervical incision is made slightly to left of midline for an anterolateral approach to the esophagus. The cervical esophagus is dissected down to the thoracic inlet, where it should meet the thoracic dissection plane. Care must be taken to avoid the recurrent laryngeal nerve as it lies in the tracheoesophageal groove. Strap muscles may be divided to provide adequate exposure if needed.

Step 4. The specimen is removed through the cervical incision, and the esophagus is divided approximately 1–2 cm below the cricopharyngeus muscle. A 25 mm EEA stapler is used to perform the esophagogastric anastomosis in a similar manner to the Ivor Lewis procedure. A slightly smaller anvil is generally used in the cervical esophagus than in the mid-thoracic esophagus.

Step 5. The abdomen is re-evaluated to assess for twisting of the conduit. The conduit is then tacked to the right crus of diaphragm to prevent herniation.

Transhiatal Esophagectomy

The transhiatal approach originates back to 1933 [26], but was returned to popularity in 1978 by Mark Orringer [27]. It is performed through cervical and abdominal incisions only, and must be performed with incisions large enough to place the surgeon's hands through for blind manual dissection of the intrathoracic esophagus. In a similar manner, the esophageal hiatus may be widened for manual esophageal dissection, followed by sutured hiatal closure if necessary. The primary advantage is avoidance of thoracotomy. The technique may not be feasible if there is significant scarring around the esophagus that has distorted or obliterated tissue planes. In cases of especially difficult dissection, en masse ligation of tissue at the hiatus may be required to prevent thoracic duct leak and subsequent chylothorax. In the same manner as the McKeown esophagectomy, specimen removal and anastomosis are performed through the left cervical incision [28].

Procedure Steps

Step 1. Upper midline incision is used to enter the abdomen. The intra-abdominal portion of the surgery is performed similarly to other esophagectomy techniques but is completed through a laparotomy incision rather than laparoscopically.

Step 2. The distal 10 cm of the esophagus is dissected through the abdomen, and this cavity is then packed to assist with hemostasis.

Step 3. A cervical incision is made in the same fashion as a McKeown esophagectomy. The esophagus is circumferentially bluntly dissected using finger fraction. A Penrose drain is then placed around the esophagus for cephalad traction.

Step 4. A hand is then placed, palm facing forward through the diaphragmatic hiatus along the posterior esophagus with the back of the hand along the spine (Fig. 20.3). If the diaphragmatic hiatus is not large enough to accommodate the surgeon's hands, it must be widened at this step.

Step 5. The esophagus is bluntly dissected from the cervical incision toward the hand placed at the previously dissected lower thorax.

Step 6. This maneuver is repeated to clear the anterior and lateral surfaces of the esophagus.

Step 7. The cervical esophagus is divided with a GIA stapler, and the specimen is withdrawn cephalad and removed through the cervical incision. The mediastinum is then packed from each direction.

Step 8. The gastric conduit is then laid across the anterior chest to evaluate for proper length. It is then manually advanced through the hiatus and brought through the cervical incision (Fig. 20.4). The anastomosis may be performed using an EEA or GIA stapler (as described by Orringer [28]). The diaphragmatic hiatus may be closed with crural stitches at this time if hiatal widening was required.

Fig. 20.3 Manual transhiatal esophageal mobilization. (Adapted with permission from Kim et al. [29])

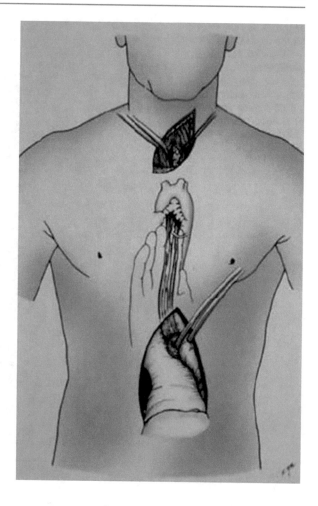

Conclusion

Caustic ingestion is a common occurrence in the United States, especially in the pediatric and adolescent population. Early management of caustic ingestion is primarily medical in the absence of esophageal perforation. Unfortunately, one of the frequent long-term sequelae is esophageal stricture. This pathology may be treated first by medical and endoscopic management, but for persistent or refractory strictures esophagectomy is indicated. There are multiple techniques used for esophagectomy, with the primary indications for each being the location of the stricture and the surgeon's comfort with the technical steps and experience in minimally invasive or robotic surgery.

Fig. 20.4 Evaluation of
gastric conduit length. The
cervical dissection site
(outlined arrow),
pyloromyotomy site
(arrowhead), and the
gastric division line (short
black arrow) are illustrated.
(Adapted with permission
from Kim et al. [29])

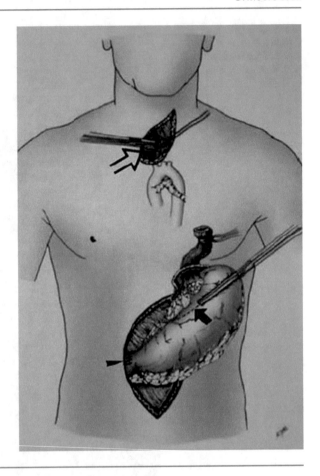

References

1. Gummin DD, Mowry JB, Spyker DA, Brooks DE, Fraser MO, Banner W. 2016 Annual Report of the American Association of Poison Control Centers' National Poison Data System (NPDS): 34th annual report. Clin Toxicol (Phila). 2017;55(10):1072–252.
2. De Lusong MAA, Timbol ABG, Tuazon DJS. Management of esophageal caustic injury. World J Gastrointest Pharmacol Ther. 2017;8(2):90–8.
3. Ramasamy K, Gumaste VV. Corrosive ingestion in adults. J Clin Gastroenterol. 2003;37(2):119–24.
4. Contini S, Scarpignato C. Caustic injury of the upper gastrointestinal tract: a comprehensive review. World J Gastroenterol. 2013;19(25):3918–30.
5. Zargar SA, Kochhar R, Mehta S, Mehta SK. The role of fiberoptic endoscopy in the management of corrosive ingestion and modified endoscopic classification of burns. Gastrointest Endosc. 1991;37(2):165–9.
6. Chibishev A, Pereska Z, Simonovska N, Chibisheva V, Glasnovic M, Chitkushev LT. Conservative therapeutic approach to corrosive poisonings in adults. J Gastrointest Surg. 2013;17(6):1044–9.
7. Cakal B, Akbal E, Köklü S, Babalı A, Koçak E, Taş A. Acute therapy with intravenous omeprazole on caustic esophageal injury: a prospective case series. Dis Esophagus. 2013;26(1):22–6.
8. Gümürdülü Y, Karakoç E, Kara B, Taşdoğan BE, Parsak CK, Sakman G. The efficiency of sucralfate in corrosive esophagitis: a randomized, prospective study. Turk J Gastroenterol. 2010;21(1):7–11.

9. Howell JM, Dalsey WC, Hartsell FW, Butzin CA. Steroids for the treatment of corrosive esophageal injury: a statistical analysis of past studies. Am J Emerg Med. 1992;10(5):421–5.
10. Kochhar R, Ray JD, Sriram PV, Kumar S, Singh K. Intralesional steroids augment the effects of endoscopic dilation in corrosive esophageal strictures. Gastrointest Endosc. 1999;49(4 Pt 1):509–13.
11. Kochhar R, Poornachandra KS. Intralesional steroid injection therapy in the management of resistant gastrointestinal strictures. World J Gastrointest Endosc. 2010;2(2):61–8.
12. El-Asmar KM, Hassan MA, Abdelkader HM, Hamza AF. Topical mitomycin C can effectively alleviate dysphagia in children with long-segment caustic esophageal strictures. Dis Esophagus. 2015;28(5):422–7.
13. Usta M, Erkan T, Cokugras FC, Urganci N, Onal Z, Gulcan M, et al. High doses of methylprednisolone in the management of caustic esophageal burns. Pediatrics. 2014;133(6):E1518–24.
14. Bautista A, Varela R, Villanueva A, Estevez E, Tojo R, Cadranel S. Effects of prednisolone and dexamethasone in children with alkali burns of the oesophagus. Eur J Pediatr Surg. 1996;6(4):198–203.
15. Anderson KD, Rouse TM, Randolph JG. A controlled trial of corticosteroids in children with corrosive injury of the esophagus. N Engl J Med. 1990;323(10):637–40.
16. Fulton JA, Hoffman RS. Steroids in second degree caustic burns of the esophagus: a systematic pooled analysis of fifty years of human data: 1956-2006. Clin Toxicol (Phila). 2007;45(4):402–8.
17. Kluger Y, Ishay OB, Sartelli M, Katz A, Ansaloni L, Gomez CA, et al. Caustic ingestion management: world society of emergency surgery preliminary survey of expert opinion. World J Emerg Surg. 2015;10:48.
18. Lewis I. The surgical treatment of carcinoma of the esophagus with special reference to a new operation for growths of the middle third. Br J Surg. 1946;34:18–31.
19. Pennathur A, Awais O, Luketich JD. Technique of minimally invasive Ivor Lewis esophagectomy. Ann Thorac Surg. 2010;89(6):S2159–62.
20. Broussard B, Evans J, Wei B, Cerfolio R. Robotic esophagectomy. J Vis Surg. 2016;2:139.
21. Mikulicz. Archiv für klinische Chirurgie. 1888;xxxvii:79.
22. Fuchs HF, Broderick RC, Harnsberger CR, Divo FA, Coker AM, Jacobsen GR, Sandler BJ, Bouvet M, Horgan S. Intraoperative endoscopic Botox injection during total esophagectomy prevents the need for pyloromyotomy or dilatation. J Laparoendosc Adv Surg Tech A. 2016;26(6):433–8.
23. Witzel O. Zur Technik der Magenfistelanlegung. Zentralbl Chir. 1891;18:601–4.
24. McKeown KC. Total three-stage oesophagectomy for cancer of the oesophagus. Br J Surg. 1976;63-4:259–62.
25. Luketich JD, Alvelo-Rivera M, Buenaventura PO, Christie NA, McCaughan JS, Litle VR, et al. Minimally invasive esophagectomy: outcomes in 222 patients. Ann Surg. 2003;238(4):486–94; discussion 94–5.
26. Turner GG. Excision of thoracic esophagus for carcinoma with construction of extrathoracic gullet. Lancet. 1933;2:1315–6.
27. Orringer MB, Sloan H. Esophagectomy without thoracotomy. J Thorac Cardiovasc Surg. 1978;76:643–54.
28. Orringer MB. Transhiatal esophagectomy: how I teach it. Ann Thorac Surg. 2016;102(5):1432–7.
29. Kim SH, et al. Esophageal resection: indications, techniques, and radiologic assessment. Radiographics. 2001;21(5):1119–37.

Endoscopic Management of Esophageal Perforations

21

Naomi Berezin

Introduction

The past 10 years have seen a paradigm shift in the management of esophageal perforations. Whereas perforations were previously managed either conservatively or aggressively with surgical intervention depending on various criteria, endoscopic therapy and wide drainage have now become the mainstays of treatment. This has resulted in considerable improvement in patient morbidity and mortality. Yet, despite this shift in therapeutic approach, esophageal perforation remains a highly morbid and mortal diagnosis. The following chapter discusses the etiologies of esophageal perforations, presentation, workup, therapy, and outcomes.

Etiology

The incidence of esophageal perforation is largely unknown. The literature varies widely and is mostly estimated based on single-center studies or isolated populations due to the relative rarity of this condition. In Canada, for instance, the incidence is approximately 3.1 per 1,000,000 per year [1]. This number is on the rise yearly in proportion with the increased number of upper endoscopies [2].

Iatrogenic injury is the leading cause of esophageal perforation globally and most commonly occurs during endoscopy, which accounts for 60% of all perforations [3]. On the whole, upper endoscopy carries a 0.033% risk of perforation, with therapeutic endoscopy more frequently resulting in perforation than diagnostic [4]. Other iatrogenic causes such as intraoperative injuries during foregut surgery or

N. Berezin (✉)
General Surgery, Montefiore Medical Center/Albert Einstein College of Medicine, Bronx, NY, USA

© Springer Nature Switzerland AG 2021
N. Zundel et al. (eds.), *Benign Esophageal Disease*,
https://doi.org/10.1007/978-3-030-51489-1_21

unrelated surgeries in the abdomen, chest, neck, and spine have been described, as well as from other instrumentation such as nasogastric tube placement.

Ingested foreign bodies such as fish or poultry bones account for 80% of cervical esophageal perforations [5].

Penetrating trauma is another well-described cause of esophageal perforation that is most frequently caused by either stabbing (15–20%) or gunshot (70–80%) [6].

Boerhaave syndrome, the most common cause of spontaneous perforation, is the second leading cause of esophageal rupture, representing between 8% and 56% of perforations [3]. Other etiologies of spontaneous perforations have been described related to various medical diagnoses and treatments including achalasia, infection, inflammatory and autoimmune diseases, radiation, and medications. Malignancy accounts for approximately 1% of perforations [5].

Finally, caustic ingestion is a leading cause of perforation among the pediatric population where this injury is almost always accidental [7]. Conversely, in the adult population, caustic ingestion is relatively rare and is more often seen as the result of an intentional ingestion during attempted suicide [8]. Household cleaning products are the most common culprit, accounting for 80% of cases, with alkali solutions more likely to cause perforation than acidic solutions [9].

Location

In terms of both therapeutic approach and outcomes, the location of an esophageal perforation is paramount. The esophagus is stratified into three regions based on its relation to anatomical compartments: the cervical esophagus, the thoracic esophagus, and the abdominal esophagus. Perforations of the thoracic esophagus account for 72.6% overall, followed by cervical at 15.2% and finally abdominal at 12.5% [10].

Perforations due to instrumentation are most likely to be thoracic (45%), whereas spontaneous and operative perforations are more commonly abdominal (60% and 75%, respectively), and trauma and foreign body perforations are predominantly cervical (80% and 85%, respectively) [5].

Signs and Symptoms

Presenting signs and symptoms are dependent on the location of esophageal perforation as well as time elapsed. Often patients with esophageal perforations will relay an inciting event. Patients with cervical perforations will present with neck pain, aerodigestive symptoms, or subcutaneous emphysema [10].

By and large, patients with thoracic esophageal perforations will present with chest pain that is pleuritic in nature and radiates to the back or shoulder [10]. Patients with Boerhaave syndrome, in particular, may present with Mackler's triad: emesis followed by chest pain and then subcutaneous emphysema, though this is seen only 14% of the time [11].

Finally, patients with abdominal esophageal perforations will present with abdominal pain, typically epigastric, or frank peritonitis [12]. Due to the rapidly progressive natural course of this disease, late presentation (>24 h) is often nonspecific with progressive findings of pneumonia, sepsis, multiorgan dysfunction, and shock [13, 14].

Diagnosis

A high index of suspicion is critical for the diagnosis of esophageal perforation. Careful history and physical exam will commonly reveal instigating events such as recent endoscopy, emesis, bone ingestion, choking, or trauma, or physical findings such as subcutaneous emphysema or peritonitis [15]. Laboratory exams may show a leukocytosis with left shift consistent with infectious process. Chest X-ray may reveal pneumomediastinum, pneumonia, or pneumothorax. In thoracic perforations, standard lung X-ray is abnormal in 90% of patients, though this is often nonspecific [3].

More specifically, there are three imaging modalities commonly used to definitively diagnose esophageal perforations. Computed tomography (CT) is the initial diagnostic test of choice as it is quick and easily obtainable in any institution. CT may reveal stigmata of perforation such as extraluminal air adjacent to the esophagus in the neck, thorax or abdomen, pneumomediastinum or pneumothorax, or pleural or mediastinal fluid. Sensitivity can be increased up to 92–100% with the addition of oral contrast [16]. This should always be water soluble in the setting of suspected perforation as barium can cause irreversible mediastinitis/fibrosis. Additionally, CT aids in ruling out other confounding diagnoses.

Fluoroscopy, or oral contrast esophagogram, similarly may reveal extravasation of oral contrast; however, it is more difficult to obtain in smaller centers. While some studies advocate fluoroscopy over CT, others show that oral contrast-enhanced CT is far superior, with fluoroscopy demonstrating only 50% sensitivity for cervical perforations and 75–80% for thoracic perforations [5, 17].

Finally, endoscopy is an excellent modality as it allows for both diagnosis and therapy. Endoscopy allows for direct visualization of the defect, and enables characterization and planning to address both the acute problem and any underlying issue [18].

Treatment and Outcomes

Early diagnosis and treatment of esophageal perforations are essential in reducing morbidity and mortality. Overall mortality for esophageal perforations is approximately 11.9%; however, for patients who necessitate operative intervention, the mortality is 20% [3, 19]. Diagnosis and treatment within 24 h, however, reduce mortality by up to 50% [20, 21].

Cervical perforations carry an overall mortality of 5.9%, thoracic perforations 10.9%, and intraabdominal perforations 13.2%. By cause, mortality after esophageal perforation secondary to foreign body was 2.1%, iatrogenic perforation 13.2%, and spontaneous perforation 14.8% [19].

First and foremost, supportive care, nil per os status, and broad-spectrum antibiotics should be initiated on presentation. Antibiotics should cover upper gastrointestinal (GI) flora including gram-positive bacteria, gram-negative bacteria, and yeast, and should be narrowed based on cultures [13]. Intervention should be performed as early as reasonably possible to shorten the length of ongoing contamination and should be focused on source control with closure or coverage of the defect where possible as well as drainage of the affected cavity when indicated [20, 21]. Perforations recognized at the time of endoscopy or surgery should be treated immediately. Intuitively, patients with small defects that are diagnosed and treated expeditiously have the best outcomes [22].

At the time of intervention, consideration for enteral feeding access should be given, as many patients will remain nil per os for extended periods of time [22].

Management of malignant perforations requires special consideration and is not discussed in this chapter.

Endoscopy Versus Surgery

There is no better opportunity to diagnose and treat simultaneously than with upper endoscopy. Surgery is far more invasive, necessitating neck dissection, thoracotomy, laparoscopy, or possibly laparotomy. Therefore, with appropriate patient selection, endoscopy should be considered the initial intervention of choice [18]. The number of patients with esophageal perforations that are managed nonoperatively has dramatically risen in the past 10 years, such that surgical intervention now is used in less than half of all cases, and this number continues to decline annually [10]. Should operative intervention be required either acutely or due to failure of nonoperative or endoscopic management, the general principles of esophageal repair apply. Regardless of location, these include: exposure, debridement of nonviable tissue, closure of defect in two layers, the use of buttress, and tube drainage [6].

Surgical approaches and technique will be discussed in the next chapter.

Endoscopic Techniques

Endoscopic management of esophageal perforations is an evolving field and techniques vary from center to center based on the availability and comfort of specialists. These injuries should only be handled in high-volume specialty centers with access to endoscopic experts as well as a thoracic or foregut surgeon who is familiar with the management and operative repair of esophageal perforations. In centers that lack these resources, patients should be stabilized and transferred expeditiously. Endoscopy, though an excellent standalone therapy when an esophageal perforation is immediately recognized, often must be combined with drainage procedures in the setting of gross contamination in order to achieve appropriate source control. Predictors of successful endoscopic therapy are smaller defect and shorter time to diagnosis and therapy [23, 24].

Clips

Endoscopic clip placement is an excellent means of managing small perforations with minimal surrounding inflammation. There are two types of clips that are used. Small clips are deployable via the working port of the endoscope, whereas the bear-trap-like over-the-scope clip (OTSC®) system (Ovesco Endoscopy AG, Tubingen, Germany) offers larger clips with fewer limitations. The latter clips are useful for lesions up to 30 mm and exert greater force on the closure [25]. When compared to through-the-scope clips, OTSCs are associated with lower rates of surgical intervention [26]. There are few unique complications of endoscopic clip use other than malfunction and failure.

Overall, clips are successful in closing 56–100% of perforations for which they are attempted, without the need for any surgical intervention or repeat endoscopy [18]. Furthermore, when clips are used as first line therapy, there is a higher rate of success than when applied after another therapy has failed [27]. Limitations include the size of the perforation, and the quality of the surrounding tissue. Along these lines, risk of failure is greater with chronic perforations and fistulae [28]. The average size lesion that results in successful closure with endoscopic clips is 8 mm, with a significantly increased rate of failure for defects greater than 13 mm [29, 30].

Stents

Endoscopic stents have become the mainstay of therapy for esophageal perforations that are too large or long standing to be amenable to endoscopic clipping. Stents are indicated in almost any type of esophageal injury but have varying rates of success depending on the size and location of injury. Overall, technical success rate is ~91% and clinical success rate ~81% with endoscopic stenting. The rate of stent migration is significantly higher with plastic stents than metal stents, 27% versus 11%, respectively, whereas metal stents are more prone to causing postprocedural strictures. Due to the differences in stent migration, patients with plastic stents need far more reintervention [31]. Bare metal stents are prone to mucosal ingrowth, and therefore are excellent for permanent placement such as for patients with malignancy. Covered stents are retrievable, and because of this, self-expanding covered metal stents should be used preferentially.

There are four factors that are most predictive of stent failure: injury to the proximal cervical esophagus, injury that traverses the gastroesophageal junction, length of injury greater than 6 cm, and anastomotic leak associated with more distal conduit leak [32].

Despite initial technical success, some patients will still require surgery upon stent removal due to persistent leak. Several studies have shown various outcomes with self-expanding metal stents with ranges from 77% to 100% success. Stent failure either mandates repeat stenting for long-term course or operation [33, 34].

Not surprisingly, stent migration is the most common complication, 8.8–40%, with other complications including tissue overgrowth, erosions/ulcerations, bleeding, aspiration, perforation, fistula, and reflux being relatively rare [35, 36]. When compared to open repair, stent placement is associated with a 4% morbidity as opposed to 43%. Length of stay, time to oral intake, and cost are also significantly decreased [32].

Endoluminal Vacuum Therapy

In light of the improved outcomes with nonoperative treatment of esophageal perforations, new techniques are on the horizon that could potentially obviate the need for surgery even in patients who would otherwise not meet the criteria for endoscopic management. One such therapy is endoluminal vacuum therapy, which utilizes a vacuum sponge that is endoscopically placed into the perforation cavity. The Endo-SPONGE® is not yet FDA approved for esophageal perforations, and studies are still underway regarding its efficacy. Currently, it is approved only for the treatment of rectal anastomotic leaks.

References

1. Bhatia P, et al. Current concepts in the management of esophageal perforations: a twenty-seven year Canadian experience. Ann Thorac Surg. 2011;92(1):209–15.
2. Peery AF, et al. Burden of gastrointestinal disease in the United States: 2012 update. Gastroenterology. 2012;143(5):1179–1187. e3.
3. Chirica M, et al. Esophageal perforations. J Visc Surg. 2010;147(3):e117–28.
4. Merchea A, et al. Esophagogastroduodenoscopy-associated gastrointestinal perforations: a single-center experience. Surgery. 2010;148(4):876–82.
5. Brinster CJ, et al. Evolving options in the management of esophageal perforation. Ann Thorac Surg. 2004;77(4):1475–83.
6. Sudarshan M, Cassivi SD. Management of traumatic esophageal injuries. J Thorac Dis. 2019;11(Suppl 2):S172.
7. Betalli P, et al. Update on management of caustic and foreign body ingestion in children. Diagn Ther Endosc. 2009;2009:969868.
8. Cheng H-T, et al. Caustic ingestion in adults: the role of endoscopic classification in predicting outcome. BMC Gastroenterol. 2008;8(1):31.
9. Chirica M, et al. Caustic ingestion. Lancet. 2017;389(10083):2041–52.
10. Sdralis EIK, et al. Epidemiology, diagnosis, and management of esophageal perforations: systematic review. Dis Esophagus. 2017;30(8):1–6.
11. Mackler SA. Spontaneous rupture of the esophagus; an experimental and clinical study. Surg Gynecol Obstet. 1952;95(3):345–56.
12. Aronberg RM, et al. Esophageal perforation caused by edible foreign bodies: a systematic review of the literature. Laryngoscope. 2015;125(2):371–8.

13. Shaker H, et al. The influence of the "golden 24-h rule" on the prognosis of oesophageal perforation in the modern era. Eur J Cardiothorac Surg. 2010;38(2):216–22.
14. Søreide JA, Viste A. Esophageal perforation: diagnostic work-up and clinical decision-making in the first 24 hours. Scand J Trauma Resusc Emerg Med. 2011;19(1):66.
15. Herrera A, Freeman RK. The evolution and current utility of esophageal stent placement for the treatment of acute esophageal perforation. Thorac Surg Clin. 2016;26(3):305–14.
16. di Castelguidone EdL, et al. Esophageal injuries: spectrum of multidetector row CT findings. Eur J Radiol. 2006;59(3):344–8.
17. Makhani M, et al. Pathogenesis and outcomes of traumatic injuries of the esophagus. Dis Esophagus. 2014;27(7):630–6.
18. Watkins JR, Farivar AS. Endoluminal therapies for esophageal perforations and leaks. Thorac Surg Clin. 2018;28(4):541–54.
19. Biancari F, et al. Current treatment and outcome of esophageal perforations in adults: systematic review and meta-analysis of 75 studies. World J Surg. 2013;37(5):1051–9.
20. Onat S, et al. Factors affecting the outcome of surgically treated non-iatrogenic traumatic cervical esophageal perforation: 28 years experience at a single center. J Cardiothorac Surg. 2010;5(1):46.
21. Vallbohmer D, et al. Options in the management of esophageal perforation: analysis over a 12-year period. Dis Esophagus. 2010;23(3):185–90.
22. Madanick RD. Medical management of iatrogenic esophageal perforations. Curr Treat Options Gastroenterol. 2008;11(1):54–63.
23. van Halsema EE, et al. Stent placement for benign esophageal leaks, perforations, and fistulae: a clinical prediction rule for successful leakage control. Endoscopy. 2018;50(2):98–108.
24. El H II, et al. Treatment of esophageal leaks, fistulae, and perforations with temporary stents: evaluation of efficacy, adverse events, and factors associated with successful outcomes. Gastrointest Endosc. 2014;79(4):589–98.
25. Gubler C, Bauerfeind P. Endoscopic closure of iatrogenic gastrointestinal tract perforations with the over-the-scope clip. Digestion. 2012;85(4):302–7.
26. Khater S, et al. Over-the-scope clip (OTSC) reduces surgery rate in the management of iatrogenic gastrointestinal perforations. Endosc Int Open. 2017;5(5):E389–94.
27. Haito-Chavez Y, et al. International multicenter experience with an over-the-scope clipping device for endoscopic management of GI defects (with video). Gastrointest Endosc. 2014;80(4):610–22.
28. Disibeyaz S, et al. Endoscopic closure of gastrointestinal defects with an over-the-scope clip device. A case series and review of the literature. Clin Res Hepatol Gastroenterol. 2012;36(6):614–21.
29. Sulz MC, et al. Multipurpose use of the over-the-scope-clip system ("Bear claw") in the gastrointestinal tract: Swiss experience in a tertiary center. World J Gastroenterol. 2014;20(43):16287–92.
30. Hagel AF, et al. Over-the-scope clip application yields a high rate of closure in gastrointestinal perforations and may reduce emergency surgery. J Gastrointest Surg. 2012;16(11):2132–8.
31. Dasari BV, et al. The role of esophageal stents in the management of esophageal anastomotic leaks and benign esophageal perforations. Ann Surg. 2014;259(5):852–60.
32. Freeman RK, et al. Analysis of unsuccessful esophageal stent placements for esophageal perforation, fistula, or anastomotic leak. Ann Thorac Surg. 2012;94(3):959–64; discussion 964–5.
33. Johnsson E, Lundell L, Liedman B. Sealing of esophageal perforation or ruptures with expandable metallic stents: a prospective controlled study on treatment efficacy and limitations. Dis Esophagus. 2005;18(4):262–6.
34. Fischer A, et al. Nonoperative treatment of 15 benign esophageal perforations with self-expandable covered metal stents. Ann Thorac Surg. 2006;81(2):467–72.
35. Speer E, et al. Covered stents in cervical anastomoses following esophagectomy. Surg Endosc. 2016;30(8):3297–303.
36. Turkyilmaz A, et al. Complications of metallic stent placement in malignant esophageal stricture and their management. Surg Laparosc Endosc Percutan Tech. 2010;20(1):10–5.

Surgical Treatment of Esophageal Perforation

22

Thomas C. Tsai, Christopher R. Morse, and David W. Rattner

Introduction

Esophageal perforation is a rare but potentially highly morbid event. The hallmark of management of esophageal perforation remains expeditious diagnosis and management. Delay in identification and treatment usually results in high rates of morbidity and mortality due to mediastinitis. Management of esophageal perforations should be individualized by anatomic location, timing of diagnosis, size of defect, and degree of sepsis. Although management of esophageal leaks from cervical or thoracic anastomoses is a well-known complication following esophagectomy, this chapter will focus on perforations rather than anastomotic leaks. While recent advances in endoscopic techniques such as clips, stents, and vacuum-assisted sponges have broadened the options for management, surgical repair remains an essential procedural option for the treatment of benign esophageal perforation.

Etiology

The esophagus has three anatomic areas of narrowing: the cricopharyngeus muscle (approximately 14–16 cm from the incisors), the bronchoaortic narrowing (approximately 22–24 cm from the incisors), and the gastroesophageal junction

T. C. Tsai · D. W. Rattner (✉)
Division of General and Gastrointestinal Surgery, Massachusetts General Hospital, Boston, MA, USA
e-mail: drattner@mgh.harvard.edu

C. R. Morse
Division of Thoracic Surgery, Department of Surgery, Massachusetts General Hospital, Boston, MA, USA

© Springer Nature Switzerland AG 2021
N. Zundel et al. (eds.), *Benign Esophageal Disease*,
https://doi.org/10.1007/978-3-030-51489-1_22

(approximately 40–45 cm from the incisors). While perforations can occur any-where along the esophagus, most iatrogenic injuries are related to these three ana-tomic areas of narrowing. Classically, for esophagogastroduodenoscopy (EGD), perforations are associated with Killian's triangle that is the posterior space bor-dered by the cricopharyngeus muscle inferiorly and the inferior constrictor muscle superiorly. Especially as this area represents the upper esophageal sphincter, exces-sive force passing the endoscope through this area during intubation of the esopha-gus can lead to perforation.

Iatrogenic causes include those occurring during routine upper endoscopy as well as those during therapeutic interventions. Upper endoscopy perforations occur from 1 in 2500 to 1 in 11,000 cases [1, 2]. Additional factors that increase the risk of perforation include the presence of Zenker's diverticulum, esophageal strictures, and malignancies. Perforation during therapeutic interventions is typi-cally associated with dilations of benign strictures. Dilation of complex stric-tures with Maloney dilators have been associated with perforation rates of 2–10% [3]. With the increasing use of endoscopic mucosal resection for Barrett's esoph-agus as well as endoscopic submucosal dissection (ESD) for benign lesions, there has been an increase in the frequency of esophageal perforations, with esophageal perforations occurring approximately in 2% of ESD cases even at expert, high-volume centers [4]. Prior surgical procedures in the vicinity of the esophagus such as cervical spine surgery, resection of pulmonary and mediasti-nal masses, antireflux surgery, esophagogastric myotomy for achalasia all have associated risks of esophageal perforation.

The classic noniatrogenic cause of benign esophageal perforation is Boerhaave syndrome. Boerhaave syndrome can be considered a form of barotrauma to the esophagus. Less common noniatrogenic causes include ingestion of foreign bodies and both blunt and penetrating trauma.

Diagnosis

High clinical suspicion is needed in the management of esophageal perforation. Patients typically present with symptoms of pain related to the anatomic location of the perforation in the neck, chest, or upper abdomen. Fever and tachycardia are early signs of perforation. While cervical perforations rarely progress to sepsis, intrathoracic and intraabdominal esophageal perforations, if uncontained, can rap-idly progress to sepsis when diagnosis and treatment is delayed for more than 24 h. Classically, radiographic diagnosis entails the use of a water-soluble upper gastro-intestinal series. If no perforation is seen, a follow-up upper gastrointestinal series with dilute barium is recommended (Fig. 22.1, panel a). In the modern era, IV and oral contrast-enhanced esophageal protocol-computed tomography (CT) scans have emerged as either an adjunct or even primary diagnostic modality (Fig. 22.1, panel b). Prompt EGD can also be beneficial, but in the setting of surgical management, this can be performed intraoperatively to aid localization and treatment of the perforation.

Fig. 22.1 Radiographic findings of thoracic esophageal perforation. A 62-year-old gentleman with a history of alcohol abuse presented to our institution with acute esophageal perforation consistent with Boerhaave syndrome. (**a**) Barium swallow revealed linear pooling of contrast posteriorly (arrow). (**b**) CT scan demonstrated significant left pleural effusion, mediastinal fluid, and extraluminal air in the mediastinum (arrow). This patient was managed with surgical drainage and esophageal stenting

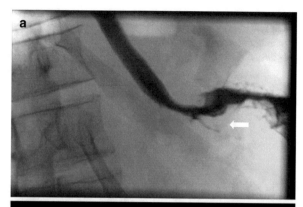

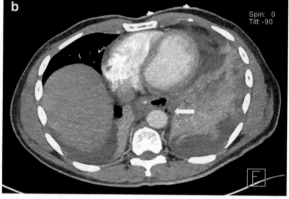

Principles of Surgical Management

The mainstay of the surgical management of esophageal perforation is prompt diagnosis, stabilization of the patient and administration of IV antibiotics, and decision to proceed with surgical or nonsurgical management. In historical series, delay in diagnosis greater than 24 h was associated with an increase in overall mortality from 14% to 27% (Table 22.1) [5]. Initial management includes making the patient nil per os (NPO); broad-spectrum antibiotics such as piperacillin/tazobactam (3.375 g every 6 h); antifungal coverage (fluconazole 400 mg daily); and transfer to intensive care unit if the patient manifests any hemodynamic instability or early sepsis.

Primary repair of the perforation is preferred in most situations. Getting to the OR promptly is essential because the tissue around the perforation rapidly becomes friable and tissue planes become distorted due to inflammation. The greater the interval between perforation and repair, the less the chance of finding useable tissue to reapproximate successfully. Principles of primary repair include debridement of devitalized tissues; longitudinal incision of the esophageal muscle fibers to fully expose the extent of mucosal injury; a two-layer closure with interrupted absorbable sutures of the mucosa and interrupted nonabsorbable sutures of the muscle layers; and buttressing with pedicled flaps (typically intercostal muscle). Exceptions

Table 22.1 Prognostic variables associated with mortality following esophageal perforation

Prognostic variable	Mortality (%)
Etiology (*n* = 431)	
Spontaneous	36
Iatrogenic	19
Traumatic	7
Anatomic location (*n* = 397)	
Cervical	6
Thoracic	27
Abdominal	21
Time to diagnosis (*n* = 396)	
<24 h	14
>24 h	27

Adapted with permission [5]. Copyright 2004

include a cervical perforation that can be managed with drainage alone or a perforation too large to be reapproximated. With large esophageal perforations in the setting of a significantly contaminated mediastinum, drainage and diversion via a cervical esophagostomy and draining gastrostomy tube may be needed to get sepsis under control. Definitive repair of the esophagus and restoration of continuity can be undertaken if the patients survive this phase of their illness. These are generally very morbid procedures and efforts to reverse the esophagostomy and re-establish esophageal continuity are associated with a postoperative complication rate of as high as 68% [6].

Perforations of the Cervical Esophagus

Given the accessibility of the cervical esophagus, perforations in this segment are often best managed with surgical drainage in the retroesophageal space. An incision in the left neck along the anterior border of the sternocleidomastoid (SCM) muscle is made unless EGD or radiographic studies localize the perforation to the right neck. Dissection proceeds to expose the cervical esophagus by retraction of the SCM and carotid sheath laterally; division of the middle thyroid vein and omohyoid muscle; and retraction of the esophagus medially and anteriorly. If a perforation is clearly visualized then it can be primarily repaired, but extensive dissection to identify the mucosal tear is not warranted in the cervical esophagus given the propensity for these injuries to heal with adequate drainage, supplemental nutrition, and antibiotic coverage. Drainage can be accomplished with either a Penrose drain in the retroesophageal space or suction Jackson–Pratt drains. Soft tissues can be closed over the drain, but in settings of gross contamination the wound can be left open and packed with wet-to-dry dressing with eventual conversion to negative pressure wound therapy (vacuum-assisted closure).

Perforations of the Thoracic Esophagus

Identification of the location of the perforation in the thoracic esophagus is critical for surgical planning. Conservative management can be considered in two situations: (1) contained perforation without signs of sepsis or (2) intramural perforation between the mucosa and muscularis [7]. For most perforations in the thoracic esophagus, the consensus is clear that early operative intervention leads to optimal clinical outcomes. A right thoracotomy via the sixth or seventh intercostal space is preferred for mid-esophageal perforations and a left thoracotomy via the eighth intercostal space is preferred for distal esophageal perforations. However, this should be modified based on the laterality of the perforation as well as the proximity to the thoracic inlet or diaphragm. Care should be made to preserve the intercostal muscle during the thoracotomy to preserve options for a muscle flap.

Once the perforation is identified, the defect is extended longitudinally in both the longitudinal and circular muscular layer to ensure full visualization of the mucosal defect (Fig. 22.2). Devitalized tissues are debrided back. The mucosa is then closed with interrupted absorbable sutures such as 4-0 Vicryl. A second layer of closure is accomplished by closing the muscularis with interrupted nonabsorbable suture such as 3-0 silk. Once the defect has been closed, bringing in healthy

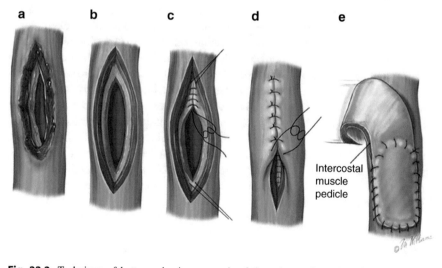

a   b   c   d   e

Intercostal
muscle
pedicle

Fig. 22.2 Technique of buttressed primary repair of thoracic esophageal perforation. (**a**) The extent of mucosal injury is often greater than the extent of the muscle injury. (**b**) The muscle tear is extended to fully expose the mucosal injury, and both are debrided back to healthy tissue. (**c**) The mucosa is closed with 4-0 absorbable sutures. (**d**) The muscle is closed with permanent suture in a second layer. (**e**) An intercostal muscle flap with its vascular supply is sutured around the circumference of the repair site to buttress the primary repair. (Reproduced with permission [7]. Copyright 2015, McGraw-Hill Education)

well-vascularized tissue to buttress the repair is very important. Most commonly, this is accomplished with an intercostal muscle flap. The intercostal muscle flap is then secured over this defect with additional interrupted nonabsorbable sutures. While pleura may also be used, it may be too thin or friable to serve as an effective flap and generally is not as well vascularized as intercostal muscle. Alternate buttressing tissues include omentum, pericardial fat, or gastric wall in a distal perforation (i.e., Thal patch).

In the setting of late perforation presenting >24 h, an alternate strategy employs the use of a T-tube inserted into the perforation in conjunction with surgical drainage and decortication [8, 9]. Either a 16F biliary T-tube or a percutaneous endoscopic gastrostomy tube can be used [9]. The T-tube is brought through the chest wall and wrapped with intercostal muscle, creating a controlled fistula. The T-tube can then be slowly backed out in an ambulatory setting 4–6 weeks after the perforation. However, with the advent of endoscopic stents the T-tube approach of late presenting thoracic esophageal perforations has largely fallen out of favor.

Perforations of the Abdominal Esophagus

Intraabdominal esophageal perforation can be approached laparoscopically if there is sufficient minimally invasive foregut experience. The pars flaccida is opened in the gastrohepatic ligament. The short gastric vessels are also taken down along the gastric fundus. The gastroesophageal junction is then fully exposed by taking down the phrenoesophageal ligament. Mediastinal dissection is then performed to mobilize an intraabdominal segment of esophagus. Similar to thoracic perforation, devitalized esophageal muscle is debrided. A longitudinal myotomy is also performed to fully expose the perforated mucosa. Repair is carried out with 4-0 Vicryl for the mucosa and 3-0 silk for the muscle. The repair can then be buttressed with either an anterior Dor fundoplication or a posterior partial fundoplication depending on the location of the perforation. Blake or Jackson–Pratt drains are then placed. In patients with achalasia, it is essential that the lower esophageal sphincter is made completely incompetent, usually by performing a myotomy on the contralateral side of the esophagus. If there is any resistance to esophageal emptying, the repair of the perforation is likely to fail to heal.

Postoperative Care

Patients are kept NPO for 5–7 days. A fluoroscopic upper gastrointestinal series is then performed to evaluate for ongoing leak or obstruction. Antibiotics are typically continued for 1 week. For thoracic and abdominal esophageal perforation, a nasogastric tube can be placed intraoperatively. Depending on the extent of the perforation, degree of contamination, and patient's preoperative nutritional status, we selectively place a jejunostomy tube for enteral feeding. In settings of early repair of a small perforation, a jejunostomy is typically not necessary. After demonstration of resolution of the perforation on UGI series, we start a clear liquid diet for 1 day, with transition to full liquid diet for the first week, followed by a soft diet. Regular diet is resumed 3 weeks after surgery.

Alternatives to Surgical Repair

Even with early diagnosis and treatment, open surgical repair of esophageal perforations is still associated with significant morbidity and mortality. Although this chapter focuses on surgical repair of esophageal perforations, recent developments in endoscopic approaches have radically changed the management paradigm for esophageal perforations. In appropriate settings, stenting is the primary treatment modality. In retrospective series, esophageal stenting has been associated with successful exclusion of the leak in up to 89% of patients [10, 11]. However, stenting often requires repeat procedures for stent changes. In the absence of a stricture, maintaining stent position can be challenging. Hence, even when stents are successfully placed, there can be a need for concurrent debridement or decortication of the lung via thoracotomy, which can obviate the benefits of the stenting only approach [12]. Risks for stent failure include cervical esophageal perforations; perforations at the gastroesophageal junction; and perforation greater than 6 cm [13]. Overall, stenting for esophageal perforation may lead to lower costs and shorter lengths of stay (5-day shorter length of stay and earlier oral alimentation) for suitable patients [14].

With the popularization of per oral endoscopic myotomy (POEM) for achalasia and complex ESD, endoscopic clipping has emerged as an alternate endoscopic approach to close mural defects. Endoscopic clipping is best suited for iatrogenic injuries diagnosed in real time with minimal extraluminal contamination. More recently, endoscopic vacuum sponge therapy has been utilized to treat both early and late esophageal perforations. Endoscopic vacuum sponge therapy remains investigational and is generally associated with lower rates of closure than with stenting or surgical approaches [15, 16]. Its advantages are that it allows good control of mediastinal sepsis and can aid in gradual closure of an abscess cavity.

Summary

Esophageal perforations represent a highly morbid condition. While endoscopic interventions have recently emerged as an important management strategy, surgical treatment remains the core treatment option for patients presenting with benign esophageal perforations. The main surgical principles include correct identification of the anatomic location of the perforation; debridement of devitalized tissues; closure in two layers where appropriate; buttressing with pedicled tissue flaps; and wide surgical drainage. The most important key to obtaining optimal outcomes for the treatment of esophageal perforation is prompt recognition and intervention to prevent unfavorable tissue conditions and the development of mediastinitis.

References

1. Sieg A, Hachmoeller-Eisenbach U, Eisenbach T. Prospective evaluation of complications in outpatient GI endoscopy: a survey among German gastroenterologists. Gastrointest Endosc. 2001;53(6):620–7.
2. Quine MA, Bell GD, McCloy RF, Matthews HR. Prospective audit of perforation rates following upper gastrointestinal endoscopy in two regions of England. Br J Surg. 1995;82(4):530–3.
3. Patterson DJ, Graham DY, Smith JL, Schwartz JT, Alpert E, Lanza FL, et al. Natural history of benign esophageal stricture treated by dilatation. Gastroenterology. 1983;85(2):346–50.
4. Sato H, Inoue H, Ikeda H, Grace RSE, Yoshida A, Onimaru M, et al. Clinical experience of esophageal perforation occurring with endoscopic submucosal dissection. Dis Esophagus. 2014;27(7):617–22. https://doi.org/10.1111/dote.12125.
5. Brinster CJ, Singhal S, Lee L, Marshall MB, Kaiser LR, Kucharczuk JC. Evolving options in the management of esophageal perforation. Ann Thorac Surg. 2004;77(4):1475–83. https://doi.org/10.1016/j.athoracsur.2003.08.037.
6. Barkley C, Orringer MB, Iannettoni MD, Yee J. Challenges in reversing esophageal discontinuity operations. Ann Thorac Surg. 2003;76(4):989–94; discussion 95.
7. Blasberg JD, Wright CD. Management of esophageal perforation. In: Sugarbaker DJ, Bueno R, Colson YL, Jaklitsch MT, Krasna MJ, Mentzer SJ, et al., editors. Adult chest surgery. 2nd ed. New York: McGraw-Hill Education; 2015.
8. Bufkin BL, Miller JI Jr, Mansour KA. Esophageal perforation: emphasis on management. Ann Thorac Surg. 1996;61(5):1447–51; discussion 51–2. https://doi.org/10.1016/0003-4975(96)00053-7.
9. Linden PA, Bueno R, Mentzer SJ, Zellos L, Lebenthal A, Colson YL, et al. Modified T-tube repair of delayed esophageal perforation results in a low mortality rate similar to that seen with acute perforations. Ann Thorac Surg. 2007;83(3):1129–33. https://doi.org/10.1016/j.athoracsur.2006.11.012.
10. Freeman RK, Van Woerkom JM, Vyverberg A, Ascioti AJ. Esophageal stent placement for the treatment of spontaneous esophageal perforations. Ann Thorac Surg. 2009;88(1):194–8. https://doi.org/10.1016/j.athoracsur.2009.04.004.
11. D'Cunha J, Rueth NM, Groth SS, Maddaus MA, Andrade RS. Esophageal stents for anastomotic leaks and perforations. J Thorac Cardiovasc Surg. 2011;142(1):39–46 e1. https://doi.org/10.1016/j.jtcvs.2011.04.027.
12. Koivukangas V, Biancari F, Merilainen S, Ala-Kokko T, Saarnio J. Esophageal stenting for spontaneous esophageal perforation. J Trauma Acute Care Surg. 2012;73(4):1011–3. https://doi.org/10.1097/TA.0b013e318265d176.
13. Freeman RK, Ascioti AJ, Giannini T, Mahidhara RJ. Analysis of unsuccessful esophageal stent placements for esophageal perforation, fistula, or anastomotic leak. Ann Thorac Surg. 2012;94(3):959–64; discussion 64–5. https://doi.org/10.1016/j.athoracsur.2012.05.047.
14. Freeman RK, Herrera A, Ascioti AJ, Dake M, Mahidhara RS. A propensity-matched comparison of cost and outcomes after esophageal stent placement or primary surgical repair for iatrogenic esophageal perforation. J Thorac Cardiovasc Surg. 2015;149(6):1550–5. https://doi.org/10.1016/j.jtcvs.2015.01.066.
15. Kuehn F, Loske G, Schiffmann L, Gock M, Klar E. Endoscopic vacuum therapy for various defects of the upper gastrointestinal tract. Surg Endosc. 2017;31(9):3449–58. https://doi.org/10.1007/s00464-016-5404-x.
16. Heits N, Stapel L, Reichert B, Schafmayer C, Schniewind B, Becker T, et al. Endoscopic endoluminal vacuum therapy in esophageal perforation. Ann Thorac Surg. 2014;97(3):1029–35. https://doi.org/10.1016/j.athoracsur.2013.11.014.

Index

A

Abnormal pH-impedance, 7
Abnormal tests, 99
Absent contractility, 97, 98, 108, 109
Absorbable onlay mesh, 81
Achalasia, 95, 118–120, 138, 149, 151, 152
    botulinum toxin (BTx) injection, 138, 139
    diagnosis of, 93, 94
    endoscopic surgical treatment, 125
    endoscopic treatment for, 124, 125
    esophagogastric junction outflow
        obstruction, 106
    incidence, 93
    neuronal damage, 92
    phosphodiesterase inhibitors, 105, 106
    surgical Heller's myotomy, 138
    surgical/endoscopic therapies, 106
    symptoms, 93
    type 1, 104
    type 2, 104
    type 3, 105
Acid suppression medications, 25
Anti-reflux mechanism, 32
Anti-reflux mucosectomy (ARMS), 19
Anti-reflux surgery, 31, 44
    diaphragmatic relaxing Incision, 82
    early failure, 74, 75
    fundoplication failure, 72
    hiatal hernia repair, 80
    late failure, 75
    magnetic sphincter augmentation
        device, 86
    minimally invasive esophagectomy, 84, 85
    outcomes, 87
    presentation, 75
    redo-fundoplication, 78, 79
    Roux-en-Y Gastrojejunostomy, 82–84
    surgical options and techniques, 78
    transoral incisionless fundoplication
        procedure, 85
    work-up, 76, 77
Argon plasma coagulation, 228
Aspiration pneumonia, 71

B

Barium esophagogram, 94
Barium swallow, 3, 4, 34, 53, 62, 116
Barrett's esophagus, 11, 51, 233
    argon plasma coagulation, 228
    chronic inflammation, 219
    cryotherapy, 228
    definition, 220
    epidemiology, 225
    esophageal mucosa, 219
    excessive, 219
    gastroesophageal reflux disease, 226
    management, 226
    medical treatment, 221, 222
    radiofrequency ablation, 227
    risk factors, 221
    surveillance, 221, 222
Boerhaave syndrome, 260
Botulinum toxin (BTx) injection, 138, 139

C

Calcium channel blockers, 105
Capnothorax, 36
Cardia ligation anti-reflux procedure
    (CLEAR), 19
Caustic ingestion
    abdominal portion, 249, 250
    acidic, 243
    alkaline, 243
    antibiotics, 247

© Springer Nature Switzerland AG 2021
N. Zundel et al. (eds.), *Benign Esophageal Disease*,
https://doi.org/10.1007/978-3-030-51489-1

Caustic ingestion (*cont.*)
  clinical presentation, 244, 245
  conduit completion, 251
  diagnosis, 245, 246
  endoscopy, 248
  esophageal mobilization, 252
  esophageal stricture, 248
  gastric conduit, 251
  gastric mobilization, 250
  intra-thoracic anastomosis, 252
  ivor lewis esophagectomy, 249
  jejunostomy tube, 251
  liver retraction, 250
  McKeown esophagectomy, 253
  mitomycin-C, 247
  nasogastric tube, 246
  neutralizing agents, 246
  pyloroplasty, 250
  systemic steroids, 247, 248
  thoracic portion, 252
  transhiatal esophagectomy, 253, 254
  triamcinolone, 247
Chagas disease, 120, 121
Chicago classification, 119, 122
Chicago classification v3.0 system, 117
Chronic reflux, 11
Clostridium difficile infections, 71
Collis gastroplasty, 36, 81
Collis-Nissen technique, 56
Computed tomography, 62
Contractility, 103
Contrast-enhanced video fluoroscopy, 115

D
DeMeester score, 35
Diffuse esophageal spasm (DES)
  diagnosis, 96
  symptoms, 96
Distal esophageal spasm, 107, 109, 117, 122
Distal latency (DL), 103
Dysphagia, 74, 76, 114

E
Eckardt scoring system, 114
Electrical lower sphincter augmentation, 38
Endoluminal vacuum therapy, 264
Endoscopic submucosal resection (EMR)
  advantages, 239
  Barrett's esophagus, 233
  complete eradication, 237, 238
  complications, 239
  indications, 234
  injection-assisted EMR, 238

  limitations, 239
  multiband mucosectomy, 237
  oncologic efficacy, 240
  post-procedural considerations, 239
  pre-procedural preparation, 234
  single-band EMR, 237
Endoscopic techniques, 262
Endoscopy, 2, 33, 62
Enlarged hiatal defect, 86
Epiphrenic diverticula
  diagnosis, 199
  emerging trans-oral endoscopic
    treatment, 204
  surgical treatment, 200
  symptoms, 199
Epiphrenic diverticulum (ED)
  clinical presentation, 167, 168
  evaluation, 169, 170
  laparoscopic approach, 212, 213
  postoperative care, 216
  robotic approach, 215, 216
  surgical treatment, 201–203
  thoracoscopic approach, 214, 215
Esophageal
  acid exposure, 36
  adenocarcinoma, 220
  diverticula
    incidence, 174
    Zenker's diverticulum, 173
  dysmotility, 35
  food transport, 137
  hiatus, 67
  lengthening procedures, 36, 37
  manometry, 3, 62
Esophageal diverticulum (ED)
  abdominal esophagus, 165
  cervical esophagus, 165
  epiphrenic diverticulum
    clinical presentation, 167, 168
    evaluation, 169, 170
  inner circular layer, 165
  intramural pseudodiverticulosis
    clinical presentation, 168
    evaluation, 171
  midthoracic diverticulum
    clinical presentation, 167
    evaluation, 169
  outer longitudinal muscles, 165
  prevalence, 166
  thoracic esophagus, 165
  Zenker diverticulum
    clinical presentation, 166, 167
    evaluation, 169
Esophageal motility disorders
  achalasia, 118–120, 138

Chagas disease, 120, 121
conversion from LHM to POEM, 159
conversion from POEM to Heller
    Myotomy, 160
distal esophageal spasm, 122
EGD, 155
esophageal cancer development, 153
esophagectomy, 160
esophagogastroduodenoscopy, 115
failed fundoplication, 153
gastric emptying study, 157
gastroesophageal reflux disease, 152, 153
high resolution manometry, 155
history and physical exam, 114, 115
hypercontractile esophagus, 123
hypertensive lower esophageal
    sphincter, 122
incomplete myotomy, 152
incorrect indication for initial surgery, 151
ineffective esophageal motility, 153
manometry, 116–118
motility treatment failure, 150
new fundoplication, 160
pH/Impedance, 156
pharmacological treatment, 124
pneumatic dilation, 157
primary surgical failure, 152
Re-do Fundoplication, 159
Re-do Heller myotomy, 158
Re-do POEM, 158
robotics, 161
symptoms motility treatment failure, 150
systemic sclerosis, 121, 122
upper gastrointestinal series, 154, 155
upper GI fluoroscopy, 115
Esophageal perforation
abdominal esophagus, 272
alternatives to surgical repair, 273
cervical esophagus, 270
clips, 263
diagnosis, 261, 268
endoluminal vacuum therapy, 264
endoscopic techniques, 262
endoscopy vs. surgery, 262
etiology, 259, 260, 267, 268
location, 260
postoperative care, 272
signs and symptoms, 260, 261
stents, 263, 264
surgical management, 269
thoracic esophagus, 271, 272
treatment, 261, 262
Esophagectomy, 128, 129
Esophagitis, 3
Esophagocardioplasty, 121

Esophagogastric junction outflow obstruction
    (EGJO), 106, 151
diagnosis, 96
symptoms, 95
Esophagogastric outlet obstruction, 107
Esophagogastroduodenoscopy (EGD), 115
Esophagus, 52, 65
EsophyX device, 12
EsophyX2 device, 14

F
Fragmented peristalsis, 110, 111
Fundoplication, 34–36, 56, 67, 80
herniation, 73
procedure, 26

G
Gastric bypass, 38
Gastric cardia, 12
Gastric polyposis, 71
Gastroesophageal reflux disease (GERD), 39,
    219, 226
acid production, 32
acid suppression medications, 25
algorithm for treatment, 56, 57
ambulatory pH monitoring, 3, 4, 6
barium swallow, 3
clinical presentation, 11
complications, 6, 25
differential diagnosis, 6
electrical lower sphincter augmentation, 38
endoscopy, 2
esophageal lengthening procedures, 36, 37
esophageal manometry, 3
esophageal motility and acid clearance, 33
fundoplication, 34–36
gastric bypass, 38
gastric emptying study, 6
GEJ incompetence, 32
incidence, 1
laparoscopic magnetic sphincter
    augmentation, 37
laparoscopic Nissen fundoplication, 25
magnetic sphincter augmentation, 26
obesity, 33
preoperative workup, 33, 34
prevalence, 25
proton pump inhibitors, 25
sleeve gastrectomy, 33
symptom, 1, 2
transoral incisionless fundoplication
    procedure, 13, 15

Gastroesophageal reflux disease health-related
        quality of life (GERD-HRQL)
        scores, 87
Gastroesophageal reflux symptom scale
        (GERSS), 87

H
Handheld manometer, 140
Heller, 150, 153, 157
Heller's myotomy, 138
Hernia sac dissection, 66
Hiatal hernia, 4, 50
        barium swallow, 62
        closure of diaphragmatic crura, 66
        computed tomography, 62
        endoscopy, 62
        esophageal manometry, 62
        evaluation, 62
        fundoplication, 67
        patient positioning, 63
        pH monitoring, 62
        repair, 80
        surgical treatment, 63
        symptoms and complications, 60, 62
        trocar placement, 63
        type I HH, 59, 60
        type II HH, 59
        type III HH, 60, 61
        type IV HH, 60, 61
High resolution manometry (HRM), 62,
        103–105, 122
        findings, 137
        treatment options, 143–145
Hypercontractile esophagus, 106–108, 123
Hypertrophic lower esophageal sphincter, 117
Hypopharyngeal diverticula
        cricopharyngeal myotomy, 182
        diagnosis, 177
        diverticulectomy, 182
        flexible endoscopic approach, 196
        open cricopharyngeal myotomy, 182
        open hypo-pharyngeal diverticulectomy,
                180, 181
        open hypopharyngeal invagination, 181
        pathophysiology, 174–176
        postoperative care, 194
        preoperative assessment, 194
        rigid transoral approach, 195, 196
        symptoms, 177
        trans-oral flexible endoscopic submucosal
                approach hypo-pharyngeal
                diverticulae, 194
        trans-oral flexiblendoscopic hypo-
                pharyngeal diverticulotomy, 186,
                188, 193
        trans-oral hypo-pharyngeal
                diverticulotomy, 183
        trans-oral hypo-pharyngeal diverticulotomy
                with thermal devices, 184, 185
        trans-oral stapled hypo-pharyngeal
                diverticulotomy, 185, 186
        treatment, 179, 180
Hypotensive lower esophageal sphincter
        (LES), 32

I
Ineffective esophageal motility, 110
Inhibitory neurotransmitter nitric oxide, 105
Injection-assisted EMR, 238
Intra-abdominal esophageal segment, 54
Intramural pseudodiverticulosis (IP)
        clinical presentation, 168
        evaluation, 171

J
Jackhammer esophagus (JHE), 96, 97

K
Killian's triangle, 173, 176

L
Laparoscopic magnetic sphincter
        augmentation, 37
Laparoscopic Nissen fundoplication (LNF),
        36, 43, 44
LINX® MSA device
        early research and development, 27
        indication and contraindication, 26
LINX® reflux management system, 26, 37
Los Angeles classification system, 3
Lower esophageal sphincter (LES)
        pneumatic dilation, 139, 141
        relaxation, 104

M
Magnetic sphincter augmentation (MSA),
        12, 26, 86
        post-market experience and long term
                follow-up, 27–29
        surgical placement, 26
Manometry, 51, 53, 116, 117
McKeown, 254
Medigus ultrasonic surgical endostapler
        (MUSE), 16
        contraindications, 16
        endolumenal fundoplication, 16

GERD-HRQL scores, 17
  multicenter prospective study, 17
Mid esophageal diverticula
  diagnosis, 198
  surgical treatment, 198
  symptoms, 197
Midthoracic diverticulum (MD)
  clinical presentation, 167
  evaluation, 169
Minimally invasive esophagectomy
    (MIE), 84, 85
Monopolar energy, 86
Motility disorders, 123
  absent contractility, 97, 98
  achalasia (see Achalasia)
  DES
    diagnosis, 96
    symptoms, 96
  EGJO, 106, 151
    diagnosis, 96
    symptoms, 95
  high resolution manometry, 103, 104
  jackhammer esophagus, 96, 97
  minor disorders of peristalsis, 98, 99
Multiband mucosectomy, 237

N
Nationwide inpatient sample (NIS), 31
Neoesophagus, 37
Neutralizing agents, 246
Nissen fundoplication, 67, 78
Normal esophageal motility, 104
Normal pH-impedance, 7

O
Obesity, 33
Osteoporosis, 71

P
Paraesophageal hernia, 65
Patient positioning hiatal hernia, 63
Penrose drain placement, 66
Peroral endoscopic myotomy (POEM),
    125–127, 138, 142–144, 157, 159
  experimental procedure, 126, 141
  mucosal incision, 141
  randomized trial, 142
pH monitoring, 62
Phosphodiesterase inhibitors, 105, 106
Pinstripe pattern, 118
Pneumatic dilation, 124, 139–141, 157
Popularization of per oral endoscopic
    myotomy, 273

Postoperative pseudoachalasia, 138
Proton pump inhibitors (PPI), 11, 25, 71
Provocative tests, 99

R
Radiofrequency ablation, 227
Radiofrequency therapies, 12
Randomized control trial, 43
Recurrent dysphagia, 127, 128
Recurrent hiatal hernias, 81
Re-do Heller myotomy, 158
Re-do POEM, 158
Reflux episodes, 5
Reflux recurrence, 43
Reoperative gastroesophageal surgery, 71
RESPECT trial, 13
Rezende classification, 115, 117
Roux-en-Y Gastrojejunostomy, 82–84

S
Scleroderma, 98
Secondary antireflux surgery, 44
Short esophagus, 81
  anatomy, 49, 50
  chronic inflammatory process, 48
  Collis Nissen gastroplasty, 56
  endoscopy, 50, 51
  evaluation and diagnosis, 49
  history of, 47, 48
  incidence, 55
  intraoperative measurement, 54
  manometry, 51, 53
  pathophysiology, 48
  post-fundoplication failure, 55
  prevalence of, 81
  radiology, 53
  reported incidence, 55
Single-band EMR, 237
Sleeve gastrectomy, 33
Spastic paralysis, 117
Sternocleidomastoid (SCM), 270
Stretta
  contraindications, 18
  esophageal acid exposure, 19
  esophageal pH values, 19
  GERD-HRQL scores, 19
  outpatient setting, 17
  procedure, 18
  radiofrequency energy, 17
  randomized trials, 18
  transient LES relaxations, 18
Surgical Nissen fundoplication, 44
Suturing, 66
Symptoms and short-segment BE (SSBE), 226

Systemic sclerosis, 121, 122

T
TEMPO study, 13
Transhiatal, 249, 253
Transient lower esophageal sphincter
    relaxations (TLESRs), 32
Transoral fundoplication procedure, 12, 14
Transoral incisionless fundoplication
    (TIF), 43, 44
  procedure, 12, 13, 15, 85
Transthoracic approach, 36
Trocar placement, 63
Trocar positioning, 64
Trypanosoma cruzi, 138

U
Unsedated transnasal endoscopy (uTNE), 222
US Food and Drug Administration (FDA), 12

V
Verapamil, 105
Verres needle, 63

Z
Zenker diverticulum (ZD), 173, 185
  clinical presentation, 166, 167
  evaluation, 169

Printed in the United States
by Baker & Taylor Publisher Services